T0253727

MANAGING
INNOVATION
IN HEALTHCARE

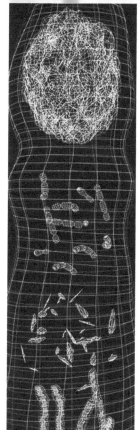

MANAGING
INNOVATION
IN HEALTHCARE

James Barlow
Imperial College London, UK

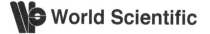

World Scientific

NEW JERSEY · LONDON · SINGAPORE · BEIJING · SHANGHAI · HONG KONG · TAIPEI · CHENNAI · TOKYO

Published by

World Scientific Publishing Europe Ltd.

57 Shelton Street, Covent Garden, London WC2H 9HE

Head office: 5 Toh Tuck Link, Singapore 596224

USA office: 27 Warren Street, Suite 401-402, Hackensack, NJ 07601

Library of Congress Cataloging-in-Publication Data
Names: Barlow, James, 1957–   author.
Title: Managing innovation in healthcare / James Barlow (Imperial College London, UK)
Description: New Jersey : World Scientific, [2017] |
    Includes bibliographical references and index.
Identifiers: LCCN 2016033505| ISBN 9781786341518 (hc : alk. paper) |
    ISBN 9781786341525 (pbk : alk. paper)
Subjects: | MESH: Technology Assessment, Biomedical--trends | Delivery of Health Care--trends |
    Biomedical Technology--organization & administration
Classification: LCC R855.3 | NLM W 82 | DDC 610.28--dc23
LC record available at https://lccn.loc.gov/2016033505

British Library Cataloguing-in-Publication Data
A catalogue record for this book is available from the British Library.

Copyright © 2017 by World Scientific Publishing Europe Ltd.

All rights reserved. This book, or parts thereof, may not be reproduced in any form or by any means, electronic or mechanical, including photocopying, recording or any information storage and retrieval system now known or to be invented, without written permission from the Publisher.

For photocopying of material in this volume, please pay a copying fee through the Copyright Clearance Center, Inc., 222 Rosewood Drive, Danvers, MA 01923, USA. In this case permission to photocopy is not required from the publisher.

Desk Editors: Suraj Kumar/Mary Simpson

Typeset by Stallion Press
Email: enquiries@stallionpress.com

Printed in Singapore

PREFACE AND ACKNOWLEDGEMENTS

Why write a book on managing innovation in healthcare? There are plenty of books on technology and innovation management, some written by my colleagues, so what's different about healthcare that means it needs its own dedicated textbook?

Like many, the origins of this textbook lay in a university course which lacked a single source of material to support its lectures. After developing and teaching an Imperial College Business School MSc module on managing change and innovation in healthcare, and being greeted by new students every year asking 'what's the course book?', I decided it was time to produce one.

The time seemed right for several reasons. Travelling around the world speaking at conferences, sitting on expert panels and attending research workshops and meetings, I found the same questions coming up again and again. Why do seemingly good healthcare innovations fail to be taken up? What is it about the health system that makes innovation so hard, whether you look at it from the perspective of those who are creating new innovations — drugs, devices, processes — or the perspective of those who are adopting them into everyday healthcare practice? Why is the science of health and medicine forging ahead at such a dramatic pace, but the process of translating this science into actual healthcare innovations so slow?

I found that the responses to those questions, at least in countries with highly developed health systems, seemed to be fairly consistent even though the emphasis varied. People typically said: it's to do with the complexity of healthcare, there are organisational, financial, political challenges, the economics are tricky, it's all the fault of our government, our doctors, the managers, the public, the health technology industries, the market, the lack of a market, market failure, and more.

Another constant was that the nature of innovation in healthcare was seen as somehow 'different' from other parts of the economy and society. Seemingly well-understood concepts from the research and practice of technology and innovation management didn't necessarily hold true when looking at innovation in healthcare. So while many general textbooks and guides on technology and innovation management certainly provide an extremely useful grounding, it's important to look beyond them at the specificities of healthcare which do seem to make it rather different when it comes to innovation.

Apart from providing my students with the course book they wanted, the time also felt right for a book on innovation management in healthcare because the debate on how to design health systems and pay for them in the 21st century is growing more intense. This is in response to funding and resource constraints in the developed countries and the need to provide universal care in developing ones. Technological innovation is continuing apace, though, changing the way we think about care and opening up opportunities for new ways of providing it. Innovations in diagnostics and telecommunications are allowing countries with underdeveloped health systems to potentially leapfrog the increasingly outdated and expensive models of developed ones. Innovations in data science and life sciences are beginning to revolutionise the process of creating new drugs. And it's not all about high-tech, high cost innovation. New business models for providing affordable care, combined with new technology, are helping to improve access in poorer parts of the world. New organisational models are placing people at the centre of integrated services. All this is also beginning to have an effect on the built infrastructure for healthcare, the kinds of hospitals and other buildings that support it and where they need to be located.

Healthcare is a hugely important part of all our lives, whether we live in developed countries with highly advanced health systems or countries where many people don't have adequate access to healthcare. It's also a substantial part of the economy in many countries. A better understanding of how to manage innovation and lead the changes that are required to create an efficient and effective healthcare system is more important now than ever before.

Many people have inspired my thinking and contributed in different ways to this book. Over the last fifteen years and more, I have been involved in a wide range of research projects on healthcare innovation issues. The book has benefited from the long hours of discussion with colleagues working on these projects and it also makes use of their outputs and original material. Chapter 5 draws especially on work carried out with Inger Abma, Steffen Bayer, Theti Chrysanthaki, Richard Curry, Jas Gill, Kyriakos Hatzaras, Jane Hendy, Anja Kern, Martina Köberle-Gaiser, Elena Pizzo, Jens Roehrich, Dimitrios Spyridonidis, and Danielle Tucker. I must give special thanks to Brice Dattée. Many hours of discussion in Paris and Lyon helped knock my fairly rudimentary knowledge of complexity theory into shape, and Chapter 7 is in no small way the result of his insight and help.

Some of the original research used by the book was based on projects funded by the EPSRC, the Department of Health (England), and the National Institute Health Research.

The enthusiasm, insights and world view of my PhD students over the last few years have helped inspire me: Paola Boscolo Chio Bisto, Valentina Cisnetto, Fawaz Fram, Tiago Cravo Oliveira and Linda Pomeroy. Other students from MSc courses at Imperial College London have both contributed background research and acted as guinea pigs, reading some of the chapters: Sami Agush, Omar Bhakri, Talha Haroon, Mohammad Kobrosly, Meric Oztap, Vainius Rakauskas, Carolyn Sharpe, Tiffany Robyn Soetiknom, Mukunda Somisetti, Amrita Viswambaram, and Juan Vargas.

Many people have helped formed my ideas over the years. Some have contributed insights, others have read and commented on parts of the book. They include: Rifat Atun, Richard Baldwin, Eliana Barrenho, Derek Bell, Adrian Bull, John Cole, Andy Davies, Alan Dilani, Mark Dodgson, Barrie Dowdeswell, Henry Feldman, Stan Finkelstein, Giovanna Forte, David Gann, Colin Gray, Adrian King, Chris Harty, Axel Heitmueller, Jeremy Huddy, Prashant Jha, Mike Kagioglou, Loy Lobo, Nick Mays, Melody Ni, Shirlene Oh, Andrew Price, Julie Reed, Hugo Tewson, Oliver

Wells, Steve Wright, and my colleagues from HaCIRIC, PIRU and North West London CLAHRC — they know who they are and what the acronyms stand for.

The tables and figures were produced by Tom Barlow-Brown.

Finally I must also thank Hilary and my family for their patience and support over the two years it took to put the book together.

ABOUT THE AUTHOR

James Barlow is Professor of Technology and Innovation Management (Healthcare) at Imperial College Business School. Previous appointments include SPRU (Science Policy Research Unit, University of Sussex) and the Policy Studies Institute. He was educated at the London School of Economics and Political Science.

His research, teaching and consultancy focuses on the adoption, implementation and sustainability of innovation in healthcare systems. He has also worked extensively on innovation in housing provision and other housing policy issues.

James was a founder and co-director of Imperial College Business School's Innovation Studies Centre and during 2006–2013 was Principal Investigator and director of HaCIRIC, the world's largest research programme on innovation in healthcare infrastructure.

He has been a member of many expert panels on healthcare innovation, both in the UK and internationally, and has worked with a wide range of companies from the medical technology, pharmaceutical, ICT and construction sectors.

CONTENTS

LIST OF CASE STUDIES

LIST OF TABLES

LIST OF FIGURES

LIST OF BOXES

WHY DO WE NEED TO UNDERSTAND HEALTHCARE INNOVATION?

01

We all need healthcare but despite the huge advances made over the last century, healthcare remains a problem — a problem for those who do not receive the care they need, a problem for those who barely receive it at all, and a problem for all who have to pay for it. Healthcare is also the most complex and fast moving industry that exists. Developments in life sciences are revolutionising our understanding of diseases and the challenges of ageing, and how we can tackle them. New technologies are constantly being developed, all with the potential to support new approaches to medicine and clinical practice.

So why the problem? If research and development (R&D) is delivering so much new science and technology, why do we need to understand healthcare innovation? And what do we mean by healthcare innovation, anyway? Aren't there already books and large volumes of research papers on technology and innovation management? There are two answers to these questions.

First, not all the science and technology is taken up into everyday, mainstream healthcare practice. Much of the effort around technological innovation is not targeted at the poorest people in the world and is either unaffordable or unsuitable for their health systems. But even in the advanced health systems, there is a disconnection between the research effort and the proportion that makes it into mainstream practice.

1

Moreover, the advanced health systems are facing an onslaught from an ageing population and the growing incidence of chronic disease, so the search is on for ways of providing the best quality healthcare as afford-ably as possible. Innovation in its various guises has an important part to play in tackling these challenges.

The second answer is that while innovation — thinking creatively about what healthcare is and how we deliver it — is needed more than ever, innovation can itself be a problem. As we will see later, unlike other areas of the economy, new technologies often increase costs because they allow us to 'do more' healthcare. And even when there is good evidence for the benefits of a new technology it may be hard to introduce, leaving patchy adoption and differences in access to it across the population.

This book introduces you to the latest thinking on healthcare innova-tion. It is about how you *create*, *implement*, *embed*, and *sustain* innova-tions in healthcare systems. We explore what 'technology' and 'innovation' mean in relation to healthcare:

- How researchers and companies develop new healthcare products such as medical devices or new drugs, and how they are commercial-ised, and how they are taken up into mainstream practice.
- How to manage innovation from the perspective of governments responsible for shaping policy, from the perspective of healthcare organisations providing services and juggling competing demands, and from the perspective of the industries that supply new products and services.

Using examples and cases from around the world, you will learn why innovation in healthcare services and policy is critical, you will learn about the strategic and organisational skills needed to manage innovation processes in healthcare, and you will learn why embedding innovation within everyday practice is so hard in healthcare.

There is no single approach to managing technology and innovation that works best in all situations in healthcare. While many of the processes of technology and innovation management are largely generic, techno-logical, organisational, policy and market specific factors within health-care may well constrain the choices and actions of those involved. Successful innovation requires an understanding of how these factors interact and the way in which the local context, whether at the level of individual hospitals, other healthcare providers or national health systems, influences the outcomes of innovation efforts.

This book is about how healthcare organisations cope with the mass of new products, technologies and novel business and service models they face, how the companies trying to sell new products and services cope with the challenges of shepherding them into the healthcare market, and how government and regulators shape the environment within which all this takes place.

This book was written with the needs of postgraduate and MBA students studying healthcare services, management, and innovation issues. But it is also relevant to managers, clinicians, policymakers, and entrepreneurs involved in healthcare. There is a lot of received wisdom about healthcare innovation, but the reality is often more complex than we think and frustrating for those involved. Understanding why this is the case is essential for healthcare to move forwards and take advantage of all the new ideas that are emerging from R&D. This book helps you do this, but it is not a primer — you will need to draw from it the lessons that are relevant to you and find your own ways to best apply them to meet your needs.

Each chapter is informed by the latest research, as well as my own experience researching, teaching, and consulting over many years. In such a fast moving domain, research can become dated quickly. Future editions will be updated with the latest thinking. There are, however, a number of enduring studies which underpin our basic understanding of technology and innovation management, both in healthcare and elsewhere. You are encouraged to seek out and read the sources for this book when you feel it is necessary — they will give you a much deeper understanding of the points being made. Useful background reading has been identified at the end of each chapter.

Three innovation challenges for 21st century healthcare

Why do we need to understand healthcare innovation better? Aren't there already books and research papers that can help us? Can't we just apply the lessons about technology and innovation management from other industries? As you will find out as you read this book, you will see that the answer is that healthcare is not like other industries. While those concerned with healthcare can certainly learn from the voluminous literature on technology and innovation management, the lessons need to be adapted to its highly complex and fast-moving context. And within healthcare, there is huge variability in the way health systems are organised, in the challenges they face and in the resources at their disposal. What is common across health systems, though, is that new thinking — innovation — is needed more now than ever to ensure that in the 21st century, the best possible care is available to as many people as possible and as affordably as possible. There are three big issues in healthcare that require innovative thinking.

Resources, costs, and demand — the challenges for advanced health systems

In 2010, around USD 6.5 trillion was spent on healthcare around the world, rising by a few percentage points a year (EIU, 2013). Expenditure per capita ranged from USD 12 per person a year in Eritrea to over USD 8000 in the USA (WHO, 2012). As a percentage of GDP healthcare spending ranges from 6.4% in the Middle East and Africa to 10.7% in Western Europe and 17.4% in the USA (EIU, 2013). And healthcare is big business for some countries — around 11% of all employment in Germany works in its 'medical-industrial complex', accounting for over EUR 330 billion of the economy (Busse, 2014).

Across the developed world, in the high- and middle-income countries with advanced health systems, healthcare is consuming an ever-increasing share of GDP. Driven by an ageing population, the rising incidence of non-communicable diseases such as diabetes and a continual flow of new technology, the share of GDP spent on healthcare could grow to over 25% in the USA and 20% in several European countries by 2040 (Kibasi *et al.*, 2012).

Decisions about how much we spend on healthcare over the next few decades will partly be shaped by political choices about how we allocate national resources. In the wealthiest countries spending a fifth of GDP on healthcare may not be a problem provided there is sustained economic growth. But in the medium term — in the next few years at least — healthcare providers, payers such as insurance companies, governments and the public may be facing a perfect storm of escalating demand, rising expectations for better care, and concerns over the need to control public expenditure.

There is much discussion about the sustainability of health systems in the face of these demographic, economic and other pressures. Finding new ways of coping, including innovating in the models of healthcare delivery, is generally regarded as essential. Many countries with long-established health systems are therefore trying to redesign them — adopting new payment and reimbursement models to incentivise innovation and improve performance, moving from a paradigm that emphasises sickness and treatment to one which is more about wellness and prevention, reforming the organisational architecture by integrating primary, secondary and social care, and trying to find new ways of involving the private and voluntary sectors. There is much interest 'disruptive innovation', moving towards cheaper, simpler organisational, and technological solutions which emphasise the importance of individuals taking more responsibility for their own care and shifting services away from expensive hospitals to community settings.

> ➜ *Chapter 5 provides more information on ways incentive systems are being used to promote innovation and performance improvement in health systems*

> ➜ *Chapter 6 discusses the impact of disruptive innovation on health systems*

New technologies such as 'big data', innovative medical devices and new drugs products all play a role in supporting these efforts to modernise healthcare delivery models. Yet, technological innovation is something of a double-edged sword; it has the potential to greatly improve the performance of healthcare systems and health outcomes for individuals, but it also requires upfront financial investment by healthcare organisations for a possible payoff further down the line. And it has a tendency to increase overall healthcare costs. New drugs and other

> ➜ *Go to Chapter 3 to find out more about the economics of healthcare innovation*

technologies extend life expectancy, better diagnostics allow more medical conditions to be picked up and more people need to be treated. Some estimates suggest that technology-based costs have accounted for as much as half the total cost inflation in US healthcare since the 1960s. For this reason, Atul Gawande, Professor in the Department of Health Policy and Management at Harvard University, argues that a focus on redesigning healthcare systems outweighs science and technology when it comes to delivering possible solutions.

"Research on our healthcare systems can save more lives in the next ten years than bench science, research on the genome, stem cell research, cancer vaccine research and everything else we hear about on the news." (Atul Gawande in NHS Confederation, 2008)

Governments want healthcare systems to be innovative — they are concerned with how innovation can be stimulated and how new technologies and management, process or service innovations can be rapidly and sustainably embedded within the health system and its organisations. One problem that especially exercises policy makers is the substantial time lag that often exists between research being conducted and its lessons (and innovations) being taken up into everyday practice (Seddon *et al.*, 2001). This has been the subject of debate since the 1950s (Lomas, 2007; Niccolini *et al.*, 2008). As well as consequences for clinical outcomes and healthcare quality, this 'research translation

→*Chapters 4 and 5 discuss how governments try to support healthcare innovation*

gap' potentially wastes some of the huge financial resources spent each year on R&D. In the UK, the efforts of successive government have tried to put in place the organisational and funding infrastructure to make innovation and its spread central to the National Health Service (Barlow, 2015).

Healthcare technology innovation is big business — but it needs to evolve

It is not surprising that governments are concerned to support the healthcare technology industries. These upstream players in the health system, the producers of the innovative technologies that underpin global healthcare provision, are big business. Healthcare is supported by four major industrial sectors: pharmaceuticals and biotechnology ('biopharma'), medical devices, information technology (IT) and the built environment (design, engineering, and construction). Collectively the companies that make up the healthcare industries have global revenues in the order of USD 2 trillion a year, about a quarter of overall global spending on healthcare. But they are experiencing a changing landscape — an evolving market for their products, a changing balance of power across the healthcare value chain and pressures on their business models:

- The pharmaceutical industry is the largest of the four. Total global sales of prescription drugs are touching USD 1 trillion annually and growing at around 2.4% a year. In addition, sales of pharmaceuticals based on biotechnology are now around USD 233 billion annually and growing at almost 10% per year (DTT, 2014; BIS, 2013).
- The medical devices sector is considerably smaller. Its sales are around USD 350 billion per year, but its growth rate is faster than pharmaceuticals, at 2.6% a year (DTT, 2014; BIS, 2013). Global spending on healthcare IT is much harder to pin down due to the fragmented structure of the industry, both in product and corporate terms. One estimate suggests total global sales were about USD 105 billion in 2015 (Gartner, 2015), while another projects that the global healthcare IT market will only reach USD 66 billion by 2020 (Gold, 2014) — much depends on the definitions of healthcare IT.
- Often overlooked in research and policy debates, the built environment industries that provide the large fixed capital infrastructure to support healthcare services — the hospitals and other facilities — are about the same size as the medical devices industry, with sales of USD 300–400 billion a year (PwC, 2010). This can be expected to grow at least in line with rising global healthcare spending.

Of these four core industries, biopharma has been the most turbulent. The innovation model for the pharmaceutical industry has faced a slowdown in the development of new drugs at the same time that a 'patent cliff' — the loss of drug sales as patent

➜*Go to Chapter 4 for more on the challenges faced by the drug and medical devices industries*

protection expires — has been most acute. Innovation has also become harder partly due to the increasingly complex science underlying the drug discovery process, as the industry shifts its attention towards people with chronic diseases. At the same time, the regulatory and economic context has become more demanding as governments and healthcare payers such as insurance companies have exerted downward pressure on prices and tightened regulations around the drug development process (Deloitte, 2013). Pharmaceutical companies are therefore rethinking how to generate and capture the benefits of innovation, and generally improve the productivity of their R&D models.

The medical devices industry has also experienced challenges to its rate of innovation and the market environment for its products. Previously important engines of growth such as the cardiovascular and orthopaedic markets have slowed and have not been replaced by alternatives. And like the pharmaceutical industry, medical technology has increasingly come under the scrutiny of governments and payers. The approval process has grown longer and its products are subject to the same concerns over cost effectiveness as those experienced by the pharmaceutical industry (Kruger and Kruger, 2012).

Innovations in the healthcare IT sector have been slower to take-off for several reasons (Powell and Goldsmith, 2012). Many healthcare IT investments are designed to improve back-office processes and are often seen by healthcare providers as something that can be deferred. Innovation in healthcare IT fails to get recognition because it is hard to clearly demonstrate its benefits, unlike a new drug or medical device. The industry is also fragmented, with products that include hardware, software and system integration services, addressing both the front- and back-ends of healthcare (i.e. the patient-facing versus the back-office activities). Meanwhile new players are emerging in the healthcare IT sector such as developers of 'mobile health' ('mHealth') applications for both the consumer and healthcare provider markets, stimulated by the spread of smartphones. The IT industry is also poised to play a part in radically changing the science and practice of healthcare in the form of 'big data'. This has implications for the drug industry, policy-makers and regulators, and for us as patients and consumers of healthcare. Big data allows the more complete collection and analysis of data to support far more personalised decision-making around medical care. It also opens up opportunities for integrating data to advance our understanding of the underlying basis of diseases, potentially helping the pharmaceutical industry tackle some of its innovation productivity problems. And governments and regulators could gain a deeper and speedier understanding — at the individual patient level — of the implications of their interventions in the health system.

The future is likely to increasingly involve technological convergence — combinations of technology across manufacturing and service sectors resulting in new hybrid products and combinations of products and services. Examples include point-of-care testing devices that can be used by patients or healthcare workers outside hospitals and therapeutically active devices such as drug eluting stents that slowly release a drug. This has implications for incumbent firms in the health technology industries because the blurring of these different product sectors means they may have to develop new technological capabilities and abandon their familiar old ones (Burns *et al.*, 2012).

Delivering universal high quality healthcare in lower-income countries

Achieving the UN's Sustainable Development Goals (see Box 1.1) will require innovation. As well as the demands from a growing population and the need to address many basic health needs, WHO estimates that the shortage of healthcare workers may grow from 7.2 million today to 12.9 million by 2035 (WHO, 2014). Technological innovation can play a part, not only in the form of new drugs and devices, but also through advances in sanitation and agriculture. But as Howitt *et al.* (2012) and others have pointed out, *where* the R&D effort is directed is important. There is an inverse relationship between availability of health technology and health need — people in the world's poorest countries often lack the most fundamental drugs and devices, let alone the latest advances in science and technology. Tackling this gap requires the development of appropriate and affordable health technologies, and ensuring their availability to the poorest people in the world — the 'bottom of the pyramid'. Innovative thinking is therefore needed to achieve this, as we explore in Chapter 6.

Box 1.1   BACKGROUND: Sustainable development goals: good health and well-being

The UN Sustainable Development Goals, launched in September 2015, replaced the Millennium Development Goals. The good health and well-being targets in the SDGs are listed below. Other SDGs are inextricably tied to with healthcare, such as those relating to poverty, hunger and food security, gender equality and learning. Tackling health and well-being therefore requires a system-wide perspective.

- By 2030, reduce the global maternal mortality ratio to less than 70 per 100,000 live births.
- By 2030, end preventable deaths of newborns and children under 5 years of age, with all countries aiming to reduce neonatal mortality to at least as low as 12 per 1,000 live births and under-5 mortality to at least as low as 25 per 1,000 live births.
- By 2030, end the epidemics of AIDS, tuberculosis, malaria, and neglected tropical diseases and combat hepatitis, water-borne diseases and other communicable diseases.
- By 2030, reduce by one third premature mortality from non-communicable diseases through prevention and treatment and promote mental health and well-being.
- Strengthen the prevention and treatment of substance abuse, including narcotic drug abuse and harmful use of alcohol.
- By 2020, halve the number of global deaths and injuries from road traffic accidents.
- By 2030, ensure universal access to sexual and reproductive healthcare services, including for family planning, information and education, and the integration of reproductive health into national strategies and programmes.
- Achieve universal health coverage, including financial risk protection, access to quality essential healthcare services and access to safe, effective, quality, and affordable essential medicines and vaccines for all.
- By 2030, substantially reduce the number of deaths and illnesses from hazardous chemicals and air, water and soil pollution and contamination.
- Strengthen the implementation of the World Health Organisation Framework Convention on Tobacco Control in all countries, as appropriate.

(Continued)

Box 1.1 (*Continued*)

- Support the R&D of vaccines and medicines for the communicable and non-communicable diseases that primarily affect developing countries, provide access to affordable essential medicines and vaccines.
- Substantially increase health financing and the recruitment, development, training, and retention of the health workforce in developing countries.
- Strengthen the capacity of all countries, in particular developing countries, for early warning, risk reduction and management of national and global health risks.

Source: UN Sustainable Development Knowledge Platform.[1]

But developing new technology alone is not enough. To many in the global health community, the word 'innovation' carries baggage associated with restrictive patents and high cost medicines (Gardner *et al.*, 2007). Global health experts stress that technology should not be considered in isolation from the local context or health system within which it is being introduced. Health technologies are frequently inaccessible not simply because they are too expensive — a host of other constraints play a part, including inadequate distribution networks, unreliable energy or water supply, and a lack of trained human resources. Introducing a new health technology is often only successful when it is combined with innovative thinking in funding models, organisational and business models, and ways of implementing, and scaling it up from small pilot projects. Broadening what we mean by innovation to embrace the whole process from initial idea to implementation and diffusion is therefore essential, whether we are talking of new products, services, processes, practices, and policies. Gardner *et al.* (2007) argue that effort is therefore necessary both in terms of:

- Technological innovation, to create affordable new drugs, devices, diagnostics, and vaccines that are more cost-effective than existing interventions; and
- Social innovation, to ensure the distribution of essential goods and services, including new technologies.

[1] https://sustainabledevelopment.un.org/?menu=1300

We therefore need to think carefully about how healthcare providers and local communities can work together to implement innovations in their particular local setting, by building local capacity for innovation to ensure lower income countries can improve the effectiveness and equity of their own health systems.

Efforts to address all these areas for innovative thinking in global health are growing (Gardner *et al.*, 2007):

- 'Product development partnerships' have been developed to acquire and manage portfolios of new technologies — largely drugs — to speed them through the development process.
- Large procurement funds such as the GAVI Alliance have been created.
- 'Advance market commitments', where donors offer binding contracts to guarantee future procurement and stimulate new drugs for neglected diseases, have been established.

Across the low- and middle-income countries, organisational, and financial innovations are helping to maximise use of current health technologies and create novel ways of improving access to healthcare. Sometimes the innovation can seemingly be minor, but it still has a significant

> ➔ *Chapter 6 describes how how frugal and disruptive innovations are helping to increase access to healthcare in lower-income countries*

impact. The ColaLife project uses existing distribution networks and the space between Coca-Cola bottles in crates to ensure that essential medicines reach those who need them, even in remote areas. To tackle malaria in sub-Saharan Africa, the colour of bed nets treated with insecticide was changed from white to green because white bed nets, in the eyes of many recipients, looked like funeral shrouds; this led to increased use (Howitt *et al.*, 2012).

Innovative technologies do not have to be specifically designed for health purposes to have an effect. A distinction needs to be made between healthcare technologies such as drugs and medical devices, and other technologies which potentially have health benefits — for example, the spread of mobile phones and the internet is helping to ensure that health advice or support reach the greatest number of people. Innovative thinking in other domains such as road safety, sanitation, and the supply of food has huge global health benefits.

The flow of innovation need not be one-way, from rich countries to poorer ones. 'Frugal technology' and other innovations designed for resource poor contexts offer opportunities that might help mitigate escalating healthcare costs in the advanced health systems. The trick is to find ways of managing the disruption when such innovations are introduced in developed countries.

How this book is organised

The book is designed to provide you with an accessible and structured introduction to technology and innovation management in healthcare. It leads you through an understanding of the key concepts to their

---

Box 1.2   SUMMARY: Key questions tackled in each chapter

Chapter 2: What do we know about technology and innovation processes in general? The fundamentals from research and management practice.

Chapter 3: Is healthcare different from other sectors of the economy and does this impact on its innovation processes?

Chapter 4: How do the main industries involved in healthcare — biopharma and medical devices — create and bring to the market new products and services? What challenges do they face?

Chapter 5: Why is it so hard to ensure that innovations are embedded into healthcare organisations and practices? What measures can be adopted to help?

Chapter 6: What is 'disruptive' and 'frugal' innovation in healthcare and why is it important for tackling the healthcare challenges, both in developed and developing health systems?

Chapter 7: Why do we need to view healthcare innovation from a complex systems perspective? How can we understand and manage the system-wide impacts of healthcare innovation?

Chapter 8: The lessons for tackling future healthcare challenges.

---

application to the big challenges faced by governments, healthcare providers and industry. Some prior knowledge of healthcare systems and policies is assumed — the book does not describe the basics of how different countries organise the way they finance and provide healthcare services (Britnell, 2015).

In Chapter 2, we start by considering what we mean by the terms 'technology' and 'innovation'. Both are much used, but also much abused, so it is important to understand their meanings. Until relatively recently research, policy and industry attention was largely focused on the non-healthcare sectors of the economy. 'Technology' was often seen in terms of physical, tangible products — a tablet computer, a medical instrument —

"Organisations, by their very nature are designed to promote order and routine. They are inhospitable environments for innovation." (Ted Levitt, former editor Harvard Business Review)

"What we've done to encourage innovation is make it ordinary." (Craig Wynett, Procter & Gamble)

while 'innovation' was seen as something related to new products coming out of creative organisations or companies. But technology can have both 'hard' (physical) and 'soft' (knowledge) features. It may be a physical product or a new service, process or an app on a smartphone. And innovation is both an *outcome* and a *process* — it involves creating a new idea *and* turning it into something that can be used in practice. Innovation is often associated with risk taking and entrepreneurship, and questioning the *status quo* — a well-known quote, which may or may not be by Albert Einstein, says 'If at first the idea is not absurd, then there is no hope for it'. Innovation is also about embedding creative thinking in organisations. A quick search on the internet will reveal many quotes on this; two wellknown ones are above on the right.

So how do these ideas apply to healthcare? In Chapter 3, we start to look at why it might be different from other industries. We see how hard and soft technologies come together in healthcare as a part of corporate and research ecosystems for drugs or medical devices. The way these innovative products are created and commercialised is therefore often complex, involving many stakeholders and interaction with tough regulatory requirements. Innovations are usually introduced into a payment and decision-making environment which comprises many organisations, with possibly competing interests and which are capable of vetoing decisions. The sheer complexity of healthcare systems, emerging over generations, therefore exerts an influence over innovation processes that is quite unlike that found in other sectors. Another distinctive feature of healthcare is its pace of scientific and technological change (see Box 1.3). As we will see,

---

Box 1.3 BACKGROUND: The pace of scientific and technological change in healthcare

How quickly does science change the knowledge base of healthcare? Of course, this all depends on definitions, but some have tried to work out how rapidly healthcare knowledge doubles. One widely cited estimate is Jim Carroll's:

'(new genetic) knowledge reorients the entire medical system, from one where patients are treated once they are sick to one where patients are treated for what they are likely to develop as a result of their genetic makeup. The volume of medical knowledge is doubling every eight years ...'

Source: http://www.jimcarroll.com/2011/10/trend-the-future-of-knowledge/#. Utlkt_bFK2w

There are many other estimates, helpfully summarised by Geoff Nunberg, UC Berkeley School of Information (*The Organisation of Knowledge. Concepts of Information* i218, 17 February, 2009):

- Medical information doubles every 19 years.
- Medical knowledge doubles every 19 years — a physician needs 2 million facts to practice.
- Medical knowledge doubles every 17 years.
- Volume of new medical information doubles every 10–15 years and increases tenfold in 23–50 years.
- Medical knowledge doubles every seven years.
- Medical knowledge doubles every six to eight years, with new medical procedures emerging everyday.
- There are about 20,000–30,000 medical journals published and the amount of medical information doubles every fifth year.
- Medical information doubles every four years.
- Medical information doubles every three years.
- Medical knowledge doubles every two years.

this poses big challenges for managers and policymakers responsible for planning and delivering healthcare services, not least because the economics of technological innovation in healthcare often mean that overall costs are driven up rather than reduced, as is generally the case in other sectors. Given that the financial resources available for health systems are not infinite, changing the volume and intensity of clinical practice — including its technological inputs — is the main lever by which policy makers can control costs. As David Eddy pointed out almost a quarter of a century ago, this means that every innovation, no matter how small, needs to have its introduction carefully managed (Eddy, 1993).

Chapter 4 is the first of two chapters that explore the healthcare innovation process from the initial development and commercialisation of new technologies to their adoption, implementation, and diffusion. Healthcare is regarded by the developers of technological innovations as a difficult market — commercialising new products is fraught with risks and the market has peculiarities compared to other sectors. We look at the different phases of the new product development process from the perspective of the pharmaceutical, medical biotechnology and medical device industries, and learn why many companies are turning to 'open' and 'user-led' models of innovation. We also discuss why support from government may be needed to help companies developing new healthcare technologies.

In Chapter 5, we turn to the challenges healthcare organisations face in implementing and embedding innovations they have either adopted from elsewhere or have developed themselves. We see that a fundamental issue in healthcare is the question of evidence for the benefits of innovations and how this enables or constrains adoption. Sometimes the evidence is not accepted by certain stakeholders who can influence adoption decisions. Problems in identifying how the impact of an innovation falls across different parts of the healthcare system can also mean that even when there is robust evidence for its benefits, it may still fail to be adopted. This is especially the case when the innovation is complex and involves a mix of technological, organisational, and service delivery change, typical of many examples in healthcare. We look at the measures taken by government to help stimulate the adoption of innovation.

In Chapter 6, we explore the characteristics of 'disruptive' and 'frugal' innovation and its application to healthcare. Since it was first introduced in the late 1990s, the idea of disruptive innovation has become increasingly common, both in the context of healthcare and more widely across business and government. But the concept is often misunderstood and used uncritically to describe many different kinds of innovation that are seen as somehow radical or potentially disruptive of existing ways of working. A growing interest in the notion of frugal innovation — cheaper, simpler technology designed for resource poor environments — is further muddying the waters.

Chapter 7 turns to the question of complexity. We know that health systems are usually big and complex, with many stakeholders, professional and organisational cultures, unusual economics and convoluted politics. To give people the care they need and keep costs down, everything has to work well and work together as a system. However, efforts to improve healthcare through innovation can unfortunately result in progress in one area but make things worse in another. There is much talk of a 'whole systems approach' to improvement, which draws either explicitly or implicitly on concepts from theory on complex adaptive systems. We see how lessons from this theory can help to inform organisations, policy makers, and companies how to better design and introduce innovations into health systems.

Finally, in Chapter 8, we draw conclusions on the role of technology and innovation in tackling the big healthcare challenges facing the world, and the lessons for innovation management.

Throughout the book, there are examples to provide you with more information. These are organised into:

- *background information* boxes, expanding on the points in the main text,
- *concepts* boxes, containing more information on a theory or concept discussed in the main text,
- *innovation in action* boxes, describing an example of an application of healthcare innovation or illustrating an innovation challenge noted in the main text, and
- *case studies*, longer discussions of an example of healthcare innovation, to help you understand the concepts more easily and demonstrate what they mean in a real-life context.

Each chapter and longer case study also provides a number of questions for discussion, which encourage you to review and apply the knowledge you have acquired and test your understanding of the theories and points covered.

All references are listed at the end of the book, but selected further reading is highlighted after each chapter.

There are a number of good general textbooks on technology and innovation management. They provide very useful background on the key concepts that underpin thinking in the field. Those I have found useful in preparing this book are by Smith (2010), Bessant and Tidd (2007), Tidd and Bessant (2014), and Dodgson *et al.* (2008).

Among the leading academic journals that focus on technology and innovation management, and economics are: *Research Policy, Technovation, International Journal of Innovation Management, Technology Analysis and Strategic Management, R&D Management, Industry and Innovation, Journal of Product Innovation Management, European Journal of Innovation Management.*

Selected further reading

Britnell M (2015) *In Search of the Perfect Health System.* United Kingdom: Palgrave.

Howitt P, Darzi A, Yang G-Z, Ashrafian H, Atun R, Barlow J, *et al.* (2012) Technologies for global health. *The Lancet Commissions.* http://dx.doi. org/10.1016/S0140-6736(12)61127-1

02

TECHNOLOGY AND INNOVATION MANAGEMENT: THE NUTS AND BOLTS

THIS CHAPTER WILL HELP YOU TO:

- Understand what we mean by technology.
- Understand the nature of innovation and be able to distinguish between invention and innovation.
- Distinguish between the different forms that innovation can take, such as product, process and service innovation.
- Distinguish between different types of innovation such as radical and incremental innovation.
- Understand the links between innovation and technology performance improvement.
- Describe the main activities associated with innovation.
- Understand the ways in which innovations are adopted and diffused.

Both in research and in popular imagination, 'technology' and 'innovation' are often seen as something related to new products coming out of creative companies. Words like 'R&D', 'entrepreneurship', 'competitiveness' — and faster, better, cheaper products — are all conjured up in our minds when we talk about innovation. But what do we actually mean when we think of technology and innovation? It is important to have a grounding in the core concepts from the extremely large and diverse literature on technology and innovation management if we are to understand how they can be applied to the healthcare sector.

Fundamentally innovation is both an outcome and a process. It involves the act of turning an idea or invention into something that can be sold to customers or somehow made practical use of. Lewis Duncan, former Dean of Engineering at Dartmouth University, succinctly described innovation as 'the ability to convert ideas into invoices.' Innovation is also sometimes associated with individuals who have particular characteristics — inventors, entrepreneurs, risk takers. Taking a risk and failing is seen as an essential part both of the innovation process and entrepreneurship. Many commentators believe that to successfully innovate it is necessary to take risks, make mistakes and occasionally fail.

There is a wealth of research and experience on managing technology and innovation. This chapter discusses the nuts and bolts — the most important lessons that provide insight into how innovation works. Most of the research and debate about technology and innovation management has been rooted in the manufacturing and service sectors. We pick up the reasons why these lessons cannot always be directly applied to healthcare in the rest of the book. But lessons from other sectors of the economy are still very useful for pointing us towards explanations for particular innovation phenomena in healthcare. As you read this chapter, bear in mind the reasons why healthcare is different from manufacturing and service industries, summarised in Box 2.1 — Chapter 3 discusses them in more detail. Let us start with some definitions.

Box 2.1 SUMMARY: Some reasons why innovation processes in healthcare might be different from other sectors

- Healthcare is a system and it is very complex — there are many organisations involved, with many professional and financial silos and entrenched cultures.
- Healthcare is always evolving because of constant change in its underlying science and the development of new technologies, and because policymakers like to tinker with its funding and institutional arrangements.
- Healthcare is heavily regulated — 'taking a risk' by trying out something new does not necessarily go down well with healthcare managers, politicians or patients.
- Healthcare is usually highly politicised — for instance we may know that the most rational option to improve services might be to close a hospital or hospital department that is no longer needed, but this is almost guaranteed to result in angry voters and anxious politicians.

What is 'technology'?

The term 'technology' tends to be closely associated with 'innovation'. We talk of firms introducing a new technology in the same way that we talk of firms being innovative. But technology and innovation are not the same. It is important to develop a working understanding of technology and its various dimensions. Most writers come to the conclusion that technology is a slippery concept (Roberts and Grabowski, 1996; Orlikowski, 1992). The consensus is that technology is concerned with the application of knowledge to solve problems. Mitcham (1994) argues that technology has four dimensions: knowledge, activity, objects and volition. Some define it very broadly. For example, Schon (1967) described technology as 'Any tool or technique: any product or process, any physical equipment or method of doing or making by which human capability is extended.' An early edition of the OECD's *Oslo Manual* (on the measurement of scientific and technological activities) suggests that technology is 'the whole complex of knowledge, skills, routines, competence, equipment, and engineering practice' (OECD/EUROSTAT, 2005).

> "*By aggregating task, technique, knowledge, and tools into a single construct — technology — interaction among these constituting components and with humans is ignored. For example, we cannot examine how different assumptions, knowledge, and techniques can be embedded in different kinds of artefacts or practices, and how these have differential consequences for human action and cognition.*"
> (Orlikowski, 1992)

Such definitions have been criticised because of their breadth. Orlikowski (1992) argues that this makes it hard to distinguish the relative impact of new knowledge, physical artefacts or practices. There are also concerns that the words 'technological' and 'technology' are imbued with particular meanings that are associated with physical, manufactured products. These may not be appropriate when used in relation to the study of innovation because many people interpret the word 'technological' to mean 'using high-technology plant and equipment', and thus something that is not applicable to service or process innovations (OECD/EUROSTAT, 2005).

For our purposes, there are some important points to extract from these discussion about technology.

Hard and soft technologies

A distinction is usually made between *hard* technology, tangible artefacts such as computers or mobile phones, and *soft* technology, the knowledge about how those artefacts work (Swamidass and Nair, 2004). Soft technology is defined by Bessant and Francis (2005) as 'systems of thought, practice, and action that facilitate the achievement of explicit aims' — in other words, soft technology enables the application of hard technology to a problem. Orlikowski (1992) argues that a particular technology will be inscribed with ways of working that reflect individual values, world views, and organisational procedures and processes. How we understand a technology such as some software may therefore be heavily influenced by the knowledge encoded within it (Kogut and Zander, 1992; Blackler 1995; Fernandes and Melo Mendes, 2003).

There is a large literature on the relationship between knowledge and technology and innovation. This focuses on questions such as how 'explicit', 'tacit' or 'situated' it is, whether it is 'codified' or 'embodied', what capabilities organisations need to select, adopt or abandon technology, or support performance improvement (Box 2.2). Some knowledge — such as software to operate a device — is explicit, but tacit or situated knowledge may also be present and will influence its adoption and use (Suchman, 1987). This type of knowledge develops as the result of learning about a technology as it is used

---

Box 2.2   CONCEPTS: Types of knowledge

- **Explicit knowledge** can be readily articulated, codified and accessed.
- **Tacit knowledge** is the opposite of explicit knowledge; it cannot be adequately articulated by verbal means.
- **Codified knowledge** is tacit knowledge converted to explicit knowledge in a usable form.
- **Embodied knowledge** is the routines, habits, tasks, and information we understand without conscious thought.
- **Situated knowledge** is knowledge affected by the history, language, and values of the person knowing it.

in a specific context, and is therefore hard to capture or transfer to another individual or context or organisation (Lave and Wenger, 1991; Sole and Edmondson, 2002).

"The tools themselves are not the technology; it is the use to which they have been put that marks them out as a technology, and it is people who do the putting to some use for some purpose."
(Teich, 2003)

It is important to recognise that hard and soft technologies are not simply two ends of a continuum with physical artefacts at one end and intangible artefacts at the other. They are distinct types of technological entity, but entities which are bound together to a greater or lesser extent. An important implication of this is that human agency influences our actions and understanding of technology. We use technology both in a habitual and unconscious, and in a planned and deliberative way. We also make strategic choices about the application of technology and its future development. In short, we affect the way technology is used and evolves, and thus the factors that enable or inhibit technological innovation. The consensus is that technologies are not neutral in how they relate to both human agency and to the institutions in a society.

Researchers therefore suggest that technology forms part of a 'socio-technical system' — a system where people, organisations, institutions, and technologies interact (Trist, 1981; Teich, 2003) — and its role is subject to processes of 'social construction', where understandings of the world and shared assumptions about reality are jointly constructed by individuals (Orlikowski, 1992). It cannot be treated as a given (Weick, 2001), nor can its implementation be viewed in a deterministic fashion (see below). Many have studied how technology is 'socially constructed' (e.g. Bijker *et al.*, 1987; Bijker, 1995; Garud and Rappa, 1994). This highlights the way meanings associated with diverse technologies affects their development — for example, trade-offs made between traction, speed, and aesthetics influenced the bicycle tyre.

As we will see in later chapters, these distinctions about hard and soft technology and the nature of knowledge are important for understanding why innovation processes in healthcare are different from other sectors of the economy. In particular, healthcare technology cannot be defined solely in terms of physical artefacts. Its power lies in the soft

➔*Go to Chapter 5 to find out more about how this can make it hard to gather and interpret evidence about the impact of some kinds of healthcare innovation* knowledge associated with technology — in the skills and techniques involved and how these are put to use. This knowledge is adaptable to specific conditions — customised around the needs of individual patients and the local organisational context, such as a specific hospital in a particular national health system. It is also subject to evolution because of the reflexive nature of healthcare professions (i.e. practitioners learn from experience about themselves and their work). It may therefore be shaped by a process of social construction. This is why the implementation and impact of healthcare technology and healthcare innovation can be both challenging and unpredictable.

Technology determinism

While the implementation of technology cannot be treated deterministically, technology nevertheless has some deterministic qualities, in the sense that once it has started it may not be easy to reverse a particular technology trajectory. The internal combustion engine, developed in the late 19th century, still shapes the motor vehicle industry in the 21st century. A wholly new infrastructure of charging stations and battery recycling needs to be created to support electric vehicles. The continued use of the QWERTY arrangement on keyboards — not necessarily the most efficient for English speakers — is another well-known example (David, 1985).

Because technology is socially constructed and forms part of a wider socio-technical system, it is therefore important to recognise that there is nothing inevitable about a technological trajectory. This applies as much to a technology's general direction of

> "*Technology is built and used within certain social and historical circumstances and its form and functioning will bear the imprint of these conditions.*"
> (Orlikowski, 1992)

travel as it does to the relationship between a technology and society, since there is no guarantee that it will be adopted or its use will result in a specific outcome (Barley, 1986; Edgerton, 1999). How a technology is currently configured — its hard and soft elements, and the assumptions, values and knowledge that are embedded within it — is therefore closely shaped by its starting point and subsequent historical evolution (Clark, 1985).

A technology or technology system will therefore embody legacy elements as well as features associated with contemporary influences. Morison (1966) describes how old practices — soft technology — were embodied in contemporary artillery — hard technology — during the Second World War in the form of a short pause before firing: a routine introduced in the past to 'hold the horses' was followed without question, despite the very different circumstances of modern warfare.

Why we need to be more precise in our definitions of 'innovation'

The term 'innovation' is overloaded with meaning. It can refer to an *outcome* — we often implicitly use it in relation to physical objects or products — and it can refer to the *processes* by which these are developed. The outcomes of innovation can be physical objects, but new services or business models

> "*Innovation is 'an idea, practice, or object that is perceived as new by an individual or other unit of adoption'.*" (Rogers, 2003)
>
> "*Innovation is 'the process of bringing inventions into use'.*" (Schon, 1967)

can also be described as innovations — the new business model of a low cost airline, for example. Viewing innovation as a discrete product is often characteristic of the research literature on adoption, while viewing it as a process is more associated with research on implementation (Rye and Kimberly, 2007). As we will see later, in healthcare this separation can be somewhat artificial.

Until relatively recently business model or service innovation was generally overlooked in research, debate and teaching. Although things have improved, arguably there is still an overemphasis on the aspects of innovation that relate to the creation of new products and bringing them to a commercial market. There remains relatively little work on public sector innovation, the development and application of new ideas in a non-commercial setting. This is important because much of the provision of healthcare lies in the not-for-profit or public sector, even if the pharmaceutical, medical devices and other companies that supply its inputs are in the private sector.

Box 2.3   CONCEPTS: Defining innovation

Department of Trade and Industry, UK, definition of innovation (DTI, 2004):

- The action or process of innovating.
- A new method, idea, product.
- The successful exploitation of new ideas.

Some other definitions:

- 'Anything that creates new resources, processes or values, or improves a company's existing resources, processes or values' (Christensen *et al.*, 2004).
- 'The effort to create purposeful, focused change in an enterprise's economic or social potential' (Drucker, 1985).
- 'Innovation is a slow process of accretion, building small insight upon interesting fact upon tried-and-true process' (Rae-Dupree, 2008).
- 'Innovation is ... a new patterning of our experiences of being together, as new meaning emerges from ordinary, everyday work conversations ... a challenging, exciting process of participating with others in the evolution of work' (Fonseca, 2002).

Innovation has both a *creative* dimension (often described as 'invention') and a *commercial* or *practical* dimension that involves the exploitation of the invention. Only when both these dimensions are effectively managed does one have an innovation. It is therefore important not to confuse innovation and invention — they are related, but they are not the same. Many ideas fail to make it beyond the invention stage. The pathway to adoption can be long and hard. And even when a decision to adopt has been made, implementation into everyday practice and diffusion across a population can be hard. Perhaps nowhere is this more the case than in healthcare.

Can we be more robust and analytical in how we categorise innovations? This is important because the influence of technology can differ enormously depending on whether it changes *individual components* of a product (or service or business model), or *whole systems* of components, such as the shift from analogue to digital telephones. If we want to better understand the evolutionary process associated with innovation — how

---

Box 2.4   SUMMARY: Defining innovation — the key points

- *New ideas* — a new (or improved) product, process or service, or a whole new business or business model.
- *Exploitation* — the idea must be implementable and potentially value generating (i.e. innovation = invention + exploitation).
- *Successful* — the innovation is adopted by the target audience.
- *'New'* is a relative term — it can mean 'new to the world', 'new to the market' or 'new to the firm'.

A strict definition of the term 'innovation' might restrict its use to first-of-a-kind breakthroughs (e.g. the jet engine), but it also commonly used in connection with more modest incremental improvements to existing innovations.

Source: University of Cambridge Institute for Manufacturing.

---

innovation might change a product or service in the future — we need to make judgments about the degree of technological change embodied in that product or service.

Innovations (rather than the innovation process itself) have been categorised in various ways. One distinction is according to where the demand for the innovation is originating — is it *pushed* by the developers of a new technology or service, where there was previously no demand, such as the e-book. Or it is *pulled* by some kind of expressed demand, perhaps the need to reduce production costs or address a safety or quality issue. In practice, innovation is rarely a simple matter of 'push' or 'pull'. It tends to result from an interaction between the two, in which innovators simultaneously create ('push') new possibilities and at the same time identify evolving consumer or other needs ('pull') (Tidd and Bessant, 2014). For innovators, it is important to maintain a balance between keeping an eye on the market to ensure that their good ideas are actually potential innovations that people might want, and ensuring they are not so close to the market and its short term demands that they are blinkered in their search for truly radical ideas.

Another distinction that is often made is between *'incremental'* and *'radical'* innovation. For much of the time innovation is about exploiting and elaborating ideas, creating variations on a theme within an established technical or market trajectory (Tidd and Bessant, 2014). Occasionally, however, breakthroughs occur, creating a new technology trajectory, at which point the cycle repeats itself.

For our purposes, it is sufficient to classify innovations in three ways, according to:

- their *scope*, i.e. their degree of novelty (how new they are),
- their *form* or *application* (whether they are product, process, service) and
- their *innovativeness* (how much change there is in their components, compared to the current norm).

Scope: how new is new?

How we conceptualise the relationship between innovation and newness is essentially a question of judgement. Whether something is new or not depends on someone's perception of 'newness'. The perspective in innovation research is often that of the adopter. Novelty is seen in relation to the perception of adopters, whether they are individuals, companies or other kinds of organisation. An innovative product or process may already be in existence elsewhere. But its novelty may be in relation to a particular industry sector or a technology ecosystem such as a national healthcare service. Thus a new drug could be an innovation in one health system but not in another, where it is already widely used.

The definition of 'newness' can be subtle. One meaning of newness used in the innovation literature is 'differentness', the extent of departure from the *status quo*. Often this refers to some form of embodied knowledge, such as a prevailing technological norm or an external standard such as commonly accepted 'best practice' (Rye and Kimberly, 2007) (see Box 2.5). Thus medical innovation has been defined as a significant departure from previous techniques in a field, as determined by the collective judgments of experts (Meyer and Goes, 1988). Another definition of newness relates to 'recency', either the actual or perceived time that something has been in the world (Rye and Kimberly, 2007).

A well-known model is that of Cooper (2001), who classified innovations according to the degree to which they are *new to a market* or *new to*

Box 2.5 CONCEPTS: The ambiguity of 'newness' and 'differentness'

In their systematic review of the literature on healthcare innovation adoption, Rye and Kimberly (2007) argue that researchers are often rather casual in their use of alternative definitions of 'newness'. This is a problem because how we view newness influences both the definition of an external standard and the perceptions of potential adopters. They describe various options in a simple table:

		External standard	
		Innovation	**Not an innovation**
Adopter perceptions:	**Innovation**	1. Innovation	2. *Ambiguity*
	Not an innovation	3. *Ambiguity*	4. Not an innovation

In cell 1, there is clearly 'innovation' both in terms of adopter perceptions and external standards, but it is unclear whether this is because the innovation is novel in relation to an external standard, novel in relation to the adopter's perception, or a mix of these. Conversely, in cell 4, we can say that something is not an innovation but we cannot say precisely why. And there is more ambiguity when, for example, something is not an innovation from the perspective of an adopter but it is innovative in relation to an external standard (or vice versa). Rye and Kimberly argue that:

'The distinctions between definitions of innovation extend well beyond the level of semantics ... (They) reveal often deep-seated differences in the fundamental assumptions and viewpoints of researchers, differences that influence the character of research questions and analyses.'

We therefore need to be cautious when comparing the results of innovation adoption studies, because they may be talking about quite different things. It is important to identify clear boundaries between different types of study, because they may be built on quite different conceptualisations of innovation.

a company operating in the market. A new product line may be new to a particular company, requiring it to engage internally in innovative development, but for other companies that product may already be well established. Or a company may develop an old product to reposition it, creating

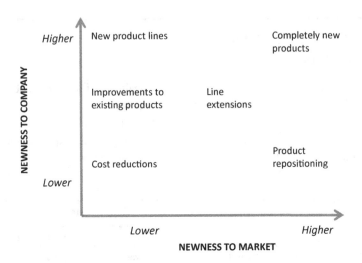

Figure 2.1.   Innovation 'newness'.
Source: Cooper (2001).

something new to the market, for example the repositioning of the drink Lucozade from something for people convalescing from illness to an energy drink for the growing fitness market. Really innovative products (or services) are new both to companies and markets. According to Cooper (2013), since the 1990s improvements and modifications to existing products — 'incremental innovations' — have grown substantially at the expense of innovations those are new to the world and new to the market (see Figure 2.1).

Freel and de Jong (2009) categorise innovations according to the *novelty of innovation outcomes* and the extent to which innovation activities mean an organisation or company has to *acquire new capabilities* — expertise, equipment or knowledge. An innovation that is new to a firm but not to the market may simply require enhancement in its capabilities and competence; radical innovations are not only new to the market but also require a firm to develop completely new capabilities (Figure 2.2).

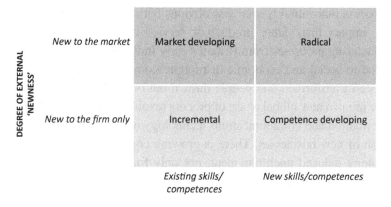

Figure 2.2.   'Newness' in relation to company-level capabilities.
Source: Freel and de Jong (2009).

Form: product, process or service?

We can also look at the *form* of an innovation. The three principal forms of innovation are:

* Products — tangible physical objects (e.g. mobile phone) that are acquired and then used by consumers.
* Services — intangible things (e.g. banking, education, and health-care), where the consumer benefits from the service, but does not actually acquire an object.
* Processes — the equipment, methods, systems used by producers of products or services.

Service innovations are often overlooked because they may be less eye-catching. The public imagination tends to identify with inventions and tangible products, but service innovations also have a huge impact on our lives — think FaceBook, ebay, Google. Service innovation can be subtle, emerging incrementally through the development of individual skills or collaborative relationships between organisations (Tether, 2005).

Process innovation is even less obvious but in the long run may have a bigger impact than either product or service innovation. Innovations in manufacturing processes from Britain's early Industrial Revolution onwards have led to social and economic disruption around the world, as industries have been transformed and people thrown out of work. Some have argued that we are in a new global phase of process revolution because of the impact of information and communications technology on business models and the creation of new businesses. There is growing concern over the prospect of technology-induced unemployment, not only for lower-skilled jobs in the manufacturing and services sectors but increasingly amongst parts of the professional workforce such as accountancy or law.

It has been argued that products or industries typically display lifecycles where the
emphasis of innovation shifts between products or processes at different stages. William
Abernathy and James Utterback (1975) developed a model in which the early stages are
marked by an emphasis on product innovation

> → *Chapter 6 discusses*
> *how disruptive innovation*
> *is impacting on the*
> *healthcare workforce and*
> *on incumbent companies*

and uncertainty. After some time, a 'dominant design' becomes established, which matches the market's needs and aspirations but may not be the best design in technical terms (in other words, creating a particular technology trajectory — see above). The emphasis then shifts from the product or product variety towards process innovation, improving manufacturing processes to deliver volume and consistent quality at the right price. Finally, a mature phase emerges, characterised by incremental innovation in both product and process, and extensive competition with other firms. Further breakthroughs eventually return the cycle to its fluid stage again and then moves forwards. From the perspective of companies seeking competitive advantage, this model means that the emphasis of their effort should be on searching for radical product innovation ideas in the early fluid phase and incremental improvements in the mature stage. However, disruption can occur in this stage as incumbent companies' products are displaced by cheaper versions by competitors.

The idea that innovations involve technology 'push' and 'pull' stimuli is also associated with this perspective. The focus of mature industries tends to be on pull as they respond to different market needs and try to differentiate themselves by incremental innovation. New industries, on the other hand, are often dominated by push stimuli, sometimes described as 'solutions looking for a problem'.

Types of innovation — radical, incremental and others

We also need to think about the 'innovativeness' of an innovation — how much R&D, design or engineering effort has gone into its creation and how does this affect performance? This is important because differences in the rate of performance change are partly related to the way innovation takes place, with implications for the kind of capabilities companies and organisations need to acquire as cycles of innovation unfold.

Rebecca Henderson and Kim Clark (1990) draw on the concepts of dominant design and the idea that different kinds of innovations can

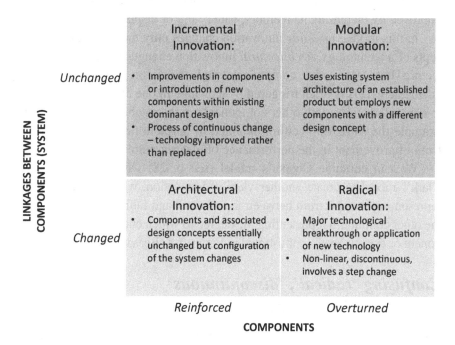

Figure 2.3.   Types of innovation.

Source: Henderson and Clark (1990).

be characterised in terms of their impact on the established capabilities of the firm. They outline a model with two dimensions. One captures the impact of innovation on the knowledge underlying the components of a product (or a service or process); the other captures its impact on the linkages between these components, i.e. the 'architectural' knowledge about the way components are linked together to make the product work. Four types of innovation are therefore possible, shown in Figure 2.3, with *radical* and *incremental* innovation representing extreme points in the innovation space. According to Henderson and Clark radical innovation establishes a new dominant design and, hence, a new set of core design concepts embodied in the components that are linked together in a new architecture. The shift from a portable cassette player such as the Sony Walkman to an MP3 player or an iPod is one example. Incremental innovation, on the other hand, refines and extends an established design. Improvement occurs in individual components, but the underlying core concepts, and the links between them, remain the same. So, once introduced, the MP3 player or IPod is subsequently improved by increasing its memory, battery life or display quality.

In this model, *modular* innovation changes only the core design concepts of a technology. *Architectural* innovation changes a product's architecture but leaves the components and their core design concepts unchanged. This is often triggered by a change in one component leading to new interactions with other components in the established product, for example the shift from ceiling mounted to portable fans, which resulted from improvement in the performance of electric motors and blades.

We can combine Cooper's model (see p. 28) with Henderson and Clark's model to create another view of innovation, with one continuum representing the spectrum between incremental and radical innovation and the other continuum representing the degree to which changes are at a component or system level, as illustrated in Figure 2.4 (Bessant and Tidd, 2007).

Confusing 'radical', 'discontinuous' and 'disruptive' innovation

There is often confusion about the terms that are used to describe more radical types of innovation. The terms 'discontinuous', 'radical' and 'disruptive' innovation are often used interchangeably. While *continuous* innovation improves but preserves the current way of doing things,

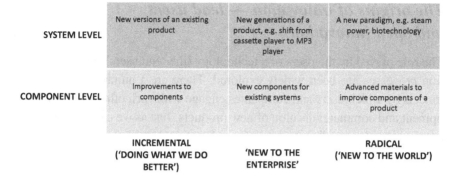

SYSTEM LEVEL	New versions of an existing product	New generations of a product, e.g. shift from cassette player to MP3 player	A new paradigm, e.g. steam power, biotechnology
COMPONENT LEVEL	Improvements to components	New components for existing systems	Advanced materials to improve components of a product
	INCREMENTAL ('DOING WHAT WE DO BETTER')	**'NEW TO THE ENTERPRISE'**	**RADICAL ('NEW TO THE WORLD')**

Figure 2.4.   Another classification of innovations.

Source: Bessant and Tidd (2007).

Box 2.6   CONCEPTS: Definition of discontinuous innovation

Discontinuous innovations cause a paradigm shift in science or technology and/or the market structure of an industry. As they are entirely new-to-the world products, made to perform a function for which no product has previously existed, discontinuous innovation requires a good deal of learning for the incumbent organisation and its value network, including the user. Discontinuous innovations disrupt established routine and may even require a very different set of capabilities and new behaviour patterns. The notion of novelty is relative so a discontinuous innovation for one organisation might be an incremental one for another. Radical innovation and discontinuous innovation are used synonymously. Disruptive innovation used to be a synonym until 1997. Since then the term has been strongly associated with Christensen's model. Incremental innovation is the opposite of radical innovation.

Source: http://lexicon.ft.com/Term?term=discontinuous-innovation

---

discontinuous innovation leads to some kind of disruption to the *status quo* (Tushman and Anderson, 1986). Radical and discontinuous innovations are essentially synonymous and describe a significant degree of change over the existing technology. But the term 'disruptive' innovation is also sometimes used interchangeably with radical innovation. The *Financial Times* has produced a simple primer, in Box 2.6. We discuss the notion of 'disruptive innovation' in detail in Chapter 6.

The origins of innovation — lead users and open innovation

The role played by the users of a technology (the 'end users') in its innovation processes has been widely explored. There are a number of different models by which users and companies engage with each other in the development and commercialisation of new products. Just as we can characterise an innovation according to its various functional attributes or degree of newness, we can also characterise it according to the processes by which it came about.

One way of doing this is to think about role end-users play in the innovation development process and the level of *openness* there is in sharing knowledge about the innovation as it is being developed, i.e. how freely the innovators reveal their intellectual property (IP). Figure 2.5 categorises different models on this basis, showing how there are different forms of innovation ranging from traditional supplier-centred, technology push models where the knowledge underpinning an innovation is either generated internally or acquired externally, through more user-centred

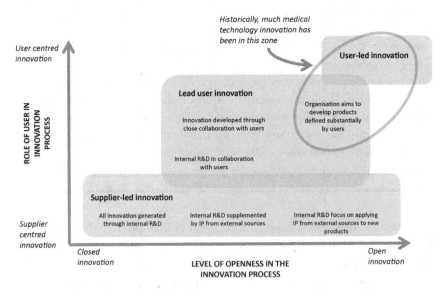

Figure 2.5. Differentiating supplier-led, lead-user and user-led innovation.

Source: Based on Savory (2009a).

models where 'lead-users' are important contributors to the innovation process, to 'open innovation' models in which users take on the prominent role in creating and developing an innovation.

Lead users are defined by Von Hippel (2005) as members of a user population who experience needs — ahead of mainstream users — that will eventually become the norm and who anticipate significant benefits from obtaining a solution to their needs. Lead users are potentially important to companies because they can provide input into the development of innovations. The difference between lead user innovation and more open or user-led models lies in who controls the development and sales process, which remains with the innovating company in the lead user case.

Another type of user needs pull is the idea of 'extreme environments' as sources of innovation. Roy Rothwell and Paul Gardiner described how 'tough customers mean good designs' (Gardiner and Rothwell, 1985), meaning that the needs of extreme environments or problems drive innovators to come up with cutting-edge ideas and radical innovations. Originally this was applied to advanced technological solutions to problems such as the need to create a radar-invisible military aircraft. More recently, the concept has overlapped with the notion of 'disruptive'

➔*Go to Chapter 6 to find out more about frugal innovation in healthcare*

and 'frugal innovation' to provide cheaper, simpler solutions to segments of a market previously not catered for, perhaps through novel business models for the 'bottom of the pyramid' population.

Different aspects of this area of research on innovation processes were brought together in the late 1980s by Henry Chesbrough into a model of open innovation (Chesbrough, 2003). The concept rejects the assumption that innovation only stems from an organisation's internal R&D capacity. Rather, some companies seek innovative ideas from outside, taking them on to develop and bring to the market, or sometimes selling on for another party to exploit them (Lichtenthaler, 2010). The emphasis in open innovation is on combining these internal and external ideas in order to advance the development of new technologies. This requires the power of actual and potential users to be harnessed to an organisation's own resources.

Essentially open innovation breaks the traditional technology-push paradigm of innovation development. While technology-push may still be the dominant model in many sectors, including much of healthcare, user-driven models have always been significant and open innovation is seen as an increasingly important way of generating new ideas.

→*Chapter 4 discusses open and other user-led innovation models in healthcare*

Some have described the shift towards open innovation as a 'democratisation' of innovation (Von Hippel, 2005) — the end-users of a product are active in its innovation process, often collaborating in communities (now assisted by social networking tools) and prepared to freely reveal their innovations.

Open innovation has been criticised for being a rather vague and prescriptive concept, and there is a lack of robust academic research on its benefits (Tidd and Bessant, 2014). While it emphasises that firms should acquire knowledge or other innovation resources from external parties, and share their own internal resources with them, when and how a firm should do this is less clear. User-innovators can be reluctant to relinquish control of their innovation projects when additional skills need to be brought in. However, if it is left too late development may have gone too far down the wrong track; too early and the innovator risks giving away their IP. Various benefits and challenges for companies embarking on an open innovation strategy are described in Table 2.1.

Box 2.7 CONCEPTS: Chesbrough's principles of open innovation

- Not all the smart people work for you.
- External ideas can help create value, but it takes internal R&D to claim a portion of that value for you.
- It is better to build a better business model than to get to market first.
- If you make the best use of internal and external ideas, you will win.
- Not only should you profit from others' use of your IP, you should also buy others' IP whenever it advances your own business model.
- You should expand the role of R&D to include both knowledge generation, and knowledge brokering.

Table 2.1. Potential benefits and challenges of applying open innovation.

Six principles of open innovation	Potential benefits	Application challenges
Tap into external knowledge.	Increase the pool of knowledge. Reduce reliance on limited internal knowledge.	How to search for and identify relevant knowledge sources. How to share or transfer such knowledge, especially tacit and systematic.
External R&D has significant value.	Can reduce the cost and uncertainty associated with internal R&D and increase depth and breadth of R&D.	Less likely to lead to distinctive capabilities and more difficult to differentiate. External R&D also available to competitors.
Do not have to originate research in order to profit from it.	Reduce costs of internal R&D, more resources on external strategies and relationships.	Need sufficient R&D capacity in order to identify, evaluate and adapt external R&D.
Building a better business model is superior to being first in the market.	Greater emphasis on capturing rather than creating value.	First mover advantages depend on technology and market context. Developing a business model demands time consuming negotiation with other actors.
Best use of internal and external ideas not generation of ideas.	Better balance of resources to search and identify ideas rather than generate them.	Generating ideas is only a small part of the innovation process. Most ideas unproven or no value so cost of evaluation and development high.
Profit from others' IP (inbound open innovation) and others user our IP (outbound open innovation).	Value of IP very sensitive to complementary capabilities such as brand, sales network, production, logistics and complimentary products and services.	Conflicts of commercial interest or strategic direction. Negotiation of acceptable forms or terms of IP licenses.

Source: Tidd and Bessant (2014).

Technology, innovation and performance improvement

Usually the performance of a product improves and unit costs fall over time. We have all experienced this with consumer goods such as laptops, tablets or mobile phones. But forecasting the future impact of innovation is often hard. We may only have limited knowledge about the rate of change in an innovation, which parameters or components are changing, or whether the effects are specific to the product or system-wide. More broadly, it is hard to accurately appraise the future because the external environment of a particular industry may be highly complex and fast changing, driven by technical, economic, social and political change.

Using 'Delphi' panels and scenario building are two approaches to exploring technological futures. We can also use historical data to tell us how a particular trend evolved in the past and extrapolate it to help guide us on its possible future evolution, or we can use heuristics — simple mental models of a phenomenon. One well-known example in innovation research is the *performance 'S curve'* (not to be confused with the *adoption and diffusion S curve*, discussed below, p. 56). Richard Foster (1986) argues that the performance of a product typically grows slowly in its early stages then speeds up before finally tailing off (Figure 2.6). This is the result of increasing, then declining, R&D productivity within a given innovation architecture. The shape of the curve implies that significant effort is needed during the early stages, but once this learning has been achieved, performance can improve with marginal effort. For some industries or products there may then be a breakthrough to a new curve, as radical innovation completely changes the innovation architecture. In other words, there is a discontinuity between the old and new

"Those who have knowledge, don't predict. Those who predict, don't have knowledge."
(Lao Tzu, 6th century BC philosopher and poet from ancient China.)

"There are two classes of people who tell us what is going to happen in the future – those who don't know, and those who don't know they don't know."
(John Kenneth Galbraith, economist, Wall Street Journal, 22 January 1993.)

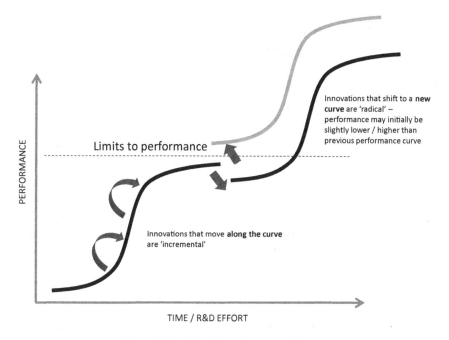

Figure 2.6. Foster's performance S curve.

curves. Understanding the nature of S curves gives us an insight into the competitive dynamics in a particular industry or technology sector. For example, in his book *The Innovator's Dilemma*, Clayton Christensen discusses how each successive computer hard drive industry was wiped out by the introduction of new technology platforms (Christensen, 1997).

This S curve model therefore helps us to assess where a technology is in its likely lifecycle and provides an indication of industry maturity. It is, however, simply a generalisation of an observed pattern of changing performance — in reality the shape of the

➜ *We return to this when we look at the pharmaceutical industry in Chapter 4.*

curve can vary considerably and we cannot infer how great the future gains are likely to be or when and how a discontinuity (i.e. radical shift) may take place. Nevertheless, performance S curves have been observed in many industries and for many technologies (e.g. Asthana, 1995).

Innovation as a process: invention, commercialisation, diffusion

The process of innovation has commonly been divided into three stages, known as 'the Schumpeterian trilogy' after the economist Joseph Schumpeter:

- The *invention phase*, where ideas are turned into workable inventions, is typically characterised by experimentation to prove the concept. Incremental innovations may involve little or no experimentation but nevertheless require a considerable amount of technical development. Much effort has gone into improving the life of mobile phone or laptop batteries as these devices have grown ever-more power hungry.

- The technological potential of an invention has to be transformed into economic value. *Commercialisation* is where the latent value of a technology is unlocked in order to generate real value. There may be many possible ways to commercialise an idea, but only a few are likely to succeed. Today the term 'commercialisation' is often used synonymously with the concept of 'business models', which are essentially enabling devices to allow inventors to profit from their ideas (Chesbrough, 2006).

- *Adoption and diffusion* is the process by which innovations are taken-up and spread through a population. This rarely takes place at a steady, linear rate. If the adoption of an innovative product is plotted over time, it frequently exhibits an S shaped curve, not to be confused with Foster's performance S curve. We come back to the adoption and diffusion curve below, p. 56.

> *"... inventiveness should not be equated with the development of novel artefacts, or indeed with novelty and innovation in general. Rather, inventiveness can be viewed as an index of the degree to which an object or practice is associated with opening up possibilities ... What is inventive is not the novelty of artefacts and devices in themselves, but the novelty of the arrangements with other objects and activities within which artefacts and instruments are situated, and might be situated in the future."*
> (Barry, 2001)

The distinction between these phases emphasises the point that successful innovation requires the entire process from invention to diffusion to be carried out. An invention is merely a nascent innovation and it may be many years before it makes it to innovation status. Equally, a nascent innovation may never make it — it may simply remain as a patented technology that is never commercialised. Failure may occur even after adoption as the implications of the innovation are more fully understood. Drugs where previously unforeseen side effects only emerge after widespread use are an example. These 'failed innovations' are rarely studied (Hadjimanolis, 2003).

There are weaknesses in this way of characterising the innovation process. In particular, the Schumpeterian trilogy has been criticised because it is seen as too linear. However, linear models are widely used by policy-makers, the business community and academics as a basic blueprint for technological innovation activities because of their simplicity (Godin, 2006). And clearly defined innovation strategies in companies — such as those relating to new product development (Cooper, 2000; Cooper *et al.*, 2000) or the development of new drugs (Northrup *et al.*, 2012) — generally make use of at least some aspects of linear innovation models.

> *"When innovation work begins, the process does not unfold in a simple linear sequence of stages and sub-stages, Instead, it proliferates into complex bundles of innovation ideas and divergent pathways of activities by different organisational units...the process diverges into multiple, parallel, and interdependent paths of activities."*
>
> (Van de Ven, 1999)

> ➜ *We see how important this is in healthcare especially in Chapters 5 and 7.*

Nevertheless, linear models hide the true complexity of the innovation process and because of this, they are seen by many as normative and deterministic. Researchers now emphasise feedback between different innovation stages and interactions between actors. Innovation — as a process — is therefore better characterised as a non-linear, dynamic system. Inventions and new ideas can occur at any point in the system, they may need to be adapted to local contextual circumstances, and their form may evolve through the process of adoption. In healthcare services especially, the innovation process tends to be iterative, problem-oriented and collaborative, starting with an issue to resolve and defining the innovations that potentially provide a solution. Either explicitly or implicitly, this process may be informed by 'design thinking' (Brown, 2008).

The innovation process is also complex because in certain industrial sectors, innovations may emerge as an output of processes within national and regional systems of innovation, sustained by an infrastructure of supporting institutions (Chapter 4) (Edquist, 2001). Other innovation systems may be sectoral, focused around a specific industrial sector and based on networks of relationships (Malerba, 2004), or technological fields (Carlsson *et al.*, 2002), or they may draw on expertise from different industrial sectors or technical disciplines defined, for example, by patent classes (Coombs *et al.,* 2003).

Technological innovation therefore needs to be seen as the result of interactions within ecosystems that bring together companies and other institutions within a particular technology or industrial sector, rather than as an output of a series of discrete processes. Different industries are characterised by different forms of innovation process, ranging from highly structured and formalised new product development processes to ones that are more evolutionary and adaptive.

New product development

From the perspective of companies producing innovative products, the ideal process is one where uncertainty is gradually reduced by tackling R&D in a series of stages in which emerging problems are systematically addressed. In this way, the product moves along a logical pathway, starting with initial scanning of potential user needs, progressing through technology development and prototyping, refining the product and finally launching it on the market. This requires firms to integrate their market- and technology-related activities along the way (Tidd and Bessant, 2014).

"*Managing new product or service development is a fine balancing act between the costs of continuing with projects which may not eventually succeed (and which represent opportunity costs in terms of other possibilities) — and the danger of closing down too soon and eliminating potentially fruitful options.*"
(Tidd and Bessant, 2014)

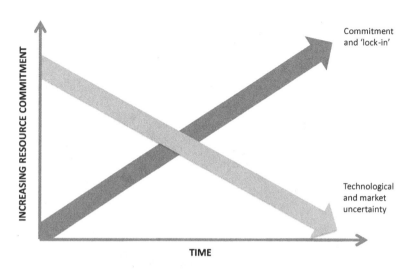

Figure 2.7.   Uncertainty and resource commitment in innovation projects.
Source: Tidd and Bessant (2014).

The model emphasises a series of planned phases of development that reduce risk and control costs to ensure final delivery of a saleable and usable product to customers. Over the life of a project, the growing commitment of resources and locked-in, sunk costs incurred by the company make it increasingly difficult to change direction (see Figure 2.7). Central to this aspect of technology and innovation management is the acquisition of knowledge obtained through market research, competitor analysis, and technological R&D. This allows uncertainty to be converted into measurable risk, an ability to take a calculated decision about whether or not to proceed with an innovation project. This process has often been described in terms of a 'development funnel', where many ideas or prototypes are progressively whittled down as uncertainty is reduced and external and internal resource constraints come into play (Cooper, 2001) (see Figure 2.8).

Actively managing the progress of technology projects from inception to development and commercialisation requires some form of structured decision-making process. This should involve clear stages and rules on which to base decisions to proceed or abandon a project. There are many variations, but the approach has been influential across a wide range of technology sectors. A well-known version is Robert Cooper's 'stage-gate' model

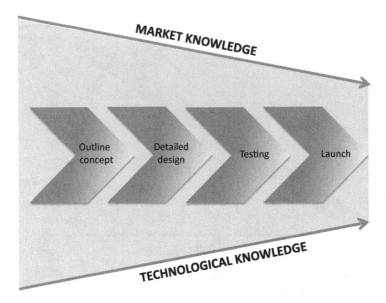

Figure 2.8.   Development funnel for new product development.
Source: Tidd and Bessant (2014).

(Cooper, 2001). Here, innovation projects have to meet specific decision criteria, 'gates', as they move through a series of discrete stages. Decisions are made according to technical, financial or marketing criteria that are appropriate to the stage (see Figure 2.9). Partly in response to criticism that the approach is too inflexible and unable to cope with more serendipitous ideas, different variations on this idea exist, such as the notion of 'fuzzy' — less rigid — gates, and the number of gates varies, but the basic stages are:

- Concept generation — identifying the opportunities for new products and services.
- Project assessment and selection — screening and choosing options which satisfy certain criteria.
- Development — translating concepts and options into a product and testing the winning ideas.
- Commercialisation — launching and marketing the new product.

In practice, new product development is not usually the simple, linear, and unidirectional process implied by these models. The reality is often

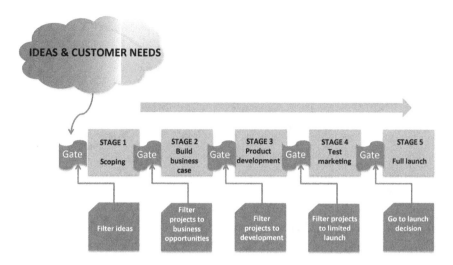

Figure 2.9.   A stage-gate process.
Source: Tidd and Bessant (2014) and others.

far messier and iterative, depending on the particular characteristics of the industry — its competitive or regulatory environment, or its sophistication in using approaches like concurrent engineering to optimise the product development process.

David Nichols (2007) has criticised of the notions of funnels and stage-gates as too rigid and constraining, because the whole emphasis is on whittling down a large number of ideas to a smaller number by culling weaker ones and picking the winners. He

➔ *Chapter 4 discusses how there are distinctive approaches to new product development within the healthcare industries, depending on the specific sector, notably the drug-development pipeline and development of medical devices.*

argues that a more constructive approach is needed to speed up the innovation process. Nichols proposes an 'innovation rocket' in which the end goal is clearly established through a full understanding of the problem, multiple ideas are generated in a process of 'combustion', potentially fruitful mixes are then subject to more detailed R&D and attention from possible funders and partners, and the best ideas are 'accelerated' through the development process (Figure 2.10).

THE INNOVATION ROCKET

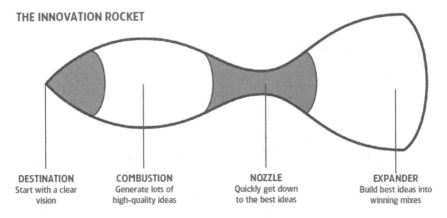

DESTINATION	COMBUSTION	NOZZLE	EXPANDER
Start with a clear vision	Generate lots of high-quality ideas	Quickly get down to the best ideas	Build best ideas into winning mixes

Figure 2.10.   Innovation rocket.

Source: Nichols (2007).

Experimentation, 'fast fail', 'safe fail'

Some companies tackle the challenge of creating new product ideas through a process of experimentation, adaptation, and evolution, using trial and error to produce a range of workable solutions in increasingly real-world situations. Experimentation might involve trying out multiple approaches or variants of an innovation, gradually focusing attention as more is understood about the innovation and its implications. This is an evolutionary approach, combining variation — pursuing a number of different options such as small-scale interventions or prototypes — and selection, where variants that work are replicated. It is essentially a *breadth* rather than *depth* first approach (Ellerman, 2004; Barder, 2010; Beinhocker, 2006).

Barder (2010) describes how a new nozzle for foam was developed by testing a set of (random) variations on the initial prototype, choosing the most effective one, testing a new set of random variations on that nozzle and so on. This approach proved far more successful than having experts try to design the optimum nozzle. One lesson is that the emphasis should not be on the need to always strive for success or ensure that failure is always avoided. Rather, ideas that are not useful should be tried and allowed to fail, but to do so in contained and tolerable ways, paving the way for those that are beneficial to be adopted — the concept of 'safe-fail experiments' (Snowden, 2010). This is all about learning quickly and learning cheaply — both in terms of costs of the innovation process itself and costs of failure — and allowing the emergent possibilities to become more visible.

For companies, therefore, safe-fail experiments are a way of tackling the critical risks first and arriving at an outcome quickly without wasting resources. Companies developing innovative products might use proxies, perhaps a single market segment or a simplified technology, to test a hypothesis and find out whether it has value, instead of pursuing an expensive idea that may lead nowhere. The goal is to try out more ideas at a lower cost, and in doing so perhaps discover unexpected new sources of value and identify possible routes to adoption.

➔ *The concept of 'safe-fail experiments' contains lessons from theories about complexity and complex systems, such as 'adaptation' and 'emergence', which we discuss in Chapter 7.*

Related to this is the notion of 'fast fail' and 'pivoting', the ability to manoeuvre very quickly during the development phase when companies realise that their product is

---

Box 2.8 BACKGROUND: Fast fail is just an excuse for poor management

The concept of fast fail has been criticised as fashionable and misplaced hype. As Rob Asghar (2014) says,

'Forget the cute mantras. No one should ever set out to fail. The key, really, shouldn't be to embrace failure, but to *embrace resilience* and the ability to bounce back. And the goal shouldn't be to glorify mistakes and errors and catastrophes, but to cultivate the ability to adapt and learn from them.'

Others go further and argue that 'failing fast' and 'pivoting' are simply excuses for explaining repeated failures, revealing that a company doesn't really know what its innovation has to do in order to address customer needs (Villon de Benveniste, 2014). What is more important than failing fast is how fast you learn from failures and successes, and quickly recognising how to modify an innovation to take advantage of the lessons.

not going the right way. Blank (2013) argues that this favours experimentation rather than elaborate planning, customer feedback over intuition, and iterative design over traditional 'big design up front' approaches. The concept of 'fast fail' has been criticised (see Box 2.8), but the principle of embracing notions of 'adaptation' and 'emergence' from complexity theory has nonetheless become an accepted part of the innovation process in many areas, including healthcare. For the drug companies, technological innovation and alliances with technology platform companies has helped them engage in large-scale experimentation in a faster, systematic process of trial and error (see Chapter 4).

Innovation adoption and diffusion

Language matters — some definitions

As with many discussions about 'innovation', there is a certain woolliness about the terms used when describing how innovations are taken up into mainstream use. Words are often used interchangeably to mean the same or very similar concepts (Box 2.9).

The *adoption* and *diffusion* of an innovation initially seem fairly clear as descriptive terms. Adoption refers to the process of making a decision to do or acquire something — the factors that are influential, the weights

---

Box 2.9   CONCEPTS: What is in a word?

All these are routinely used to describe the process of adopting and diffusing innovation:

- Adoption
- Implementation
- Normalisation
- Routinisation
- Mainstreaming

- Scaling-up
- Diffusion
- Spread
- Translation
- Transfer

we attach to them, the trade-offs that are made between them, the circumstances under which certain factors outweigh others, and so on. Diffusion is usually defined in relation to the 'spread' of an innovation through a population or perhaps geographically through a region or country — how rapidly it is taken up and factors that influence this.

But other terms are also common currency in this area of innovation research and practice — 'implementation', 'normalisation', 'routinisation', 'mainstreaming', 'scale-up', 'spread', 'translation' (or 'transfer'). The first four are frequently used more or less interchangeably, but there are subtle differences between them. These words imply a sense of action and often relate to the processes by which an innovation is taken-up by an organisation and introduced into everyday practice.

There is little consensus on the operational meaning of the other terms — 'scaling-up' or 'spread' and 'translation' or 'transfer'. These are found especially within discussions about the adoption of innovations in healthcare. We discuss this in detail in Chapter 5. Briefly, scale-up and spread capture the idea that diffusing successful trials or innovations on a wider basis can be challenging, especially in healthcare, something that researchers, practitioners and policy-makers have long wrestled with. Definitions of scaling-up include widening the geographical coverage of interventions, institutionalising practices, increasing capacity, mobilising and empowering populations, and transforming demonstrably successful pilot projects into large or mainstream programmes by going to scale (Bloom and Ainsworth, 2010).

> ➔*Go to Chapter 5 for a discussion about adoption and diffusion of innovations in healthcare and the differences between these concepts*

Technology 'translation' or 'transfer' is related to the movement of novel ideas from a research laboratory setting into the market and everyday use. It implies putting knowledge to use in some way. We will see in Chapter 4, how this is important in healthcare in relation to the commercialisation of new technologies. In contrast to diffusion, which essentially involves the spread of a product or idea through a given social system, technology transfer is a more discrete, point-to-point phenomenon (Tidd and Bessant, 2014).

Many researchers have noted that adoption is not a one-off, all-or-nothing event; it is more of a process, a sequence of decisions and actions. After initial acceptance, an innovation may need to be adapted to its local context and institutionalised within organisations and their practices (Meyer and Goes 1988; Zhu *et al.*, 2006). A distinction is therefore often made between different phases in the process of adopting an innovation within an organisation — 'evaluation', 'initiation', 'implementation' and 'routinisation' (Damanpour and Schneider, 2006). Trisha Greenhalgh, Glenn Robert, and colleagues argue that in healthcare narrow definitions of 'adoption', which fail to look beyond the initial decision to acquire an innovation, are unhelpful because in reality much of the hard work is about ensuring that innovations, once 'adopted', are assimilated into daily practice (Greenhalgh *et al.*, 2004; Robert *et al.*, 2009). Also focusing on healthcare, Carl May and his colleagues (May *et al.*, 2007; May and Finch, 2009) have developed a theory of 'normalisation' to explain the work involved in implementing, embedding and sustaining new practices in situations where the innovation and its context are marked by complexity and emergent behaviour.

Factors influencing adoption and diffusion

Adoption can be defined in terms of the processes which influence a decision to take-up an innovation, while diffusion relates to the spread of an innovation through a population. The factors which influence adoption have been much studied by a range of disciplines.

Economists often see the innovation process as the cumulative aggregation of individual, rational calculations, influenced by an assessment of the costs and benefits, under conditions of limited information and uncertainty (Tidd and Bessant, 2014). This makes the transfer of *information* about an innovation important in the adoption and diffusion process (see Box 2.10). However, this perspective has been criticised because it ignores the effects of social characteristics of adopters, of learning and feedback between them as innovations are adopted, and the impact of externalities such as the benefits of a growing population of users taking

Box 2.10   CONCEPTS: The role of information in adoption and diffusion

The importance of information flows between adopters features in various models of adoption and diffusion (Geroski, 2000):

- Probit adoption — where potential users or customers *weigh costs and benefits*. The heterogeneity of preferences means that different users or customers adopt an innovation at different paces.
- Epidemic adoption — where adoption is influenced by the *availability of information*. As potential users and customers become aware of what an innovation does and how to use it, they will adopt it.
- Information cascades and path dependence — once an innovation becomes established and its (improved) features are well known, it is legitimised and network effects take over.

'Bandwagon' effects sometimes occur. These result from pressure caused by the sheer number of people who have already adopted an innovation, rather than by individuals assessing its benefits. This can allow technically inefficient innovations to be widely adopted and sustained, such as the QWERTY keyboard (see p. 24).

To cope with the fact that adopters often have limited information on which to make decisions, Bayesian models of diffusion have been developed. These allow potential adopters to hold different beliefs about the value of an innovation, which they may revise according to the results of trials. If such trials are conducted privately, other potential adopters cannot learn from them and imitation cannot take place. This means that there is no automatic link between how well informed potential adopters are and how quickly they adopt an innovation.

up an innovation. The initial benefits of adoption may be small, but with improvement, reinvention and the effect of externalities, the benefits can increase and the costs decrease over time, as in the early days after the introduction of mobile phones as more and more people became owners.

A very influential book is Everett Rogers' *The Diffusion of Innovations,* first published in 1962. Rogers distinguishes between three types of decision-making process relevant to adoption:

- Individual: the individual is the main decision-maker. Decisions may be influenced by social characteristics and norms, and interpersonal relationships, but the individual ultimately makes the choice, independent of others. This would be typical of a consumer deciding to purchase a new product.
- Collective: choices about adoption are made jointly with others in a social system, and there is peer pressure or formal requirement to conform. An example would be the introduction of new policies to promote the recycling of domestic waste.
- Authoritative: a few individuals within a social system who have professional status or expertise have the power to make the decision to adopt. Doctors may be in this position for some types of medical technology.

Everett Rogers identified five product-based factors that govern the rate of adoption and diffusion:

- **Trialability** — the degree to which a product may be *experimented* with prior to launch.
- **Compatibility** — the degree to which a product is *consistent* with the user's context, their values and experiences.
- **Observability** — the degree to which product *usage and impact* are visible to others.
- **Relative advantage** — the degree to which a *product is better* than the product that it replaces.
- **Complexity** — the degree to which a product is *difficult* to understand and use.

However, Rogers also emphasised that simply focusing on the relative advantage of an innovation will only give us part of the story. Values and beliefs will vary with the social, economic, and cultural context. This in turn means that adopters may hold different views on the costs and benefits of an innovation, or its compatibility with their organisation, or way

Table 2.2.   *Key demand- and supply-side influences on innovation adoption.*

Demand-side factors	Supply-side factors
• Degree of direct contact with or imitation of earlier adopters • Different perceptions of benefits and risk held by adopters	• Relative advantage of an innovation • Availability of information • Technical or economic barriers to adoption • Feedback between developers and users

Source: Tidd and Bessant (2014).

of life or needs. Drawing on studies from rural sociology on agricultural innovations, Rogers characterised adoption and diffusion as an essentially social process. Actors create and share information through communication, perhaps influenced by opinion leaders, and make decisions on the basis of this. It is therefore unrealistic to assume that all potential adopters are similar and have the same needs. Nor can we assume that every potential adopter has perfect information about the innovation and its qualities. In practice, a range of demand- and supply-side factors influence adoption patterns (Table 2.2).

Opinion leaders and innovation 'champions' can be critical for adoption and diffusion, especially when an innovation requires stakeholders or consumers to change their behaviour or attitudes. Research has shown how opinion leaders and early adopters can have an important influence on the spread of certain consumer goods. In healthcare, they can be especially important in public health programmes or sex education, both in developed and developing countries' health systems. There has been much research on different forms of opinion leader and champion, and on the way they help to bridge boundaries between groups. We return to this in Chapter 5, where we look at their role in the processes of implementing healthcare innovations.

What are the implications of these ways of understanding the factors that shape the spread of an innovation through a population? How might they be translated into patterns of adoption and diffusion?

Rogers proposed a five-way classification of adopters, based on the normal distribution (bell-curve):

- Innovators (2.5% of the population of adopters)
- Early adopters (13.5%)

- Early majority (34%)
- Late majority (34%)
- Laggards (16%)

The first groups of adopters — 'technology enthusiasts' and 'visionaries' — have rather different characteristics from the other potential adopters, who simply want reliable, fool proof and finished products or services. Innovators selling to these groups therefore need different communication and sales strategies. A well-known book that elaborates on this idea is by Geoffrey Moore (1991). This focuses on the characteristics of potential adopters such as their personality, values, attitudes, interests or lifestyles. Moore argues that initial adopters may provide promising sales and enthusiastic feedback for innovating companies, but reaching the *early* and *late majority* is ultimately more important for commercial success. These groups have different perceptions of a product and its potential benefits (i.e. they want something reliable and finished), so significant changes to the product or service offer may be required. The 'chasm', for Moore, is the potential gap between the early adopters and late majority.

Cumulatively, the take-up of innovations by a population over time displays an S shaped curve. This characteristic is seen in many product innovations. The model assumes that the population of potential adopters is homogeneous. An innovation spreads because information about it is transmitted through the population by personal contact, observation and proximity to existing and potential adopters.

> ➜ *Be careful not to confuse the two types of S curve in innovation — one relates to performance improvement over time (Foster) and the other to the adoption and spread of an innovation (Rogers)*

Many innovations will, however, deviate from this neat path because of the effects of a diverse range of interactions and circumstances that are contingent on the local context for adoption — these include the policy, regulatory or economic factors that shape adoption decisions. Savory and Fortune (2013) note how assumptions about linearity in innovation development processes (see above, p. 43) are also reflected in the innovation diffusion literature. Rogers' six-phase model of diffusion is essentially a linear model, although he is careful to note how serendipitous events can knock an innovation off course and that his model is a just a general guide.

The time taken for an innovation to pass through each phase in the Rogers diffusion model varies considerably. The may be a long gap between initial adoption by enthusiasts or pioneers and mainstream use. Joe Tidd and John Bessant (2014) argue that a critical, but under-researched, question in diffusion research is what happens *before* the regular S shaped diffusion curve begins to take hold. This is very important for the creators of an inno-vation. The market introduction of a new product may be followed by an erratic pat-tern of adoption, a 'pre-diffusion phase'.

> ➔ *We will see in Chapters 4 and 5 how and why the pre-diffusion phase in healthcare innovation can be long.*

This may be the case even after an innovator has invested in the infra-structure necessary for the manufacture and distribution of the product. The market in this pre-diffusion phase is unstable. In consumer electron-ics, for example, the diffusion of new products and services often starts with the launch, withdrawal, adaptation, and reintroduction of product variants before mainstream designs appear and diffusion takes off. The length of the pre-diffusion phase varies, but research on a sample of products and industries suggests that the average length can be more than a decade.

A different, but related — perspective on adoption and diffusion, and the S shaped adoption curve, can be seen in the concept of a 'hype cycle'. This was developed by Gartner, the IT industry consultants. The hype cycle views the process of market penetration as a series of stages related to adopters' changing expectations. Initial enthusiasm gives way to disil-lusionment, realism and eventual acceptance. This model seems to work for many technological innovations. An example of the hype cycle in mid-2014 for a selection of emerging technologies can be found at http://www. gartner.com/newsroom/id/2819918

The factors that influence adoption and diffusion are therefore com-plicated. Actual or potential users or customers are usually heterogeneous in their characteristics — they have diverse needs, and they place different values on how best to meet those needs. Moreover, their needs change over time. Sometimes this is due to exogenous changes, in other words what customers want is responsive to their own changing circumstances or broad societal shifts. Sometimes they may be due to endogenous changes, where their own beliefs and behaviour change in response to technological innovation opening up new demands.

It is often hard to get people or organisations to adopt novel products or services. According to John Gourville (2006), most potential customers, most of the time, are loath to change their behaviour. They are unfamiliar with novel products, which almost always require them to make trade-offs between cost, functionality, added value and their requirements. Customers tend to be overly sensitive to the *disbenefits* of a novel product and they therefore evaluate a product on its perceived relative value. Businesses, on the other hand, often *overestimate* the potential benefits but *underestimate* switching costs for customers adopting a new product. Gourville therefore views adoption as a world populated by 'eager sellers' and 'stony buyers', with the results shown in Table 2.3.

Richard Nelson and colleagues describe four models of innovation adoption and diffusion based on two dimensions (Nelson *et al.*, 2004) — whether or not increasing returns to the adoption of an innovation exist

Table 2.3.   *Adopter behaviour change, innovation payoff and the likelihood of success.*

		Payoff	
		Low	**High**
Behaviour	*Not much*	Easy sells	Smash hits
change	*A lot*	Sure failures	Long hauls

Source: Based on Gourville (2006).

Table 2.4.   *Models of innovation diffusion.*

	Absence of dynamic increasing returns	**Presence of dynamic increasing returns**
Ability to get sharp persuasive feedback	Model I: rational choice diffusion	Model II: quasi rational choice with possibility of 'lock in'
Inability to get sharp persuasive feedback	Model IV: fads	Model III: social construction

Source: Nelson *et al.* (2004).

(i.e. the extent to which the value of adoption is increasingly enhanced as more people adopt it) and secondly the ability to receive clear feedback on the impact of an innovation (i.e. whether or not there is ambiguity in the evidence of its perfor-

➜*Nelson et al. (2004) applied their model to a healthcare innovation, polio vaccine, discussed in Chapter 5.*

mance). This follows the notion that the way a technology is perceived and understood — hence valued — may be socially constructed, as noted earlier, p. 23. In one of the options, outlined in Table 2.4, there is the possibility of 'lock in' to a sub-optimal, inefficient technology because of the presence of increasing returns as more and more people use the innovation.

Moving from a view of adoption that is focused on individual users

There is a huge volume of research on innovation processes in an industrial and consumer market context which shows that adoption and diffusion is more likely when innovations are simple, trialable, observable and so on — recall Everett Rogers' list of factors. But there are three limitations to much of this research, both as a body of knowledge on innovation in general and, as we will see later, when it is applied to healthcare. First, it has tended to focus on new *products* rather than *services* or *business models*. Second, the innovations studied have often been *single products with unambiguous characteristics* — a specific product delivering a clear benefit to the user. In the healthcare context, this is rarely the case. Finally, explanations have often stressed the aggregate effect of *independent decision-makers* making *individual* adoption decisions. Innovations involving collective or organisational decision-making have been relatively neglected. In healthcare, we are more likely to be interested in the latter, for example whether or not a hospital as an organisation decides to adopt an innovative scanner or whether it decides to embark on a series of radical changes to operational processes. So how are adoption decisions made at an organisational level?

Organisations can be highly complex entities, possibly none more so than in healthcare. Many academic and other studies have explored the

---

Box 2.11   CONCEPTS: Innovation leadership

Innovation leadership is the work of:

- Creating the right conditions for innovation to occur.
- Putting in place the infrastructure to support innovative thinking — the roles, decision-making structures, networks, physical space, equipment and so on.
- Envisioning a better future.
- Having the courage to challenge the *status quo*.
- Being comfortable with risk taking.
- Having sufficient ego strength.
- Facilitating and empowering others to be as creative as they can.

Source: Malloch (2011).

---

attributes of organisations seen as innovative. An organisation's ability to recognise, absorb and apply knowledge from outside — its 'absorptive capacity' (Cohen and Levinthal, 1990; Zahra and George, 2002) — has been closely linked to attitudes towards innovation and its adoption. This in turn rests on the right kind of organisational culture to provide a foundation for a climate in which innovation can be fostered. The important characteristics of an innovative organisational culture include:

- A climate conducive to experimentation and risk taking, and an expectation that all members challenge assumptions.
- Visionary staff in pivotal positions.
- Clear strategic vision.
- Strong leadership.

The last of these points itself requires certain cultural attributes, such as a high regard for creativity and openness to new ideas. Innovation leadership therefore requires leaders to possess the right characteristics, outlined in Box 2.11.

Being 'ready' for the adoption of innovations generated elsewhere and being 'innovative', in the sense that an organisation generates and uses new ideas internally, are not necessarily the same thing, although there is a blurring between the two; organisations prepared to scan the world for new ideas and take them on may well be more prone to generate innovations themselves.

The adoption of innovations at an organisational level is likely to be more complex than decision-making by individuals about a single product, and will be influenced by factors such as the range of stakeholders involved in adoption decisions, their goals and how powerful they are, as well the four characteristics outlined above. The *evidence* for the benefits of the innovation may be important — how clear and unambiguous are the facts about what it delivers? And the *nature* of the innovation, how radical or incremental it is, may also make a difference.

As Tidd and Bessant (2014) point out, decisions about adopting an *incremental* innovation may be fairly straightforward. A well-defined business case can be assembled, costs and benefits can be argued and the innovation's 'fit' with the organisation's current activities can be demonstrated. But the more *radical* an innovation or the greater its complexity, the higher the likely resource commitment and risks of adoption, and the more that emotional or political influences within the organisational will be influential.

Radical innovations may require organisations to reframe their mental models of the world. Organisations will ask themselves what the alternative options are ('what if we don't adopt this innovation?') and whether the strategic decisions involved are consistent with each other. Simply gathering more evidence for the benefits may be insufficient and an organisation — and the individuals within it — may need to change the 'frame' through which it sees and interprets that evidence in order for it to make sense within its specific context.

This can be especially challenging when the core competencies of a firm or organisation are strong and long established. Organisations have comfort zones beyond which they are reluctant or unable to consider innovation projects, whether as innovators or adopters. In Chapter 4, we discuss stage-gate models used by companies developing new products to decide whether to proceed or not. These work where the criteria for decisions are clearly established and perceived as appropriate by all stakeholders, and there are steady-state conditions where the world is not rapidly changing. But the higher levels of uncertainty associated with more radical innovations put pressure on these models. This may result in organisations (or individuals — see Box 2.12) rejecting ideas which do not fit their

Box 2.12   CONCEPTS: Cognitive barriers to innovation held by individuals

Our ability to accept change is also constrained by cognitive barriers that work at the level of individuals within organisations. Some of these are associated with a lack of awareness or knowledge of an innovation, but others relate to a lack of willingness to try out innovations (Lettl, 2005). In his book *Adapt*, Tim Harford (2011) describes how various psychological attributes prevent us from learning from our failures and moving forwards. One of these is denial (challenging a *status quo* of our own making) due to 'cognitive dissonance', the mind's difficulty in holding two seemingly contradictory thoughts simultaneously. Another is the way we 'chase our losses' in an attempt to make them go away, typical gambling behaviour. Finally, there is 'hedonic editing', where we convince ourselves that previous mistakes or problems don't matter, or we reinterpret past failures as successes.

mental model. There may be nothing irrational about defending an established mental model. Decisions not to proceed with an innovation project (or to adopt an innovation) may make sense in terms of the criteria associated with an organisation's dominant cognitive framework; the reasons for rejection may be clear and consistent with its own decision rules and criteria. But as Tidd and Bessant (2014) explain, organisations can cloak decisions in a shroud of 'rationality' by using empirical evidence or the lack of it as justification. Persuading such an organisation to adopt the innovation is not simply a case of gathering new information — say evidence for the benefits of an innovation — but changing the frame through which it sees and interprets that information.

Such a perspective makes it easier for us to understand the 'not invented here' syndrome common in many sectors. This is especially prevalent in healthcare where there is a problem of repeated trialling of innovations by different organisations, even when there is a good evidence base. Table 2.5

➜ *Chapter 5 discusses the relationship between evidence and trialling or piloting healthcare innovations*

shows typical reasons presented by organisations for the non-adoption of innovations.

Table 2.5.   *Examples of justifications for non-adoption of innovations.*

Argument	Underlying perceptions from within the established mental model
'It's not our business'	Recognition of an interesting new business idea but rejection because it lies far from the core competence of the firm
'It's not a business'	Evaluation suggests the business plan is flawed along some key dimension — often underestimating potential for market development and growth
'It's not big enough for us'	Emergent market size is too small to meet growth targets of large, established firm
'Not invented here'	Recognition of interesting idea with potential but rejection — often by finding flaws or mismatch to current internal trajectories
'Invented here'	Recognition of interesting idea but rejection because internally generated version is perceived to be superior
'We're not cannibals'	Recognition of potential for impact on current markets and reluctance to adopt potential competing idea
'Nice idea but doesn't fit'	Recognition of interesting idea generated from within but whose application lies outside current business areas — often leads to inventions being shelved or put in cupboard
'It ain't broke so why fix it?'	No perceived relative advantage in adopting new idea
'Great minds think alike'	'Groupthink' at strategic decision-making level — new idea lies outside the collective frame of reference
'(Existing) customers would not/ do not want it'	New idea offers little to interest or attract current customers — essentially a different value proposition
'We have never done it before'	Perception that risks involved are too high along market and technical dimensions
'We were doing OK as we are'	The success trap — lack of motivation or organisational slack to allow exploitation outside of current lines
'Let's set up a pilot'	Recognition of potential in new idea but limited and insufficient commitment to exploring and developing it — lukewarm support

Source: Tidd and Bessant (2014).

Applying lessons on technology and innovation management to healthcare

In the rest of the book, we will use these basic building blocks from the research on technology and innovation management to explore what they mean for the healthcare sector. The important question to ask at this point is how the particular features of healthcare might influence its innovation processes. How might the complexity of healthcare make a difference? How would you expect its closely regulated environment to impact on innovation adoption? What about attitudes towards the quality of evidence for the benefits of an innovation?

Two key features of healthcare are that its innovations can be often rather ambiguous in their characteristics — their technology and organisational components. The innovation itself may be multifaceted, perhaps embracing elements of hard technology mixed with a considerable degree of organisational change. It may require adopters to learn new skills (soft technology) in order to use it. An innovation may be targeting several objectives at the same time, such as improvements in quality *and* safety *and* cost. Or the evidence for improved performance may be ambiguous or contested by different types of healthcare worker. The context for their adoption may also be complex — there may be multiple users of the innovation, all of whom can be seen as 'adopters'. These may be situated in different types of organisation such as primary or secondary care providers, or they may come from different professional groups or have differing cultural characteristics. Moreover, multiple stakeholders from across primary, secondary and social care may be affected by the innovation, all with the potential to veto adoption decisions.

So often the adoption and diffusion of healthcare innovations is erratic. Conventional models, applicable widely across industries, need to be adapted. This means that not only does the adoption and use of acknowledged best practice or evidence-based innovation vary between considerably countries, it may be uneven within a country's own health system, with some healthcare providers using the leading technologies and practices but others continuing to use outmoded approaches. This can result in significant geographical differences in access to the best treatment — hence the interest of policy-makers in improving the effectiveness of healthcare innovation processes and, in particular, the spread of best practices across the system.

Chapter summary

- Definitions are important — we need to make a distinction between 'technology' (which is the application of knowledge to solve problems and not just a physical artefact) and 'innovation'.
- Innovation does not simply refer to inventions — it is both, a process which embraces different stages from initial idea to adoption and diffusion, and it is also an outcome of this process — we talk about 'an innovation' when referring to something new.
- There are different ways of looking at an innovation — we can see it in terms of its 'newness', its form (whether it is a product, process or service), or its type (is it radical, incremental or some other type, depending on the theory we use?).
- The performance improvement of a specific technology or product can often be seen as an S shaped curve, where performance initially improves slowly, but then speeds up through the application of R&D and new knowledge. Eventually it begins to tail-off as it reaches a limit.
- The adoption and diffusion of innovation is influenced by a range of factors, including the attributes of the innovation itself, the adopting individual's or organisation's context and the compatibility of the innovation with that context, and the degree to which the innovation offers the prospect of benefits.
- The processes involved in the adoption of innovations by organisations tend to be more complex and are influenced by factors like organisational culture and leadership, and the range and power of stakeholders.
- The adoption of an innovation can be plotted (typically) as an S shaped curve, with slow initial take-up followed by faster adoption by the majority of users, before tailing off.
- There are limitations to using the concepts from mainstream innovation research to explain innovation processes and adoption/diffusion in a healthcare context.

Questions for discussion

1. Why do we make a distinction between 'technology' and 'innovation'? What is the difference between 'hard' and 'soft' technology?
2. Explain the differences between 'invention' and 'innovation'. Which do you consider to be the most important and why?
3. Give examples of product, service and process innovations and describe their main characteristics.
4. Why do we categorise innovations? How might this be useful for innovators and policy-makers?
5. What is meant by 'radical innovation'? Take an example of a radical innovation and explore its impact on society. Do the same for an 'incremental innovation'.
6. Use the theory of the S-shaped technology performance curve to distinguish between radical and incremental types of innovation, using examples.
7. Using an innovation of your choice:

   • Describe the *type* of innovation using one of the models.
   • Describe the various steps in the innovation process.

8. What are the differences between 'open' and 'closed' innovation models?
9. What are the implications of open innovation as far as individual researchers and innovators are concerned?
10. Why does Eric Von Hippel describe innovation as having been 'democratised'?
11. What are the limitations of portraying innovation as a series of phases?
12. Explain what is meant by 'stage-gates' in relation to the innovation process and discuss the advantages and disadvantages.
13. Distinguish between the three main types of decision-making process in the adoption of innovations. Why might we want to focus on organisations rather than individual users when considering how adoption takes place?

Selected further reading

Chesbrough H (2003) *Open Innovation: The New Imperative for Creating and Profiting from Technology.* Cambridge: Harvard Business School Press.

Gourville J (2006) Eager sellers and stony buyers. *Harvard Business Review* 84(6): 98–106.

Henderson R, Clark K (1990) Architectural innovation. The reconfiguration of existing product technologies and the failure of established firms. *Administrative Science Quarterly* 35: 9–30.

Nelson R, Peterhansi A, Sampat B (2004) Why and how innovations get adopted: A tale of four models. *Industrial and Corporate Change* 13(5): 679–699.

Rogers E (2003) *Diffusion of Innovations.* New York: Free Press.

INNOVATION IN HEALTHCARE — A SPECIAL CASE?

03

THIS CHAPTER WILL HELP YOU TO:

- Identify characteristics of different types of healthcare innovation.
- Understand why healthcare innovations are complex.
- Learn about the unusual economics of healthcare innovation.
- Understand the adoption process for healthcare innovation.

We have looked at the important concepts from mainstream technology and innovation management research. We now need to think about how they can be applied in healthcare. In this chapter, we set out the reasons why and how innovation in healthcare might be different from other sectors of the economy. The quote from Morrisey (2008) encapsulates the key points very well. The hard and soft technologies of healthcare are created within the corporate and research

"The health care product is ill-defined, the outcome of care is uncertain, large segments of the industry are dominated by non-profit providers, and payments are made by third parties such as the government and private insurers. Many of these factors are present in other industries as well, but in no other industry are they all present. It is the interaction of these factors that tends to make health care unique." (Morrisey, 2008)

ecosystems of the pharmaceutical, medical biotechnology, and medical devices sectors. These new technologies are taken-up within an equally complex environment comprising policies and regulations, institutional and organisational structures and cultures. Healthcare innovations and healthcare services also take place within a built and telecommunications infrastructure distributed across geographies that range from low-density remote rural areas to large high-density cities. The general consensus, therefore, is that the healthcare sector is 'different' from other goods and services. Box 3.1 summarises the distinctive features of healthcare. The rest of this chapter unpacks them in more detail.

Box 3.1   SUMMARY: Distinctive features of healthcare that influence its innovation processes

- **The nature of healthcare 'technology' and 'innovation'.** The key point here is that the boundaries between the organisational and technological aspects of healthcare innovations may be very blurred. Most healthcare innovations involve some combination of 'soft' and 'hard' elements and the interplay between them means that many healthcare innovations are both 'process' and 'service' innovations (Savory and Fortune, 2013). Modern healthcare combines many sub-disciplines and requires technologically advanced equipment and drugs, yet it still very much involves human interaction. Another feature of healthcare is that what begins as one innovation can mutate into different variants as it is adopted and subsequently adapted by its users in different local, national or organisational contexts. This can be the case when the 'innovation' is a hybrid between organisational and technological changes, or it is open to interpretation by those responsible for implementation precisely what elements are adopted.
- **A risk-averse culture and extensive regulation** mean that healthcare innovations may need to follow a lengthy process of experimentation and legitimation. Gathering evidence for the benefits of an innovation is a very important part of this process. But the fuzzy nature of many healthcare

(Continued)

Box 3.1 *(Continued)*

innovations not only makes it hard to gather robust evidence, but ideas about what constitutes good quality evidence are also often contested by stakeholders from across different parts of the health and social care systems. Clinicians, nurses, GPs, and social workers may have rather different understandings of what a specific innovation is and what its defining components are (Mackenzie *et al.*, 2010).

- **The economics and politics of healthcare** are a complicating factor for the adoption of innovation. Governments in most countries play a fundamental role in shaping how healthcare is planned, regulated and financed. Politics may result in short-termism, with the result that innovations that take time to deliver their benefits are shunned in favour of quick wins. The economics surrounding healthcare innovation are influenced by the structure of national healthcare systems. The separation of payers, such as insurance companies or governments, and providers — and fragmentation of the latter into different primary, secondary and social care organisations — mean the costs and benefits of a given innovation may not fall equally across the system. The time taken for the impact of an innovation to be visible or realised may be longer than a political or planning cycle. It may be hard to identify what these impacts actually are when the innovation is complex, because they take time to realise or they are spread across the health system in an unpredictable way. Making a return from an innovation — either for the company supplying it or the adopter investing in it — can therefore be hard.

- **The environment into which new technologies and other innovations are adopted and implemented is often extremely complex**, especially in developed countries. Multiple stakeholders from across the care systems may be involved in adoption decisions. The decision-making rules and processes may be opaque. Responsibility for adopting and spreading some innovations is devolved to healthcare provider organisations or individual doctors, and for others it is centralised in organisations such as the UK's National Institute for Health and Care Excellence or the Canadian Agency for Drugs and Technologies in Health. Adoption may also be constrained by a general resistance to change due to the rigidity of a health system's institutions, professional bureaucracies, financial silos and vested interests.

What is healthcare technology and healthcare innovation?

The concept of 'healthcare technology' can be hard to grasp. When we hear these words, we tend to think of medical equipment and — possibly — drugs. We tend to associate it with the new and the high tech, rather than the eclectic range of physical products that are used everyday in healthcare, from the sticking plaster to advanced imaging equipment. And as we saw in Chapter 2, technologies are never just physical artefacts. They are used within a specific social and economic context, and we tend to imbue them with meaning and knowledge. Human agency — critical and reflective practice — shapes how individual healthcare technologies are used, as do the national and local financial, jurisdictional, ethical, and administrative governance structures surrounding healthcare systems (Webster, 2007).

The distinction between the elements of an innovation based on *tangible* artefacts ('hard' technology) and those based on knowledge and human activity involved in its use of the application of technology ('soft' technology) can be applied to healthcare technology (see Box 3.2). The power of healthcare technology lies in the way these hard and soft attributes are used in a particular context — in the knowledge and skills, techniques and practices that are embedded in them. Hard and soft healthcare technologies are therefore rarely discrete, unrelated entities. This distinction is recognised in the EU definition of a medical device (see Box 3.3).

Box 3.2 CONCEPTS: Hard and soft technologies in healthcare

- Hard technology, the physical artefacts — drugs, devices, other equipment and physical infrastructure.
- Soft technology, the practices, procedures, protocols, service designs and guidelines that are often used in conjunction with hard technologies — a protocol for carrying out an innovative surgical technique, for example, or more broadly a service design for providing 'telehealth' or 'telecare' for frail elderly people, combining sensors and other devices to monitor vital and other signs with home care services.

Box 3.3 BACKGROUND: What is a 'medical device'?

The European Union has a lengthy definition of what a 'medical device' is. Note that it recognises how an individual device may be part of a larger, more complex system:

'Medical device' means any instrument, apparatus, appliance, software, material or other article, whether used alone or in combination, together with any accessories, including the software intended by its manufacturer to be used specifically for diagnostic and/or therapeutic purposes and necessary for its proper application, intended by the manufacturer to be used for human beings for the purpose of:

- *diagnosis, prevention, monitoring, treatment or alleviation of disease,*
- *diagnosis, monitoring, treatment, alleviation of or compensation for an injury or handicap,*
- *investigation, replacement or modification of the anatomy or of a physiological process,*
- *control of conception,*

and which does not achieve its principal intended action in or on the human body by pharmacological, immunological or metabolic means, but which may be assisted in its function by such means ...'

Source: Directive 2007/47/EC of the European Parliament.

The context within which hard and soft healthcare technologies are created and deployed is very important. This can range from individual patients to healthcare organisations or whole health systems. Even clearly defined healthcare processes may be subject to a degree of customisation depending on the specific context. The meanings associated with a healthcare technology are therefore 'socially constructed' within the context and evolve over time. This has been shown in specific medical technologies. Cochlear implants (Garud and Rappa, 1994) and cataract surgery (Metcalfe *et al.*, 2005) are two examples of medical technologies which evolved during their development and use. Another well-known study, on the implementation of MRI scanners (Barley, 1986), shows how two hospitals implemented the same technology rather differently due to the effects both of the circumstances for implementation and human agency (in this case, radiologists' understanding of the technology). In the case of intraocular lenses and implantable hip joints (innovative hard technologies), the associated soft technology — procedural and tacit knowledge about their use — became established and institutionalised over time, as the new technology was adopted and diffused (Metcalfe and Pickstone, 2006). Soft technologies are potentially even more subject to adaptation and evolution because they are liable to take on properties from the institution in which they are deployed. The introduction of a continuous improvement programme in a hospital may start as a set of activities which might be fairly uncoordinated, but eventually become embedded within the organisation's structure and culture.

As well as the world of new medical technologies, innovation also takes place in healthcare organisations as they develop and adopt new ways of working, new operational processes, new protocols or standards, new payment and reimbursement models or new organisational structures. Some of these innovations will have been generated from within an organisation, others will be learnt from elsewhere, and others imposed by government or regulatory bodies. These can all be seen as innovations — 'new to the firm' or 'new to the market' as described in Chapter 2 — but how they are managed to ensure they are adopted successfully will vary according to the circumstances.

> ➔ *Chapter 2 discusses technology determinism*

Another aspect of technology noted in Chapter 2 is its deterministic quality, the way some technology trajectories can be rigid and hard to break away from. New technologies must fit within an existing legacy of hard and soft technologies, and institutional structures. The progressive development of modern healthcare over many decades means that healthcare systems are a palimpsest of past policies and past technologies, layered upon each other. How an innovation is introduced and the path it subsequently takes is therefore strongly influenced by the prevailing structural characteristics of the given health system, in the form of:

- cultural features (such as norms of practice, agreed standards of evidence, professional identities, and codes of conduct),

- physical features (such as the infrastructure of hospitals and other facilities or the existing technological architecture), and
- institutional features (the configuration of organisations, regulations, and financial systems that comprise health systems).

To be effective, the introduction of some innovative technologies may require the reconfiguration of health services, including their location and their organisational processes, job roles and skill requirements. But the choices available to those

→ *Chapter 6 discusses the impact of disruptive innovation on the infrastructure for healthcare*

seeking to introduce them may well be constrained by the rules of the game, even in situations where there is an obviously better way of delivering as aspect of healthcare.

What do healthcare innovations typically look like?

We saw in the previous chapter how innovations can be classified in different ways, for instance, according to their scope (their degree of novelty), their form (whether they are product, process, service innovation) and their 'innovativeness' (how much innovation there is in their components and from whose perspective?). These allow us to distinguish between incremental and radical — or continuous and discontinuous — innovations, along with various other subcategories.

" *... no innovation takes place or diffuses in isolation and the determinants of success for new medical procedures often reside on the development of complementary techniques, drugs and devices.* "
(Metcalfe *et al.*, 2005)

We also saw that innovation can be seen both as an outcome and as a process — the actions involved in innovating from initial idea and creation to commercial exploitation, adoption and diffusion.

One problem in healthcare is that innovation rarely takes the form of a neat physical artefact or a clearly delineated process. It has often been pointed out that both embodied (product) and disembodied (process) innovations combine, leading to changes in both the technology artefact and in practices associated with it (Bower, 2003). The way a particular health service or practice is delivered may change through a process of technological innovation, along with adjustments to work processes and organisational structures. This is very clear in the case of

> ➔*Case study 5.1 (Columba) in Chapter 5 describes the problems introducing an innovation which impacts on different parts of the health and social care systems*

'telehealth' or 'telecare', the use of sensors and other devices to monitor vital and other signs, and provide care at a distance to individuals. As the case study in Chapter 5 shows, introducing a relatively simple telecare service for elderly people involved a wide range of stakeholders from across primary, secondary and social care and considerable attention to the organisational and financial mechanisms surrounding it.

Identifying whether the scope of the innovation, its degree of novelty and even whether it is largely a product, process or service innovation can therefore be hard. A simple distinction between product innovation and service improvements (HITF, 2004), or organisational practices,

> ➔*Go to Chapter 6 for more on disruptive innovation and the impact on jobs and roles in healthcare*

organisational structures, technologies and new roles, only gives us a partial view — the reality is usually more subtle. Changes in one area can in time trigger wider changes — new hard technologies such as cheaper and simpler diagnostic devices can result in disruptive innovation where less skilled staff are able to take on roles previously occupied by specialists (Christensen *et al.*, 2000) (see Chapter 6). Research by Lansisalmi *et al.* (2006) suggested that only 13% of healthcare innovations were focused on new technology, with the rest comprising service, organisational or role innovations.

> ➔*See Chapter 4 to read more about the role of users in the development of healthcare innovations*

Although not unique to healthcare, another distinguishing feature of innovation in healthcare is the part played by end-users in developing new technologies. There is a long history of surgeons as both designers and users of surgical instruments (Kirkup, 2006). Over time, clinicians have become increasingly involved in the design of new models of health service delivery, and more recently the emphasis has been on patient and public participation in service redesign.

In healthcare, it is therefore often unclear what the 'innovation' actually is, how it originated and who was responsible. A new drug or medical device such as a better scalpel may be readily identifiable and relatively 'discrete' — the new scalpel may have an obvious inventor and does not require new training or new organisational processes to be used. However, many technological innovations in healthcare are not like this. They may require organisational changes to ensure they work effectively. Significant new training for the staff operating the innovation may be needed or the innovation may change work processes or the role of particular professional groups — for instance, cheaper, simpler imaging technology may replace the need for radiologists. A new service delivery model may have evolved over time with the input of many stakeholders and it may involve multiple changes to healthcare practices. The boundaries around many healthcare innovations, especially those targeted at service redesign, are therefore often fuzzy. They may consist of some hard technology, but a lot of soft technology such as new service delivery models or organisational changes, and they may be trying to tackle multiple objectives. Figure 3.1 classifies some healthcare innovations according to their complexity.

In subsequent chapters, we will explore how these characteristics often mean that the adoption of innovations into mainstream healthcare practice is by no means straightforward. Because an innovation may have multiple dimensions, tangible and intangible features, and several objectives, it might be understood in different ways by those involved in implementing and using it. The evidence for its efficacy may be hard to collect and interpret, and therefore contested by different stakeholders, or there may be no widely accepted criteria for judging the benefits. Implementation might involve multiple stakeholders from across the health and social care systems, all of whom need to be consulted and whose interests need to be aligned. Decisions may be subject to complex regulations. And even when an innovation is more clear cut, involves few stakeholders and has a good evidence base, adoption and diffusion can be onerous.

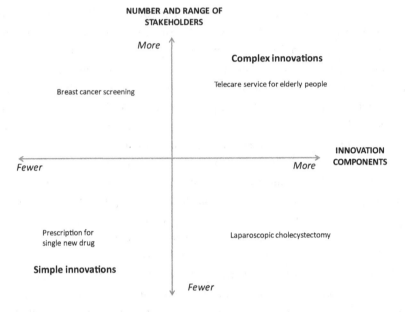

Figure 3.1.   Classifying healthcare innovations by their complexity.
Source: Based on Atun *et al.* (2010).

Box 3.4   EXERCISE: Classifying healthcare innovations

All the examples here have been recognised as 'healthcare innovations'. Two can be described as hard technology innovations and two are soft technology innovations. Scan the material and answer the following:

- Why do you think these have been described as innovations?
- What is innovative about them?
- Try to categorise them according to
  — their degree of novelty (how new?);
  — their form or application (product, process, service);
  — their 'innovativeness' (radical, incremental, architectural, modular).
- How easy do you think it will be to ensure the innovation is widely adopted? What are the organisational, cost-benefit and other acceptance issues?

(Continued)

Box 3.4 (*Continued*)

Hard technology innovations

1. **Robotic heart catheter.** Robotic surgery involves a system that can be programmed to aid the positioning and manipulation of surgical instruments to surgeons to carry out complex tasks more efficiently or remotely. It is beginning to become widely used for certain procedures, especially those involving minimally invasive surgery in the thoracic cavity and the abdominal cavity. Robotic surgery requires a different set of techniques to be adopted, with the surgeon operating from a remote console to control the equipment rather than physically operating on the patient him or herself. As well as potential benefits the patient, such as decreased risk and shorter recovery time, the wider health benefits include fewer human errors and a faster learning curve for surgeons in training. One area where robotic devices have been developed for surgical procedures is the insertion of catheters such as Hansen Medical's robotic catheter system. This allows surgeons to remotely guide a heart catheter with hand movements, while seeing a 3D view of the operation. The device allows more precise catheter movements inside the heart.

Sources:
http://www.hansenmedical.com/us/en/cardiac-arrhythmia/sensei-robotic-system/product-overview
http://www.youtube.com/watch?feature=player_embedded&v=e1aV34vlN0Q

2. **Diagnosing cataracts by smartphone.** Diagnosing cataracts typically requires a USD 5,000 piece of equipment and a physician to interpret the test results. Neither is easy to come by in rural areas and lower-income countries. A team of MIT researchers has developed a simple device, Catra, that can clip onto an ordinary smartphone and provide a diagnosis of cataracts within a few minutes. 'I like to think of this as a radar for the human eye', said one researcher. The system sweeps a beam of light across the eye to detect the cloudy patches resulting from cataracts and creates a map showing their position, size, shape and density, more detail than needed to make a decision whether or not to surgically remove the lens. Inexpensive and portable diagnostic devices such as Catra could play

(*Continued*)

Box 3.4   (*Continued*)

an important part in helping provide care for the 250 million people in the world who are blind because of preventable causes.

Sources:
http://web.mit.edu/newsoffice/2011/netra-cataracts-app-0701.html
http://www.youtube.com/watch?feature=player_embedded&v=V2BXSWuQO0M

Soft technology innovations

These are both from the *Health Services Journal* (HSJ) Best Practice Awards 2011.[1]

3. **Bupa Care Services: Improving residential care by digitalizing quality processes.** In 2010, the English health and social care regulator, the Care Quality Commission (CQC), changed its methodology for assessing quality processes in residential care homes. Bupa used this opportunity to review how they monitored its care services and re-engineer its quality assurance (QA) processes. It aimed to ensure that all QA processes were internally integrated and aligned with external regulation, to make QA simpler and less burdensome for care home managers, and to drive improved quality through better governance and more transparent reporting. Bupa moved from a paper based QA process to an online model, where compliance assessments were fully digitalised. By using a free-to-market version of Microsoft Sharepoint, Bupa was able to develop the system on a tight budget. After introduction of the system, care home managers spent less time providing their compliance assessment reports to the CQC, which meant they concentrated more on the residents and their needs. Regional managers were able to see reports before they were submitted to the CQC to ensure their accuracy. The system also resulted in more useful and actionable management information, quickly identifying concerns and allowing managers to track improvement actions between their visits.

4. **University Hospitals Southampton: Finding the missing millions and reducing admissions through medical intelligence.** Chronic obstructive pulmonary disease (COPD) is the fourth leading cause of death in the UK, with enormous social and economic implications. It is the second most common reason for an emergency hospital admission. The British Lung Foundation report *Finding The Missing Millions* highlighted the fact that

(*Continued*)

---

[1] http://www.hsj.co.uk/journals/2011/11/21/o/c/i/HSJBP2011.pdf

Box 3.4 (*Continued*)

the city of Southampton is a hotspot for COPD, yet the disease is significantly under diagnosed, leading to a higher admissions rate. It was clear that a strategy to identify undiagnosed and misdiagnosed COPD was needed. Using medical intelligence, GP practices were prioritised according to estimated undiagnosed COPD prevalence and hospital admission rates. A team from the hospital then visited and educated each GP practice. This was supported by wider educational meetings, an education package, and websites for health professionals and patients. The hospital employed a dedicated respiratory nurse to deliver the project and work closely with primary care. An audit of hospital attendances revealed that 34 patients were admitted more than three times the previous year and were responsible for 22% of admissions. These patients were looked after exclusively by the respiratory teams — reviewed in their homes by a consultant and specialist nurse to look at their health needs, optimise their current treatment and investigate the reasons why they needed to come into hospital. After implementing the project the rate of diagnosis increased from 1.5% to 2.3%, compared to an estimated 6% prevalence rate in the city. There was a 19% reduction in hospital admissions due to COPD exacerbations, and hospital readmissions within 30 days were reduced from 13% to 1.7%. Net financial savings in the first year were estimated to be GBP 301,800.

Risk and regulation

The distinctive features of healthcare also impact on the way new products (or practices, processes or services) are brought into mainstream use in healthcare. This relates partly to concerns about the risk of doing harm to patients and the consequent regulatory environment surrounding medical devices and drugs. It is also connected with the preoccupation of policy makers, payers and managers — and the general public — with the effectiveness and efficiency of healthcare. Over the last half-century or more, this has been a major force in the design of health services and the introduction of innovations. A concern with effectiveness and efficiency was greatly influenced by the work of Archie Cochrane, initially emphasising the importance of the 'randomised controlled trial' (RCT) as a support for decision-making, then arguing for the need to organise medical knowledge coherently (leading to the 'Cochrane Collaboration') and finally in 1972 publishing *Effectiveness and Efficiency. Random Reflections on Health Services* (Cochrane, 1972). Since then, the definition of effectiveness and efficiency has evolved. This is partly the result of debate over the nature of 'evidence' gathered in different ways, including through RCTs, partly because the difficulties of accurately measuring healthcare productivity have become clearer, and partly due to new notions of 'value' in delivering healthcare that have begun to emerge (see Muir Gray, 2011 for a discussion).

Gathering evidence for the impact of healthcare innovations is a crucial part of the wider framework for regulating healthcare; it forms a backdrop to their development and implementation. Depending on the context and type of innovation, this may involve a lengthy process of trial and evaluation, before medical authorities and professional groups eventually legitimise it. This is very clear in the case of new drugs, where development involves multiple phases of standardised testing and strong regulation. We discuss this in detail in the next chapter. For now, we just need to note that these different phases vary in their duration, activities, investment requirements and probability of success — a failure to progress from one phase to the next can occur at any point in the drug development pipeline and failure rates have generally increased over time. The clear development pipeline found in the pharmaceuticals industry is less characteristic of medical devices because of its heterogeneous nature, but both sectors are facing growing scrutiny by regulators, insurance companies and payers in a search for better value for money.

Evidence for the costs and benefits of the innovation is therefore a very important part of the process of selling to healthcare providers. From the perspective of companies developing innovative healthcare products, the pre-adoption phase can be costly, involving long periods of

➔*Go to Chapter 5 for a discussion on health technology assessment*

experimentation and trialling. For some innovations, formal health technology assessment (HTA) approaches are used to assess the impact and benefits. But the fuzzy nature of many healthcare innovations can make it hard to gather robust evidence that convinces all the stakeholders involved in adoption decisions, especially when they hold different views on what the innovation is or what a good standard of evidence is. For some stakeholders, experimental approaches such as RCTs may be the gold-standard for assessing certain types of healthcare technologies, and may be appropriate when the innovation is clear cut. However, they do not necessarily give the full picture because they neglect critical features of the context into which an innovation is deployed and used, or may not be appropriate when the innovation comprises multiple dimensions. Ensuring that sufficiently robust evidence, satisfactory to all stakeholders, is gathered, but not holding back implementation or stifling useful experimentation, is a goal that is rarely attained by healthcare policy makers and managers.

Innovation economics — another reason why healthcare is different?

As long ago as the late 1980s, debate about healthcare reform in the USA was concerned about a 'technological imperative' driving up the cost of medical care (Fuchs, 1986; Newhouse, 1992); in fact, studies identifying technology as a primary driver of inflation go back as far back as the 1950s (Chernew, 2010). The adoption of new medical technologies, which can improve the quality and outcomes of care, but cost more than existing treatments, is still often cited as the principal culprit behind escalating healthcare costs. The explanation for cost inflation in healthcare is not so straightforward, though.

So what is the true story? Suggesting that technological innovation is responsible for a large proportion of the total rise in real healthcare costs seems to contradict conventional wisdom in technology and innovation management (Gelijns and Rosenberg, 1994). In other sectors, technological change is seen as the primary force behind improved productivity and economic growth, making it possible to produce a given volume of output with a smaller volume of inputs.

In the past, healthcare cost inflation in the USA was at least partly the result of a lack of transparency over the real cost and benefits of medical interventions (Gelijns and Rosenberg, 1994). This was partly due to the

Box 3.5   SUMMARY: Technology-induced cost inflation in healthcare

Healthcare is unusual amongst industries because of its economics. While technological innovation is normally seen as a way of improving performance over time — by raising quality and reducing costs — many people working in healthcare or studying it have noted that this is not always the case in healthcare. There is no shortage of exciting innovations which are potentially hugely beneficial to patients and their families. Implementing them is not always easy because they can be hard to manage or accommodate within the current health system. But for policy makers and healthcare providers, there may also be a downside to technological innovation since it can raise demand and costs for governments and taxpayers.

Think about advances in medical and diagnostic equipment which increase access to care close to or at home. Patients may see this as a major advantage — they do not have to spend time or money visiting specialists in a hospital. But this may well generate new costs, which have to be borne by the primary or social care sector. Other examples include better monitoring of a patient's changing health conditions which pick up previously undiagnosed problems (which then have to be treated), advances in surgery which extend the range of patients who are eligible for a particular procedure (also increasing demand), or new drugs which may reduce the need for in-patient care (but increase demand for long term support).

way patients and doctors were insulated from the financial implications of their medical care decisions, because insurers covered the costs. It was also a result of 'over-treatment' — increased use of tests and procedures — due to concern over litigation for malpractice, and the information asymmetry between doctors and patients, which allowed doctors to influence the demand for medical services.

But technological innovation also played a part. Gelijns and Rosenberg argue that this was partly due to the USA's high rate of healthcare technology adoption compared to other countries with similar populations and disease patterns. A 'technological imperative' instilled in medical students the idea that using innovative technology was a source of professional prestige. This was compounded by hospitals' use of technology as a way of attracting patients and doctors in order to stay competitive. The USA's comparatively high proportion of medical specialists — who have been found to have a higher propensity to use new technology than generalists — further reinforced the rate of technology adoption. Once adopted, widening the use of certain technologies was common; when medical specialists acquire a new technology and the skills to use it, there is a tendency to extend its use into new treatment areas or new groups of patients. There have been a number of examples of this both in diagnostics (e.g. the use of CT and MRI technologies) and surgery (e.g. laparoscopic cholecystectomy and percutaneous coronary angioplasty, described in Chapter 6). In these cases, incremental improvements in performance began to make the technologies applicable to patients for whom it was not initially deemed appropriate (Blume, 1992; Legurreta *et al.*, 1993).

Since Gelijns and Rosenberg were writing various reforms to the USA's health system have tackled some of the factors underlying cost

---

Box 3.6 CONCEPTS: The different ways in which new technology affects healthcare costs

- 'Treatment substitution' occurs when new technologies substitute for older technologies in the therapy of established patients. The unit cost of new technologies may be higher or lower than the cost of the older technologies they replace, but they typically bring some health improvement as this is the innovation goal.
- 'Treatment expansion' occurs when new technologies lead more people to be treated. As a procedure improves, a wider range of people can be treated or more people can be diagnosed with a condition. Treatment expansion is worth it if these marginal patients benefit more than they cost. But this is not necessarily the case, so treatment expansion is often seen as a major factor in the healthcare cost inflation story.
- Patients and industry can also drive cost inflation. As new procedures enter common knowledge, strict criteria for access to them may be weakened in the face of patient demands. And medical technology industry as a whole, or individual companies, may lobby for a new treatment to be given priority.

inflation and health insurers have exerted downward pressure on prices. However, they also make the important and enduring point that long-run inflation in medical costs is strongly influenced by the way in which innovative technologies are developed, adopted and used. There is a high degree of uncertainty over the real benefits of many new healthcare technologies after their initial adoption. Often the cost consequences of what are anticipated as cost reducing innovations cannot be clearly foreseen and such innovations may have unpredictable or ambiguous effects on costs that can be resolved only after extensive use in practice. This has been seen with diagnostic tests, where the implications of widespread testing may initially be unclear. Furthermore, technological development does not necessarily end with adoption, which may only be the beginning of a prolonged process of redesign and adaptation based on feedback from users.

Various health economists have tried to disentangle the factors behind rising total expenditure on healthcare. Economists have approached the problem by looking at the residual share of cost inflation, once various measurable factors have been accounted for, such as increased demand due to demographic change, rising input costs and increased income. Demography accounts for a share of rising expenditure, as well as general movements in the overall cost of inputs such as labour and drugs. But using healthcare technologies more intensively also plays a part, although it is less clear whether this is due to increased use of old technologies, use of old technology in new contexts or use of brand new technology.

Joseph Newhouse's work in the early 1990s triggered considerable debate as it implied that in the USA as much as half the rise in healthcare expenditure since 1960 was due to technological change — or as he described it, 'the march of science' (Newhouse, 1992, 1993). Newhouse and colleagues have updated their 1992 estimate using a revised methodology (Smith *et al.*, 2009). This shows a slightly lower contribution of technology on its own to healthcare cost inflation, but they estimate it still represents between a quarter and half the observed real per capita spending growth. Of course, burgeoning use of health technology is not necessarily a problem in the context of growing economies — as Smith *et al.*

note rising GDP is in itself an important driver of growth in healthcare costs.

Other studies have identified technology-induced cost inflation in the rising cost of treating specific medical conditions. For example, Cutler and McClellan (2001) investigated five medical conditions, showing that for four of them increasing cost of technology is outweighed by improvements in health benefits. In the fifth condition (breast cancer screening and treatment), technological change brought some benefits, but these were roughly equal to the costs. Thorpe *et al.* (2004) estimated that between 43% and 61% of the total nominal change in US health spending between 1987 and 2000 was attributable to the fifteen most costly conditions. In eight of these, a rise in the cost per treated case, rather than more cases being treated, accounted for most of the growth in spending. Sometimes this was associated with technology innovation such as the availability of new drugs. However, the picture was complicated. Demographic factors accounted for about 19% to 35% of the spending increase. For some conditions, rising epidemiological prevalence or improved access to care and better recognition and diagnosis were responsible for most of the increased spending. Thorpe *et al.* therefore caution against overly simplistic explanations about the role played by technology innovation in escalating healthcare spending. New approaches may well replace less costly treatments for a particular condition, but the older treatment may have been less effective anyway.

Implications for policy makers and payers

The impact of technological innovation on healthcare costs matters for policy makers, for health service managers and for technology developers. It raises questions about the quality and level of innovation, such as what kind of innovation do we need and how much of it do we need — in other words, how do we know what the 'right' level of innovation is? The introduction of new technologies may well raise overall spending by increasing demand, but outcomes and overall societal welfare may improve by even more. And it is possible that at least some of the increase in health spending is not because of technology-induced inflation so much as recognised best practice becoming more widely adopted. This may well involve decreasing investment in innovations with low or negative value or disengaging from outmoded practices. Commentators have noted that for many technological innovations in healthcare, the benefit that is ultimately realised is limited or even negative (Rye and Kimberly, 2007). Most innovations seem to be situated in the 'cost increasing — quality comparable' cell in Table 3.1.

A key policy consideration is therefore how to squeeze innovations which deliver little or no benefit out of the health system without slowing the development and adoption of 'good innovation'. The UK government has tried to encourage hospitals to disengage from previously adopted innova-

> ➔ *Chapter 5 describes the use of financial incentives to healthcare providers to encourage them to adopt innovations*

tions and adopt beneficial innovations by using financial incentives or mandating new methods. Disengagement might involve discontinuing the use of an innovation with no therapeutic benefit without the adoption of a replacement, or substitution of one innovation for another. The processes and conditions under which either of these occur are, however, poorly understood. Disengagement is a little researched area, partly because published studies are biased towards what influences adoption and diffusion, rather than questions about why, how and under what conditions organisations disengage from innovations (Rye and Kimberly, 2007).

Table 3.1   Possible outcomes of technological innovation in healthcare and the implications for policy makers and payers.

	Quality reducing	Quality comparable	Quality improving
Cost reducing	Politically difficult	Attractive to politicians/ managers	Win–win for all
Cost comparable	Bad idea!	Most innovation is here?	Attractive to politicians, patients, taxpayers
Cost increasing	Terrible idea!	*Healthcare is unique compared to other sectors?*	Raises questions about who benefits, who pays?

When it comes to policy (or organisational) decisions about whether to adopt or abandon an innovation, much depends on the extent to which there are suitable measures of its quality and effectiveness. Both in the UK and the USA, far less funding is provided to support adoption and diffusion of healthcare innovations, and evaluation of their impact, compared to funding for R&D (Barlow and Burn, 2008).

"The United States over the past forty years has been extraordinarily successful in producing new knowledge. At the same time, there has been a deplorable failure in assessing the benefits and costs of putting this knowledge to use. A 1984 study ... found that U.S. expenditures for assessment activities were a mere 0.3 per cent of total health care expenditures."
(Gelijns and Rosenberg, 1994)

One particular problem is that the instruments for ensuring that we understand the added value of many types of healthcare innovation are poorly developed. Some countries have adopted formal HTA approaches, but use of appropriate evaluation approaches to assess interventions over their lifecycles, or to assess complex interventions, remains a challenge. We will return to this in Chapters 4 and 5.

At a wider policy level, there are also problems over the signals about where to concentrate the innovation effort. The payment and reimbursement system for healthcare to some extent provides signals and priorities for research and development. One problem, though, is that the various parts of the technology innovation ecosystem receiving these signals operate under different time horizons

➔ *Chapters 4 and 5 discuss how governments try to guide the healthcare innovation process*

and are subject to different incentives (Gelijns and Rosenberg, 1994). Contrast the non-profit research community with profit-making technology suppliers, and the differences in the latter between the medical device industry and pharmaceutical industry. All are sensitive to policy and market signals, but the R&D pipeline for drug manufacturers is usually far longer than that of device manufacturer, while the timelines for fundamental science of non-profit organisations such as universities may be even longer. Aligning these differing industrial, policy and health service needs within national research and development strategy can be challenging.

A poor relationship between signals from health policy and changing healthcare needs, compounded by inadequate mechanisms for evaluating innovations, lies behind another important policy concern. The huge waste in the health system measured by over- and under-treatment has been a major part of the currency of health system reform since the 1980s, especially in the USA (Cutler and McClellan, 2001). Over-treatment is seen partly as a result of the adoption of technological innovations which are costly and have a low marginal value. The latest estimates put the level of 'wasteful spending' in healthcare at over a quarter of total healthcare expenditure (Berwick and Hackbarth, 2012; Sahni *et al.*, 2015) — around USD 1 trillion each year. Not all of this is technology-induced. Donald Berwick and Andrew Hackbarth identify six categories of waste — over-treatment, failures of care coordination, failures in the execution of care processes, administrative complexity, pricing failures, and fraud and abuse. Even if the USA implemented all the approaches where effectiveness has been measured, they estimate that only 40% of wasteful spending would be addressed, leaving significant opportunities for new thinking and the introduction of organisational, technological and process innovation of the right type. This includes finding ways of increasing the incremental value of treatment and improving productivity.

The productivity problem in healthcare

Governments concerned with the impact of rising healthcare costs on public expenditure seem to be faced with a paradox — technological innovation potentially drives up costs but if the introduction of new technology can improve the productivity of healthcare, then surely this will help? In the eyes of politicians and managers raising productivity should free resources for high value innovations in healthcare to be introduced. In the USA, the Patient Protection and Affordable Care Act (or 'Obamacare') reforms are built on the assumption that healthcare can be more productive. In the UK, an unprecedented slowdown in the growth of government funding to the National Health Service (NHS) since 2010 has required it to pursue the most ambitious programme of productivity improvement since its foundation in 1948.

But views differ on how far this is possible. Healthcare has long been seen as 'unproductive' compared to other sectors of the economy. This is partly because the opportunities for cost efficiencies stemming from technological improvement are limited by its heavy reliance on human capital (Romley *et al.*, 2015) — we cannot expect healthcare to become any more productive because it largely involves the individualised labour of highly trained health professionals, which cannot simply be replicated by technology (Baumol, 2012). It has been argued that in itself this is not necessarily a problem. In view of the potential impact of technological innovation on levels of employment across a wide range of industries, healthcare could provide a growing source of demand for labour which is unable to find employment elsewhere in the economy (see Box 3.7).

Box 3.7   BACKGROUND: Let's be less productive

Tim Jackson from the University of Surrey explains how we may have pushed productivity to its limits, 'such that if our economies don't continue to expand, we risk putting people out of work'. One solution is to accept the productivity increases, shorten the working week and share the available work. But as Jackson argues, perhaps a more compelling solution for keeping people in work is to 'loosen our grip on the relentless pursuit of productivity'. This involves creating jobs in what are traditionally seen as low productivity sectors like healthcare, social work and education, where chasing productivity growth does not make sense since their activities rely inherently on the allocation of people's time and attention. According to Jackson,

'The care and concern of one human being for another is a peculiar "commodity." It cannot be stockpiled. It becomes degraded through trade. It isn't delivered by machines. Its quality rests entirely on the attention paid by one person to another. Even to speak of reducing the time involved is to misunderstand its value.'

It is, therefore, undesirable to focus on raising productivity when care is dependent on a carer's time and attention, because it may put the quality of the health or social care at risk. Doctors and nurses who see fewer patients per day and spend more time with them will be less 'productive' measured purely in terms of throughput, but they may be happier because they feel they have greater independence and control over their schedule, and this could be reflected in better patient outcomes.

Source: Jackson (2012).

But there is also a compelling argument that we should not assume everything currently done in healthcare is necessary and beneficial, when there are clearly inefficiencies that are the result of activities which add little or no value, or may actually be harmful. The productivity efforts of healthcare providers and governments therefore tend to concentrate on eliminating this type of waste, while streamlining healthcare processes, including the automation of certain routine tasks. Broadly, health systems and healthcare providers can achieve greater efficiencies in two ways. First, costs can be cut while improving productivity and value — in short getting more for less. Second, healthcare providers can invest their money where it really adds value by more evenly applying the evidence-based processes that are known to work. It was estimated in 2010, for example, that in England, if all parts of the country were as productive as the South West region, the NHS could cut expenditure by GBP 3.2 billion without reducing the number of patients treated (Bojke *et al.*, 2010).

One problem, though, is that accurate data on healthcare costs are lacking in most health systems and methods for measuring productivity are poorly developed. This has implications for assessing the economic impact of specific innovations and interventions designed to improve productivity. Since providers do not fully understand their costs, they are unable to link cost to process improvements or outcomes. Aggregating and analysing costs at the level of medical specialties or hospital departments — the conventional approach — tells us nothing about the costs of treating individual patients over their full cycle of care. Nor does it tell us anything about the ultimate measure of interest, added value, the amount of 'health' achieved for a given input. Although growing attention is now paid to the

> "... few acknowledge a more fundamental source of escalating costs: the system by which those costs are measured. To put it bluntly, there is an almost complete lack of understanding of how much it costs to deliver patient care, much less how those costs compare with the outcomes achieved."
> (Kaplan and Porter 2011)

→ *Case study 5.2 in Chapter 5 provides an example of the problem of using financial incentives to try to stimulate innovation in kidney care, when there is only limited knowledge of costs* measurement of health outcomes, measuring the costs required to deliver those outcomes — the other side of the value equation — has been relatively neglected.

This is one reason why the productivity story in healthcare is confused. Both in the US and UK, the most recent estimates suggest there are signs of healthcare productivity growth after years of declining productivity. Focusing just on hospitals, Romley *et al.* (2015) found evidence of cumulative annual productivity growth in certain medical conditions, although they acknowledge that the drivers of the trends are unclear. In the English NHS, much more comprehensive measurement of productivity in a very wide range of healthcare procedures shows that productivity increased by 8% between 2004 and 2010 (Street, 2013).

Why healthcare is different — the innovation adoption process

Companies involved in developing and commercialising healthcare technologies often argue that they face challenges not experienced in other industries because of the complexity of the environment into which new technologies and other innovations are adopted and implemented. Many stakeholders from different parts of the care systems may be involved in adoption decisions, and for some innovations national bodies act as gatekeepers to the health system by gathering evidence and approving new technologies. Even when technology developers have demonstrated the usefulness of their innovations, the journey to adoption and diffusion is fraught with difficulty. Firms may need to negotiate a fragmented procurement process with diverse purchasing organisations which vary greatly in size and experience. The lessons about technology and innovation management from 'mainstream' innovation research discussed in the previous chapter therefore need to be modified for healthcare.

Researchers have explored the adoption and diffusion of healthcare innovation from many different perspectives, including the attributes of the innovation itself, aspects of its organisational context such as leadership or the capacity for absorbing new knowledge, the influence of professional 'silos', how peer and expert opinion or social networks impact on knowledge about innovations, and the characteristics and attitudes of individual decision makers such as doctors.

There have been systematic reviews of the research on the factors which influence the adoption and diffusion of healthcare innovation. These include the reviews by Greenhalgh *et al.* (2004a, 2004b), Robert *et al.* (2009), Rye and Kimberly (2007), and Fleuren *et al.* (2004). The report by Savory and Fortune (2013) also contains a useful summary of the research literature. We discuss all this research in detail in Chapter 5. For now, perhaps the principal lesson is the following, outlined by Rye and Kimberly (2007):

'Examining the adoption and diffusion of organisational innovation in health care is a complex problem, and thus it is unfortunate that so few studies have taken this complexity into account.'

Rye and Kimberly argue that not only are the innovation characteristics that facilitate or impede adoption and diffusion rarely considered, there has been an overemphasis on researching the adoption of well defined, clearly bounded innovations being adopted by a single organisational unit (i.e. a new device adopted by a single hospital or team) rather than innovations that are less clear cut because they combine both technology and organisational changes. Moreover, although researchers have emphasised the important role of the wider context for shaping adoption decisions, most studies focus on a small number of causal variables such as organisation size or measures of organisational culture. Little is known about the relative effects of variables and interactions between them and contextual influences. Studies tend to explore the major theoretical categories such as innovation attributes, adopter attributes or organisational characteristics in isolation, making it impossible to shed light on their relative contribution to the likelihood of adoption. This is a particular problem for understanding the adoption and diffusion of healthcare innovations since the differing interests of management, doctors and other medical staff — along with the variety of professional groups, communities of practice and subcultures and agendas — potentially intensify conflict around resources available for innovation, the enactment of policies or the interpretation of evidence (Ferlie *et al.*, 2005). In particular, the power of professional groups to accept or reject a technology can be high, because of the way they influence accreditation and training standards, and validate evidence and new knowledge associated with it. Another problem is that the already complex organisational structures in healthcare are changing rapidly in response to technological, policy and economic factors, further complicating the dynamics in authority relationships and governance structures (Rye and Kimberly, 2007).

'Process' studies of healthcare innovation

To address these limitations, there has been a trend towards 'process' studies of adoption and diffusion. These emphasise the dynamism and complexity of innovation in healthcare. Their focus is on the characteristics of the innovation itself and the adopting organisation, the interactions with the wider context within which healthcare organisations are situated, and the innovation activities and actions which unfold over time. Key messages from this work are that:

* There is often no single adoption decision — decision-making often involves multiple stakeholders and unfolds over time as trials are conducted. It is, therefore, important to avoid rigidly separating 'adoption' and 'assimilation' in routine healthcare practice.
* The role of power and politics, and the dominance of medical professions, is vital.
* The way the decision-making process is organised is important — is it decentralised or centralised, formal or informal?
* Decisions often take a short-term perspective and fail to consider longer-term sustainability of the innovation — how likely is it to endure once the initial trial period has ended?

Process research is beginning to show how the adoption and sustainability of healthcare innovations is shaped by the structure of the healthcare system itself — the way its institutions are organised and its financial models operate. An important disincentive to adoption is the disconnection between costs and benefits. In the case

> ➔*See Case study 5.1 in Chapter 5, Case study 7.1 in Chapter 7, and the views of remote care technology suppliers (Innovation in action Box 5.3, Chapter 5)*

of innovations that have an impact across different parts of the health system, problems can arise from the uneven distribution of costs and benefits across different healthcare organisations, such that a financial investment in an innovation made by one organisation or department yields its benefits (or costs) in another organisation or someone else's budget.

Organisational fragmentation within healthcare systems tends to reinforce 'silo budgeting' — the primary, secondary and social care systems remain largely financially autonomous, although in recent years moves in the UK and elsewhere towards the delivery of some integrated primary, secondary and social care services have tried to address this situation. For example, the introduction of measures to speed up the discharge of elderly patients from hospital might reduce the average length of stay, reducing hospital costs, but raise costs in the social or primary care sectors because the elderly patients need additional support at home. Much depends on the way care services are organised and financed, but such problems can paralyse decision-making by adopting organisations. So despite creating a seemingly good idea, innovators may therefore perceive that the opportunity for their new product or service is actually rather unattractive.

Another feature of health systems which impedes innovation adoption is the time taken for the benefits of innovations to be realised, especially ones that are complex and involve multiple organisations. In the longer-term, an innovation might be cost-saving, but the short-term transition costs associated with its implementation are often unfunded, leaving little room for investment in innovations that may require significant upfront expenditure.

Healthcare also differs from other sectors in the way evidence-based medicine profoundly shapes how the adoption of new technology takes place. As we saw in Chapter 2, individuals or companies faced with the opportunity to buy an innovative new product will weigh up the pros and cons, making a judgement about its value to them. Innovations need to demonstrate unambiguous relative advantages over existing technologies, products or practices for their successful adoption and diffusion. As resources within health systems are finite, there is clearly a need to control the introduction of new technologies based on their relative clinical- and cost-effectiveness, along with a desire to practice evidence-based medicine. However, the collection and interpretation of evidence for the efficacy of healthcare innovations is problematic. The mechanisms designed to assess, trial and encourage the spread of new technologies act as a filter for the adoption of new technology. The stress on the safety and efficacy of new medical products, a highly regulated market context and a positivist scientific method — generally the primary way in which new knowledge is created and validated within healthcare — all combine to elevate 'evidence' to a rather different position than is the case in the adoption of innovations is most other industries. A lack of credible evidence, derived from

> ➔*The case study on the Whole System Demonstrators programme in Chapter 7 shows how important evidence can be in policy making, but how it can also stall the implementation of new innovations*

scientific methods, is potentially a serious blockage to the uptake of innovation if it is used to stall decisions about investment. Complex healthcare innovations that involve multiple interventions to modify a service are not usually amenable to this type of randomised controlled trial (RCT) approach, so require a more pluralist approach to gathering evidence on their impact. However, this can provide more ambiguous or hard to interpret findings, which may not be accepted by all stakeholders involved in adoption decisions. We return to this in Chapter 5.

Chapter summary

- The environment into which new healthcare technologies are adopted is complex and often quite unlike that of other industries or sectors of the economy. This is because healthcare is an immensely complex system involving interactions between a wide range of organisations, institutions, and regulations.
- In healthcare, it is often less clear what the 'innovation' is than in other industries. Many innovations do not take the form of well-defined physical products and bring together elements of new technology and organisational or service model changes.

- Healthcare innovations may lead to changes in healthcare services outside the immediate context for adoption and other unintended consequences.
- The economics of technological innovations in healthcare are unlike innovations in other industries — often costs to the health system, or payers or governments, rise because new technologies allow a larger overall 'quantity' of care to be provided.
- The role of evidence for the impact of healthcare innovations, and how it is used in adoption decisions, differs from other sectors of the economy. Positivist scientific methods such as RCTs may not appropriate for many types of complex healthcare innovation.
- There has been a trend towards 'process' studies of healthcare innovation adoption emphasising the dynamic and complex innovation processes in healthcare.

Questions for discussion

1. Compared to other industries healthcare innovations are often hard to pin down. To what extent do you think this is the case and why?
2. Using an example of a healthcare innovation, characterise it according to innovation dimensions such as product versus process, radical versus incremental, and architectural versus component. Why is it important to be able to categorise healthcare innovations?
3. There is relatively little radical innovation in healthcare compared to incremental innovation. Do you agree with this statement? Explain the reasons for your answer.
4. Choose an example of a healthcare innovation and identify some of the incremental innovations that have taken place.
5. Why has there been a trend towards 'process' studies of healthcare innovation adoption in recent years, such as those by Greenhalgh *et al.*? What are the main characteristics of these studies?
6. If you were the CEO of a healthcare provider, or a politician or minister of health, how would you explain to the public that 'more is not necessarily better'?
7. How can those who pay for technology innovation in healthcare prevent or reduce the tendency for it to increase overall healthcare expenditure?

Selected further reading

Cutler D, McClellan M (2001) Is technological change in medicine worth it? *Health Affairs* 20(5): 11–29.

Ferlie E, Fitzgerald L, Wood M, Hawkins C (2005) The nonspread of innovation: The mediating role of professionals. *Academy of Management Journal* 48(1): 117–134.

Rye C, Kimberly J (2007) The adoption of innovations by provider organisations in healthcare. *Medical Care Research Review* 64: 235–278.

INNOVATION PROCESSES PART 1 — DEVELOPING AND COMMERCIALISING HEALTHCARE TECHNOLOGIES

THIS CHAPTER WILL HELP YOU TO:

- Learn about the way new drugs and medical devices are developed and the challenges companies face in bringing new products to the market.
- Understand what is meant by open- and user-led innovation and why it is important for healthcare innovation.
- Understand how governments try to support the innovation process.

In Chapters 4 and 5, we dig deeper into the processes involved in the management of healthcare technology and innovation. We look at the challenges faced by companies developing innovations when bringing them to the market, the response of healthcare providers faced with decisions about what to adopt and how to adopt it, and the role of government in supporting an innovative healthcare economy.

This chapter focuses on the earlier stages of the innovation process for healthcare technologies. We concentrate especially on physical, tangible product innovations, but we should also recall that hard and soft technologies are intertwined and new product innovations in healthcare often also involve service or organisational changes. We explore the different phases of the new product development process from the perspective of the drug and medical device industries. We also discuss why support from government may be needed to help stimulate the flow of new technologies from initial development to commercialisation, and adoption within the healthcare system.

The chapter contains a case study of a small start-up medical devices company (Peezy Midstream), which develops low-tech, low-cost specimen collection systems. This provides an example of how start-ups need flexibility in their approaches to funding, with different sources of finance raised at different stages in what proved to be a very lengthy period of development. The company also found it necessary to pay growing attention to the collection of evidence, in order to convince potential purchasers of the product. Mini Case 4.2 is a well-known example of how a much larger medical device company, Coloplast, uses its stage-gate approach to new products development and how this has been adapted to cope with ideas that may be more radical to make it through the gates.

How do the models of new product development we discussed in Chapter 2 look in the real world of healthcare technology development? In some respects, the development and commercialisation of healthcare technologies follow the same model as those for other new products — individuals or companies come up with new ideas which are eventually turned into commercial products that are sold to hospitals, doctors and other providers of medical services. But this perspective is overly simplistic; it is generally argued that health technology is a difficult market with its own peculiarities.

To understand the creation and adoption of technological innovation within healthcare, we need to recognise the range of actors from R&D, manufacturing, policy and funding within the different value chains of the drug and medical device industries. We need to understand the interplay between them, the impact of regulation on design and safety considerations, and the role of purchasers of new technologies and the economic constraints they face. Creating new products in the drugs and medical devices sectors tends to follow the conventional new product development model described in Chapter 2, but it is important to distinguish between the two sectors. Drug development is subject to a much more structured process and is more highly regulated. Nor should we neglect innovations originating *within* healthcare providers such as hospitals. These tend to be more focused on process or service improvement. These organisations therefore have less potential for appropriating the intellectual property (IP) or any ensuing revenue from these innovations. There is, however, also a long tradition of innovative medical devices or surgical instruments being developed by the efforts of healthcare professionals, described later in this chapter.

The infrastructure of institutions that support and regulate innovation therefore fundamentally shapes the innovation processes of medical technology. Within the healthcare sector, different countries have their own particular combinations of institutions, firms and research organisations. These create and deploy the knowledge, capabilities and skills that lead to product and process innovations for diagnosis, therapy or the operation of healthcare services. Distinct innovation systems are based around networks of firms, research institution and government bodies and other institutions within a particular technological field (e.g. drugs) and bring together various underpinning technologies. These relationships help to define the process of innovation and the way in which innovations are commercialised. Geography can also be important, as clustering of firms in particular healthcare industry sectors or technologies can emerge over time, influencing the relationships and outputs of R&D (see Box 4.1).

Box 4.1   BACKGROUND: Medical technology clusters

There is no commonly accepted definition of an industry 'cluster'. Definitions include geographical closeness or proximity, concentration and interconnectedness of companies or processes. A common thread is the way the growth of all parties involved can be enhanced by physical co-location, which enables mutual exchange of knowledge and skills, or the sharing of infrastructure. Some definitions focus on the importance of linkages between firms and organisations from public and private sectors as a way of fostering innovation.

A number of studies have looked at clustering effects within the medical devices sector. Most concentrate on European countries (especially Sweden, Denmark, Germany, and the UK) and the USA, but there are now a few studies of medical technology clusters in Asia. This research generally highlights the importance of firms collaborating with research leaders such as universities,

(Continued)

Box 4.1　(*Continued*)

private research institutions, research laboratories and hospitals to stimulate innovation. For example, Wessner and William (2012) suggest that having research universities or national laboratories at the core of a cluster is an important way of leveraging regional technology advantages into companies. The transfer of knowledge between industry, universities and hospitals is one of the reasons behind the development of 'Medicon Valley', spanning Denmark and Sweden in the Skåne and Copenhagen region, as one of the leading medical technology clusters (Gestrelius and Oerum, 2006). Clustering also involves transfers of knowledge across manufacturing sectors and disciplinary boundaries (Izsak, 2014).

While a key factor underpinning successful collaborations is the strength of research linkages between industry and educational institutes, this can be problematic for financial, administrative and cultural reasons, and because timescales for planning and delivering projects in academia are often significantly longer than from those in business (Lindqvist and Sölvell, 2011). Interactions across organisational boundaries can be difficult where institutional capacity to support innovation development or adoption within the public and private sectors is weak or where is an absence of strong leadership and guidelines for co-working (Burfitt *et al.*, 2007). Strong leadership is essential for building the soft skills that are crucial for supporting formal and informal networks with potential partners and the expansion of small medical technology companies (Anderson *et al.*, 2013).

One field in which cluster formation has been especially marked is biotechnology. The number of PhDs emerging from leading universities and access to research resources and infrastructure are associated with the emergence of biotech clusters (Kim *et al.*, 2008). In the UK, the Cambridge biotech cluster has created a powerful R&D base involving collaborations between the University of Cambridge and world-leading companies such as AstraZeneca and Gilead Sciences. A nearby sub-cluster is located at Stevenage, bringing together the Wellcome Trust and GSK.

Sometimes collaboration across clusters has been driven by competition. The Tuttlingen surgical instruments cluster in Germany was under pressure from Sialkot, Pakistan, a cluster which was producing a large array of surgical instruments at low prices. Tuttlingen decided to outsource production to Sialkot (and other low-cost clusters) to enhance manufacturing productivity,

(*Continued*)

Box 4.1 (*Continued*)

transferring some technical knowledge to manufacturers in these locations (Nadvi and Halder, 2005).

Other clusters are driven by government policy. France's government has actively supported the creation of medical technology clusters in response to concerns that the country is falling behind in patent applications in the medical device sector. These offer business development and technology transfer services such as helping researchers and companies to find partners within the local network, and assisting companies wishing to set up in in the region.

New product development — the drug industries

Each year about USD 1 trillion is spent globally on prescription drugs, a figure that is growing at around 2.4 % a year. Global sales of biotechnology-based drugs add another USD 233 billion each year, with an annual growth rate of almost 10% (DTT, 2014; IMS, 2012; BIS, 2013).

The R&D process of the pharmaceutical industry is risky, time-consuming and costly. Some estimates suggest that it takes around 14 years from basic research until a new drug is licensed and brought to the market (Paul *et al.*, 2010) and it can cost over USD 1 billion to bring a new compound to initial marketing approval in the USA (Di Masi and Grabowski, 2007). The USD 1 billion figure has been in circulation for some time and has recently been subject to some scrutiny (see Box 4.2), but whatever the amount it is undeniable that developing new drugs is a very costly business. By the early 2000s, the industry was generally held to be facing an unprecedented set of challenges to its business model (PwC, 2011a, 2011b; Paul *et al.*, 2010). These were due to a combination of rising:

- *technical risk* — over time it was growing harder to develop drugs for complex disease areas, and
- *commercial risk* — an increasing number of drugs were reaching the end of their patents and were subject to competition from other manufacturers; at the same time payers were growing more unwilling to cover the cost of expensive innovative drugs.

Box 4.2   BACKGROUND: Exactly how much does it cost to develop new drugs?

Matthew Herper unpicks the USD 1 billion per new drug estimate. This figure originated in a 2003 study by Joseph Di Masi and colleagues from the Tufts Center for the Study of Drug Development (Di Masi *et al.*, 2003). The Tufts study was updated in 2014, now showing a USD 2.6 billion cost estimate, almost two and a half times their previous estimate after adjusting for inflation. This prompted yet more debate (see Di Masi *et al.*, 2015; Avorn, 2015).

Herper notes how the USD 1 billion per drug figure has been helpful to the pharmaceutical industry because it implies the development process is not so expensive an endeavour as to be ultimately futile but it can be used to justify the idea that medicines should be pricey. In fact, whether the USD 1 billion figure is too high or too low is somewhat arbitrary — it all depends on how the calculations are made. Bernard Munos of the InnoThink Center for Research In Biomedical Innovation has estimated that simply adjusting the estimate for current failure rates results in USD 4 billion cost for every approved drug. And when each drug company's R&D budget is divided by the average number of drugs approved, Munos shows the costs can be even more dramatic. Using both drug approvals and research budgets since 1997, and adjusting for inflation, Amgen spent USD 3.7 billion on research for every new drug approved (as much as the top-selling drug ever has ever generated in annual sales), while AstraZeneca spent USD 12 billion. However, as a commentator on the article, M. R. Schuppenhauer, points out, measuring the 'true' cost is not only very complex, it also depends on accounting treatments of R&D expenses, where there is considerable management discretion over what is included and the rules change over time. For example, post-approval costs and the cost of line extensions may or may not be part of the R&D budget, and acquired drug products are not fully included in R&D expenses. How the time taken for drug development and approval is measured also makes a difference to how costs are treated.

Whatever the 'true' cost, Matthew Herper argues that:

'the high cost of developing drugs shouldn't be a badge of honor for drug firms; there's no reason it has to be this expensive. And using the cost of research to justify the prices of prescription drugs was always

(Continued)

Box 4.2 (*Continued*)

a dumb move on the pharmaceutical industry's part. Just because something was expensive doesn't make it good. And another: many medicines are over-priced, but high-cost drugs are only a small part of our general health cost problem. Medicines are just among the easiest products to scapegoat because their prices are easier to track.'

Source: Herper (2012).

The effects have been described in terms of an innovation productivity crisis (Munos, 2009; Paul *et al.*, 2010; Dhankhar *et al.*, 2012; PwC, 2011b), reflected in a falling number of new drugs developed and approved, coupled with escalating R&D costs. Success in the earlier phases of the drug development pipeline was becoming less likely to predict success in the later phases — scientific success could still be accompanied by commercial failure, rejection by regulatory authorities or payers (discussed below, p. 109).

One reason for the decline in R&D productivity was the simultaneous pursuit by major pharmaceutical companies of similar blockbuster drug targets (these generate annual sales of at least USD 1 billion), resulting in duplicated and wasted effort and leading to decreasing returns. But another reason may simply be the growing complexity of the underlying science of discovery, as opportunities from 'low hanging fruit' are exhausted and attention shifts to older people with complex chronic conditions and co-morbidities. This has led pharmaceutical companies to seek new markets amongst the 6,000 rare diseases, a sector which is beginning to demonstrate superior productivity and potentially attractive future returns (Clark, 2015; Deloitte, 2014a, 2014b). Significant gaps in the development and supply of drugs remain, however, such as neglected tropical diseases and new antibiotics/antimicrobials.

Two of the key determinants of the costs of R&D in the pharmaceutical industry are drug development success rates and development times. In essence, the process of creating new drugs comprises two different value chains welded together to create a business model (Northrup *et al.*, 2012):

- The business of *scientific innovation* — discovery and early clinical development.
- The business of *innovation adoption* — creating the information that regulators and customers need and communicating it to them.

The clinical research process itself is highly structured, essentially following a stage-gate approach but with the addition of a highly formalised process of regulation

> ➔ *Chapter 2 discusses the stage-gate process for new product development*

and evidence gathering. Basic and applied research (discovery) leads to phase I and II trials to test for toxicity and clinical efficacy, then to larger phase III trials, further clinical development, registration, marketing and finally approval. After launching the drug onto the market, there may be more follow-up studies (phase IV) to monitor for any safety issues that might become apparent only when the sample size and the duration of the study are large enough.

The conventional staged trial process has now seen some evolution with the introduction of new forms of approval such as 'adaptive licensing'. Adaptive licensing is essentially a prospectively planned, flexible approach to the regulation of new drugs. A principle behind this model is that there is no single moment when a drug is proved safe and effective. Acknowledging this uncertainty means that drugs may be released before completion of a stage if there is a serious unmet need or the potential for significant medical advances, and that uncertainty will be reduced through learning and development that continues after release. Adaptive licensing therefore involves iterative phases of evidence gathering to reduce uncertainties, prior to regulatory evaluation and licensing. It seeks to balance timely access by patients to new drugs with the need to provide adequate information on benefits and harms (Eichler *et al.*, 2014).

The phase II and III stages remain important milestones for the drug development process. Failure to successfully complete the initial discovery and development stages (phase I) is largely a question of science. In itself, this can be costly but phase II trials increasingly involve larger financial commitments, i.e. sunk costs for the company (see Figure 2.7 in Chapter 2). This is partly because tougher regulatory requirements at phase III have led firms to expand the number of individuals tested in phase II, to gain a better indication of the commercial viability of proceeding to phase III (Scannell *et al.*, 2012; Mestre-Ferrandiz *et al.*, 2012).

Phase III, therefore, represents a significant shift in development philosophy for pharmaceutical firms (Northrup *et al.*, 2012). Making it to this phase means that the firm is betting on success and beginning to behave as though it has a marketable drug. Although scientific failure is still a possibility, the emphasis of R&D activity in this phase is on relationships with regulatory bodies, payers, doctors and consumers to demonstrate what the drug can do and to identify any areas of caution. Trials in this phase often involve head-to-head studies comparing the drug against current standards of care. Apart from safety, the primary interest of regulators is proving the superiority of a drug compared to existing competitors on the market, including its economic benefits.

Phase IV trials — also known as post-marketing surveillance – begin after regulatory approval and are part of the process of 'pharmacovigilance'. They are designed to monitor the safety of a drug within the general population and pick up any problems that may not have been identified in earlier stages, such as the effects of the drug on people with a variety of medical conditions or who are also taking other drugs. The USA's Food and Drug Administration (FDA) now requires mandatory post-marketing trials for fast track products and for products for which safe use in children needs to be determined.

Developing a new drug is, therefore, a multi-stage process, characterised by strong regulation to ensure drugs are safe, efficacious and accessible to consumers (see Figure 4.1). Each stage of development requires different levels of resources and scientific knowledge, and distinct competences from university and other research organisations, and pharmaceutical and other firms. The stages of the R&D process are heterogeneous in duration, scope, investment requirements and probability of success, depending on the drug target, the market characteristics and the company's strategy (Mestre-Ferrandiz *et al.*, 2012). In practice, there is no smoothly flowing development pipeline, continuously delivering new drugs to the market. Drug 'fallout' — a failure to progress to the next

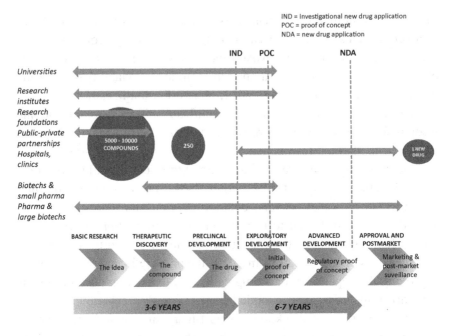

Figure 4.1.   Drug development actors and stages.

phase — can occur at any point throughout the pipeline. Failure rates have generally increased over time, although this depends on the development stage and type of therapeutic area. Some researchers estimate that only around 10% of drug candidates successfully complete the phase II mid-stage of drug discovery (Paul *et al.*, 2010; Mestre-Ferrandiz *et al.*, 2012). Others estimate that about 11% of candidate drugs pass through all three stages (Pammolli *et al.*, 2011; Di Masi *et al.*, 2010, 2015).

These characteristics mean that the innovation process of drug companies is inherently 'lumpy' (Northrup *et al.*, 2012). To cushion the blow of expensive late stage drug fallout, companies try to frontload the pipeline with potential opportunities at each stage — they try to have a large pool of phase I candidates, only some of which taken into phase II, and more viable phase II candidates than are taken into phase III. This results in a high degree of cyclicality in the output of successful drugs, a feature which may be exacerbated by spells of high late stage failure that impact on revenues and in turn constrain the early R&D effort. These characteristics translate into an R&D model where the cost of unsuccessful drug projects is far greater than the cost of the ones that succeed — perhaps two thirds of the pharmaceutical industry's long-term cost of capital may be attributable to failures.

As well as these inherent features of the drug development pipeline, the business models of the pharmaceutical companies have had to confront a series of other challenges in the last decade or so:

The rise in use of 'generics'

Those responsible for purchasing pharmaceuticals and regulatory bodies are paying more attention to incremental benefits and costs of new drugs. This has led to more widespread use of lower-cost generic drugs that are comparable to a brand or reference list drug product. Regulatory bodies such as the National Institute for Health and Care Excellence (NICE) in the UK are playing a greater role as gatekeepers to the market, and in the USA health insurance companies have exerted downward pressure on prices by seeking alternative follow-on drugs rather than branded products (see Box 4.3).

Parallel to these regulatory trends, European and US drug companies have faced greater competition from Indian and other manufacturers of

---

Box 4.3 BACKGROUND: The rise in generic drug prescribing in the UK

Since 1976, spending on primary care prescribing in the UK has grown four-fold in real terms to about GBP 8bn in 2013/14. The number of prescribed items grew from 285 million to just under 1 billion in 2013/14. But the NHS has increasingly switched to cheaper generics, leading to a significant change in the type of medicines prescribed and dispensed, along with changes in their prices. It has been estimated that NHS spending would have had to increase eight-fold in real terms (rather than four-fold) to pay for prescription drugs in 2014, assuming generic prescribing rates had remained at their 1976 levels. If generic prescribing were to rise from around 70% in 2013/14 to 90% of the total, this could allow a 51% increase in total prescriptions for a 4.4% increase in spending by 2024, other things being equal.

Source: Appleby (2015).

generics. The speed of 'genericization' has increased — a generic drug can now be produced within a few weeks of patent expiry (Burns *et al.*, 2012) — and generic drug prescriptions now capture an 84% of market share within the first year a branded drug's patent expires (Grabowski *et al.*, 2014). The total period of market exclusivity enjoyed by drug companies until competition is allowed and rival companies are able to develop 'me too' or next generation products has shrunk from up to ten years to an average of 2½ years and sometimes just 1–2 years. In the USA, this decline was initially driven by the Hatch Waxman Act 1984, which made it easier for generics to gain approval, but intense competition to be first in class has also meant that follow-on manufacturers have tended to file patents earlier and earlier, reducing the amount of time that many drugs spend on the market (Burns *et al.*, 2012).

An increasingly tight regulatory and payer environment

The pathway to a successful drug is long and tricky, from basic research to increasingly complicated trials and finally regulatory approval. As well as the increasingly complex science, the industry's profitability and growth prospects have come under pressure from payers and governments to reduce prices and from increasing regulatory costs. Pharmaceutical companies need to provide more demanding and higher quality clinical data, and the length of time taken to gain regulatory approval has been subject to much criticism. One estimate is that FDA review times grew from an average of 1–1.4 years during 2000–2009 (Northrup *et al.*, 2012).

While the regulatory approval process in both chemistry and biotechnology-based drug development is largely concerned with safety, there are some differences between the two sectors. In chemistry-based drug development, the focus is on the pharmacological profile of the end product. In biotechnology, the unpredictability of the development and manufacturing process, and ramifications of this for the stability of the end product, mean that regulators pay more attention to the earlier phases of development. The role of clinical trials in the approval of biologics is partly to demonstrate the product characteristics and similarity between them. In the USA, this is said to have slowed the introduction of 'biosimilars', generic equivalents to biologic drugs (Pfeffer, 2012). It is only relatively recently that regulatory pathways for the approval of biosimilars or follow-on biologics have been put in place in the USA — the FDA began to provide regulator pathway approval for biosimilars in 2010, whereas the European Medicines Agency (EMA), initiated its approval process in 2004. However, healthcare reform in the USA also extended the patent protection on biotechnology-produced drugs to 12 years, which may slow the development of biosimilars (Deloitte, 2014a, 2014b).

The impact on prices of the time taken to develop and approve new drugs has prompted regulators to look for ways of streamlining the approval process. New fast track reviews have been put in place both in the USA by the FDA and in Europe by the EMA. Around two-thirds of new drugs approved in the USA in 2014 went through a fast-track review designed to bring new medicines to patients faster. Similarly, in the UK the Medicines and Healthcare Products Regulatory Agency (MHRA) has established an innovation office to support companies from early in the development process, including designing clinical trials that are able to produce the evidence regulators need to make a quick decision.

The European Medicines Agency (EMA) has introduced a pilot Adaptive Pathways to Patients approach which builds on the idea of 'adaptive licensing' (see above, p. 108) and targets new drugs that address certain high unmet needs or promise significant medical advances. This aims to

> ➜ *Different approaches to speeding up adoption, such as public–private partnerships, are discussed in more detail in Chapter 5.*

find a balance between the competing demands of speed and safety in approving drugs. Drugs are made available on a conditional basis before the conventional three-stage trial process is complete, with further evidence of safety and efficacy gathered after a provisional launch. This requires elements of risk-sharing between key stakeholders — drug companies, healthcare payers and providers, and patient groups — through mechanisms such as 'coverage with evidence development' and 'non-standard authorisation'.

The drug industry's response to the productivity crisis

The initial strategy of the pharmaceutical industry partly involved a round of mergers and acquisitions (M&A). While this may have been a rational short-term strategy for firms with blockbuster drugs that were coming off patent and an insufficient development pipeline to replace them, it was not necessarily an effective response to the slowdown in R&D productivity. The research evidence for the impact of M&A on drug industry innovation is inconclusive. Some

"Often mergers beget more mergers, turning a pharmaceutical firm into a 'mass mergerer' with mergers setting off leapfrog competition with firms adopting a merger and acquisition strategy so as to be not left behind."
(Burns *et al.*, 2012)

studies suggest that it did not lead to increased R&D expenditures, nor does there seem to be a relationship between scale and R&D productivity in pharmaceutical industry (Burns *et al.*, 2012). Others have shown positive effects of M&A and alliances on R&D success rates, depending on the development pipeline phase (Danzon *et al.*, 2005), the time to drug launch (Hirai *et al.*, 2010) and internal productivity rates of firms (Higgins and Rodriguez, 2006). In fact, there have been suggestions that far from than being a solution to the pharmaceutical industry's productivity problems, M&A activity may partly be one of the causes (Burns *et al.*, 2012). This is because it diverts attention from R&D and reduces the number of firms in the market, in turn reducing competition and drivers for innovation.

Another response of pharmaceutical companies is to try to improve their innovation processes by speeding up development times, increasing R&D efficiency and reducing cost. Companies have adopted several strategies:

- Creating drug performance units focused on particular therapeutic pathways and establishing investment boards with external CEOs and venture capitalists (Burns *et al.*, 2012).
- Reducing the scale and scope of their activities, such as the number of therapeutic areas they involve themselves in, and outsourcing or out-licensing their therapeutic programmes to external firms.
- Innovation is also occurring in the drug manufacturing process as companies seek to improve their efficiency and reduce cost (see Box 4.4).

Box 4.4 BACKGROUND: Innovation in drug manufacturing processes

The drug manufacturing process is often neglected in studies of the pharmaceutical industry. However, innovation is occurring here, as companies seek to improve their efficiency and reduce cost.

There are two phases in the drug manufacturing process — manufacturing the drug substance (the active pharmaceutical ingredient) and manufacturing the drug product itself:

- Drug substance manufacturing is a process driven by science and technology. Different pharmaceutical companies have adopted different approaches: Bristol Myer Squib outsources most of these operations, while AstraZeneca conducts them itself, up to the last few steps in bulk drug synthesis.
- Drug manufacturing involves processing the active pharmaceutical ingredient into the final product. This is normally carried out at 'form-fill-finish' (FFF) sites and is typically not outsourced but situated locally, because of the variety of national regulations affecting packaging and safety.

The manufacturing process in biotechnology tends to be more expensive because bulk processes rely on biological reactions of cells to produce the active pharmaceutical ingredients and manufacturing needs to take place in a sterile operational environment. Initially this required expensive dedicated plant for each product, but flexible platforms for use by multiple products are now being introduced.

Manufacturing a drug is more than just a scaled-up version of manufacturing it for trials. This is because the process needs to be robust enough to ensure that all its steps produce the expected results and satisfy the demands of regulatory bodies. Pharmaceutical companies, therefore, need to coordinate the drug design and development stages with manufacturing, so they can make sure the chemical or biological process is optimised for manufacture. Companies have often seen development and manufacturing as different functions, but increasingly manufacturing practice is subject to regulatory scrutiny, driving pharmaceutical companies to look carefully at this aspect of drug development.

(Continued)

Box 4.4   (*Continued*)

There has been much interest in the application of 3D printing technology to the manufacture of drugs. In 2015, the Food and Drug Administration gave the go-ahead for the first 3D-printed pill to be produced, Spritam, to control seizures brought on by epilepsy. The benefits of this manufacturing approach are that layers of medication can be packaged in precise dosages, offering the potential to create bespoke drugs based on the specific needs of patients.[1]

Source: Northrup *et al.* (2012).

Over the last decade or so, innovation in the pharmaceutical industry has therefore begun to take place in an increasingly complex and segmented way. Several different R&D models have been adopted by its firms (see Box 4.5). Consensus is growing that the task of drug discovery and development has become too complex for a single firm to handle on its own, and that it must now be accomplished through inter-firm collaborative models and forms of 'open innovation'. We discuss these in detail below. Other trends include:

- Increased attention to 'drug hunting', hiring more drug discovery scientists to increase the pool of talent and expertise.
- Revisiting existing under-exploited compounds and reformulating existing products to find new uses (repurposing).
- Focusing on a smaller number of compounds selected for development in order to make fewer, but potentially larger, bets on areas that offer the prospect of breakthroughs.

More attention is also being paid to the time a drug spends in each phase of research, with speedier termination of poorly performing research projects at each stage-gate. AstraZeneca, for example, has adopted a new framework for project approval decisions. Its '5R Framework' defines five gates: *right target, right tissue/exposure, right safety, right patients* and *right commercial* application. This framework has resulted in a smaller innovation portfolio, allowing the company to focus on projects that have a higher chance of success by eliminating projects that fail to pass initial approval checkpoints (Cook *et al.*, 2015).

---

[1] http://www.bbc.co.uk/news/technology-33772692

Box 4.5   BACKGROUND: Different R&D models adopted by drug companies

Pure innovation models
Eli Lilly, Bristol-Myers-Squib, Takeda focus on new molecular entities (NMEs) developed either in their own labs or in-licensed from other firms. These generally avoid generics, and focus on pharmaceutical innovation and R&D. Pfizer, Merck, Daiichi Sankyo pursue similar focused strategy but have also moved in to generics.

Conglomerate models

Johnson & Johnson, Novartis, Roche, Abbott — large diversified companies with ability to invest on many fronts.

Innovation from a generics base

Companies such as Teva, Dr. Reddy, Cipla, Wockhardt, Torrent are typically from outside the high income countries and are diversifying from generics into innovation development.

Innovation from a service company base

Pharmaceutical service companies from Asia and Russia are expanding their innovative activities by doing their own at-risk development and starting venturing groups.

Innovation with virtual pharma models

GSK, Lilly are reorganising R&D teams, with oversight and funding similar to venture capital model.

Source: Northrup *et al.* (2012).

There are signs that the industry may be turning a corner as productivity is continuing to improve. The number of new molecular entities (NMEs) launched globally in 2014 (46) was the highest since 1997, up from 29 the previous year. The industry has also begun to see higher success rates in phase III since 2008. This has been partly explained by the shift towards specialised drugs, many for rare diseases, which tend to progress through clinical development faster (Hirschler, 2015).

The emerging role of medical biotechnology

Medical biotechnology companies are an increasingly important part of the drug industry. The more demanding regulatory and payer environment, the patent cliff for blockbuster products and the traditional pharmaceutical industry's struggles with innovation productivity have all combined to bring the pharmaceutical and biotechnology sectors closer together. Biologics are therefore now making a growing contribution to the development pipelines of pharmaceutical company and about half the top-100 product sales are expected to be generated by biologics by 2018 (Deloitte, 2014).

The drug companies' traditional core strengths include pipeline management, sales and marketing, and mobilising their financial reserves to support development and commercialisation. The biotechnology sector's strengths are rooted in discovery of new biologics. Combining the two has therefore been appealing to a pharmaceutical industry facing growing challenges in the development pipeline. The interest of traditional pharmaceutical companies in biotechnology lies both in a belief that in-licensed compounds might deliver more value than in-house research (Pfeffer, 2012) and in the prospects for combining the flexibility and entrepreneurship of small biotech companies with their own drug development expertise.

Initially, pharmaceutical companies brought in new products from biotechnology companies under license, spurred in part by evidence that such alliances helped

> ➔ *Open innovation models are discussed below and in Chapter 2*

to improve R&D productivity. There were certainly some spectacular commercial successes — Pfizer's in-licensed drug Lipitor became the first pharmaceutical product to top USD 10 billion in annual sales. However, the available pool of late-stage licensing compounds is not limitless and there are disadvantages to the in-licensing model if companies wish to maintain their own innovation capabilities, as well as the additional costs of managing such alliances (Burns *et al.*, 2012). Pharmaceutical companies are therefore turning to more open models of innovation.

Over time the relationship between the two sectors has evolved, both in terms of strategic corporate alliances and through different types of collaborative R&D relationship. The relationship between the two is symbiotic — partnerships with pharmaceutical companies enable biotech companies to access funds for research and validate their innovations, hence raising credibility amongst investors. Pharmaceutical companies gain access to new product opportunities and innovative technologies to support drug discovery and development, and some of the culture of scientific innovation found in biotech companies.

An important benefit of the relationship between biotech and pharmaceutical firms lies in the processes and technology of innovation. One of the problems underlying the pharmaceutical industry's productivity problem has been the paucity of drug targets — enzymes, biochemical pathways or ion channels — which the R&D effort could be directed at (Sammut, 2012). Research suggests that in the half century up to the late 1990s, the whole effort of the pharmaceutical industry was directed at only about 400 targets, in an essentially trial and error manner. This significantly limited the prospects for creating new drugs. The development of recombinant technology and genetics, along with other technological innovations within the biotechnology industry (see Box 4.6), has enabled the pharmaceutical industry to replace this trial and error approach with a more systematic model. But rather than creating their own capacity for doing this, which would require them to recruit new scientists and pay for new equipment, most pharmaceutical companies have opted to outsource this part of the drug development process to new genomics and proteomics companies, and to technology platform companies which provide capabilities for rapid analysis (Sammut, 2012 therapeutic areas (Sammut, 2012; Lanza,

> → *Rapid analysis of large numbers of chemical molecules can be seen as an automated form of 'fast-fail' models of new product development — see Chapter 2*

2009). Alliances between these and pharmaceutical companies have developed around particular therapeutic areas, focusing on a disease category or a combination of physiological factors such as asthma or chronic obstructive pulmonary disease. Another type of alliance involves data mining, the large-scale generation and screening of libraries of compounds, gene sequences and protein structure. There are also technology development alliances which involve a genomics company assembling a

Box 4.6   BACKGROUND: Innovation in the technologies for innovation — a key driver in the biotechnology sector

The development of medical and non-medical biotechnology has been underpinned by a wide range of product and process innovations across different areas of technology and dating back over four decades:

- Monoclonal antibodies: These have certain advantages over chemically synthesised pharmaceuticals in blocking molecular interactions because they combine to their targets more specifically and completely, may be less toxic, and can be used to block interactions that cannot be blocked with small molecules.
- Genomics and proteomics: Huge improvements in the speed of DNA sequencing have offered the prospect of more personalised drugs. New types of companies are emerging to provide the sequencing capabilities for biotechnology and pharmaceutical companies, as well as companies providing direct-to-consumer personal genetic tests and molecular diagnostic companies using personalised genetic information to diagnose and guide treatment. Proteomics is about understanding the specific function of protein in healthy and diseased animal systems to help scientists determine its role as possible drug target.
- Combinatorial chemistry: This speeds up the creation of new chemical entities (NCEs) by combining chemical building blocks of molecules in all possible ways. The cost of this technology fell rapidly over a relatively short time, meaning that companies established to do this were driven out as pharmaceutical companies developed their own capabilities.
- High throughput screening: Automated robotic platform for rapidly testing and synthesising large numbers of chemical molecules, which also became a standard drug discovery tool for all pharmaceutical companies. High throughput screening techniques use DNA microarrays or DNA chips to search for molecules that bind to specific forms of DNA.
- Gene therapy: A range of technique that use genes to treat or prevent disease, first conceptualised in 1972. Several approaches to gene therapy are being developed. The first commercial gene therapy, Gendicine, was approved in China in 2003 and in 2012 a treatment for a rare inherited disorder (Glybera) became the first treatment to be approved for clinical

(Continued)

Box 4.6 (*Continued*)

use in Europe and the USA. Epigenetics is the study of how genes are turned on and off by different enzymes.

- Antisense RNA (asRNA) and RNA interference (RNAi): Approaches to drug development using ribonucleic acid (RNA) to block gene expression for therapeutic benefit. RNAi can be used in large-scale screening to systematically shut down each gene in the cell, helping to identify the components behind particular cellular processes. Two antisense drugs were approved by the FDA in 2014.
- Systems biology: The computational and mathematical modelling of complex biological systems. By incorporating data about interactions, the outcomes of interventions such as those resulting from a new drug may be predicted at a whole organism level. The concept refers to a number of overlapping disciplines rather than a single well-delineated field, such as bioinformatics.
- Rational drug design: This uses computer-based molecular modelling and other techniques to design molecules with very specific shapes to fit a drug target.

Source: Draws on various sources, including Pfeffer (2012).

range of speciality partners in order to produce compounds that can be licensed to pharmaceutical companies or brought to market by other specialists. Sometimes these arrangements are sponsored by a pharmaceutical company.

The biotechnology innovation ecosystem is, therefore, more dynamic and complex than that of the traditional pharmaceutical industry, with different players experimenting with different roles and relationships in the innovation process. For drug companies, a key question is which innovation models to pick from. Different firms have adopted different approaches (see Box 4.5). Broadly companies have responded to the pressures they face by reducing their effort on discovery and increasing efforts at surveying research activity from universities to keep abreast of potential valuable new discoveries. They then aim to supplement their own R&D activities by partnering with the best teams from universities or smaller specialist companies. The management challenge is to ensure that they make informed decisions about what part of the research process to carry out in-house and what to outsource.

Developing new medical devices

Industry structure and innovation trends

Medical devices are broadly defined as products used to prevent, diagnose, monitor or treat diseases and medical conditions. As many as 500,000 different medical devices are currently available (Eucomed, 2012). They range from simple disposable syringes to complex implantable and hybrid devices, which combine innovation in engineering and pharmaceuticals, such as drug eluting stents that slowly release a drug to block cell proliferation.

· Around 4% of annual global healthcare expenditure is spent on medical devices (Eucomed, 2012). Sales are about a third of the value of the biopharma sector, at around USD 350 billion per year, but are growing faster (DTT, 2014; BIS, 2013). Around 62% of the sector's worldwide sales in 2009 were of medical devices and the remainder were commodity supplies such as splints or scalpels (Kruger and Kruger, 2012).

Perhaps because of its broad scope, the medical devices sector has been rather neglected within academic and policy discussions about healthcare. Pannenborg (2010) makes the point that the sector could be described as 'emerging' for over half a century, but despite its potential for helping to deliver a wide range of health benefits, medical devices remain a comparatively low priority for national governments and global bodies, unlike the drug industry. Historically, though, the industry has been highly innovative, creating new devices which require significant R&D activity in mechanical and electrical engineering, new materials and design. And as we will see later, the relationship between medical devices developers and suppliers and medical professionals can be close.

Given the diversity of the sector, when thinking about innovation processes and future industry growth rates, it is important to distinguish between those products which are established and display moderate growth (like heart pacemakers), and innovations likely to contribute to the sector's growth in years to come. Our main interest in this chapter is in the parts of the industry that are most technology-rich.

Kruger and Kruger (2012) describe some defining characteristics of the medical devices sector which make its economics unlike that of other industries. In particular, the industry has been protected from downward price pressure from purchasers and regulators by certain features:

- Parts of it are not subject to the conventional laws of supply and demand and pricing, in that demand is highly elastic (i.e. it does not depend on price) and higher profits on particular products can be sustained for long periods. This may in part be due to the fact that the industry is much smaller than the pharmaceutical industry and has therefore been less subject to attention by regulatory bodies and government pricing policy. High profitability has also been sustained by incremental innovation, i.e. the regular introduction of new versions of a product with minor product changes.
- The heterogeneous nature of medical devices, even within the same functional category, makes it hard for purchasers to compare brands (see Box 4.7). There may also be relatively high switching costs, such that once a hospital has invested in a particular brand and the training and infrastructure associated with it, changing to another product can incur significant costs.
- Demand has been fuelled by the need for devices that save time and money and improve the outcome of procedures for patients. Companies have been able to market products on the basis of performance,

---

Box 4.7 BACKGROUND: The heterogeneity of the knee replacement industry

The knee replacement market, worth USD 8.4 billion globally in 2011 is dominated by four companies — B. Braun, Smith and Nephew, Stryker, Zimmer and DePuy Synthes — which together accounted for almost 80% of the total market. In 2013, the American Academy of Orthopaedic Surgeons recorded over 150 different knee replacement designs.

Source: Transparency Market Research (2012).

enabling them to secure higher profit margins than they could through cost-plus pricing models.

- Parts of the medical device sector are protected from the shift towards consumer-product models that have partly affected the pharmaceutical industry — while many drugs can be self-administered by consumers, patients are clearly not in a position to implant their own pacemakers or stents.

The medical devices industry is dominated by large diversified companies, many of which are from the USA. This has been explained by the presence of a medical profession dominated by specialists, relatively high consumer pressure for the latest innovative products, and the absence of government controls over reimbursement and other impediments that are said to hinder the adoption of health technology innovations in European or some Asian health systems. The medical technology market in the USA is certainly attractive — per capita expenditure is more than 13 times that of the rest of the world (Kruger and Kruger, 2012).

The European medical devices sector is the second largest market in the world. The industry is extremely innovative — in the top tier of industries for investment in R&D and filing more patent applications than any other sector (Eucomed, 2012). But medical device companies find harder to gain critical mass because of the frag-

"If we change the supplier, as it stands we'd have to change pretty much everything. So we'd have a huge job on our hands. It's not interchangeable ... the devices in the patient's home wouldn't therefore work with the software back in the base, so it'll be a big issue. You can't feasibly mix and match telecare equipment ... Every now and again it improves and then there's another advance and there's lock down again ... and it goes around in circles. Two purchasers from healthcare providers, talking about telehealth."
(Barlow *et al.*, 2012)

mented nature of Europe's national health systems, the diversity in their approaches to technology procurement, and the lower level of patient choice. This in turn affects their ability to achieve economies of scale. The European industry is dominated by thousands of mainly small and medium sized firms — approximately 500,000 people are employed in

22,500 companies, 80% of which are small and medium enterprises (SMEs) (Eucomed, 2012).

European and US medical device manufacturers are not immune from competitive pressures and other challenges. In recent years, the industry has been going through a period of economic and structural change not unlike that of the pharmaceutical industry. Although demand for *in-vitro* diagnostics is growing rapidly and it is anticipated this will become the industry's largest segment by 2018 (Deloitte, 2014a), overall industry growth rates have declined. This is partly due to a slowdown in the large cardiology, imaging and orthopaedic sectors (Kruger and Kruger, 2012). Medical device suppliers from lower cost countries in Asia have also exerted downward pressure on prices in some sectors, although the regulatory and safety frameworks in the developed countries' health systems establish some barriers to entry by new players.

Another problem for medical device companies is increased scrutiny by regulators, insurance companies and purchasing authorities. Regulations for new medical device approvals are tightening in the USA and Europe, meaning that manufacturers are being required to meet higher standards to sell their products (Deloitte, 2014a). Moreover, purchasers have begun to apply more rigorous health technology assessments in a search for value for money. In the USA, hospitals are employing more sophisticated buyers who are better able to bid suppliers against one another to lower costs, while doctors are increasingly unwilling to push for a specific manufacturer's products because they are either now directly employed by a hospital or the hospital is responsible for negotiations with technology suppliers (Monheim, 2011).

"The days of selling on features and relying largely on relationships [with physicians] is coming to an end. Value-based purchasing is here and will grow for both payers as well as hospitals." (Provines, 2010).

In the UK, benchmarking of prices for certain products has highlighted significant variations in prices paid by hospitals and is changing the balance of power between purchasers and suppliers (see Box 4.8). Pressure on large medical devices firms to

➔ *Open- and user-driven innovation, and the role of clinicians, is discussed below*

Box 4.8   BACKGROUND: Price benchmarking of medical devices in the UK

The Price Benchmarking project in the NHS in England and Wales is designed to highlight variation in price of orthopaedic implants. These are purchased locally or regionally, with each purchasing authority (i.e. a hospital trust) negotiating pricing with suppliers according to local conditions and purchase volumes. Early indications were that the volume of purchases did not attract appropriate discounts and significant price variations existed for some prostheses. A successful pilot scheme in 2012/13 with three purchasing authorities demonstrated that savings ranging from GBP 50,000 to GBP 200,000 per year could be made. As well as an online reporting tool, in 2014 the National Joint Registry launched a price-benchmarking service for procurement teams and healthcare management.

Source: National Joint Registry (2013).

---

reduce field sales forces — the main point where interaction with doctors takes place — may also be impacting on the rates of innovation, since doctors represent an important source of new product ideas (Kruger and Kruger, 2012).

Medical device companies are therefore increasingly seeking new avenues for their businesses, away from manufacturing. One trend is the adoption of disease areas, rather than focusing on a single stage of a condition (MIT Technology Review, 2013) — an example might be insulin delivery for diabetes patients, where a medical device company might offer a continuum of care, from wellness and obesity-prevention measures to glucose monitoring and medication delivery. This allows firms to better understand and demonstrate the cost/benefit potential of their products, and develop new business models. One company, Medtronic, has undergone a fundamental transformation, described by one commentator (Parmar, 2015a):

'Terms like continuum of care, disease management, population management and integrated care that would have been absent from its lexicon even five years ago are popping up in presentations by its CEO, in its communication to investors and analysts and yes, in rationales for doing business.'

In 2013, Medtronic launched its catheterisation laboratory management programme for cardiovascular disease (see Innovation In Action 4.1) and also purchased Cardiocom, a provider of remote monitoring for heart failure and other chronic disease patients. The company stated that its aim was to transform itself from being a primarily device provider into 'the premier global medical technology solutions partner of tomorrow.' It subsequently acquired a Dutch diabetes clinic

---

INNOVATION IN ACTION 4.1: Moving from a device manufacturing to service provision model: Medtronic's Cath Lab Programme

Medtronic realised it needed to move from being a *medical device* company to a *healthcare* company in order to remain a leading player in the sector. This would require the company to expand its role in the overall healthcare continuum by integrating information and services for diagnosis, treatment, and disease management. In turn, it needed a new risk-sharing model for the development of new products and associated services, including a higher tolerance for risk and failure.

One outcome of this shift in approach was to establish a new business unit to work closely with hospitals in the development and introduction of new products. In 2013, The Hospital Solutions unit launched the catheterisation laboratory ('cath lab') management programme for cardiovascular disease, which included a risk-sharing approach to efficiency savings and clinical outcomes arising from the introduction of new technology. Medtronic also helps the partner hospital implement Lean Six Sigma efficiency programmes, as well as supply chain management, benchmarking and quality reporting, and the introduction of cardiovascular information systems.

On average, efficiency savings are said to range from 20% to 25% at partner hospitals, patient throughput times and waiting lists have decreased, physician and nurse satisfaction have improved, and patients are more satisfied. The programme is now being expanded globally and has evolved to include post-therapy, home care and monitoring. By 2015, Medtronic had 50 long-term agreements with hospitals, generating USD 1.5 billion in revenue over the average 5–6 year life of the contracts.

Sources: PwC (2013), Parmar (2015b).

and research centre to move into integrated diabetes care. These moves led some to question whether Medtronic could still be called a device manufacturer (Parmar, 2015a). To respond to concerns about possible conflicts of interest, because Medtronic doctors may feel pressured to prescribe the company's medical equipment, Medtronic is allowing clinical decision making to remain autonomous (Parmar, 2015b).

The medical devices innovation pathway

For the large medical device companies, the process for developing new products is not unlike that of the drug industry — market research precedes technological R&D, product development and testing, and so on. As with the development of certain drugs, smaller entrepreneurial companies or academic researchers might initiate a new idea and specialise in the earlier phases of R&D before established firms take on the later R&D stages and commercialisation. But the diversity of the medical devices sector makes the pathway from the initial idea through product development to commercialisation and adoption more varied and less formalised than that for drugs and biologics. The same is true for the way academic, industry and government researchers collaborate (Corr and Williams, 2009). The complexity of many medical devices, and the regulatory and safety framework that surrounds them, mean that specialist input from a range of disciplines is often needed.

For large medical device companies the development pipeline for a new product follows a typical stage-gate process. The example of Coloplast is well known (see Innovation In Action 4.2). How far safety and efficacy regulation is involved depends on the type of medical product and the risks associated with it. In the USA, manufacturers may need to seek either pre-market clearance or pre-market approval from the FDA. Clinical data are generally not required for pre-market clearance, which is the most common route; pre-market approval is needed for certain devices, such as implantables, and requires clinical data. As in the case of drugs,

> ➔ *Stage-gate models for managing development risk and progressing new products from initial selection to the strategic commitment of resources for production and marketing are essential for companies with multiple product and process innovation projects, and are described in Chapter 2.*

INNOVATION IN ACTION 4.2: Coloplast's evolving framework for progressing ideas into products

Coloplast is an innovative Danish manufacturer of medical products. Its origins in 1954 lie in the development of the first self-adhering ostomy bag by a nurse for her sister, a stomach cancer patient. The way in which Coloplast manages its innovation process has been widely reported. The company's AIM ('accelerating ideas to market') process is designed to clarify the rules and responsibilities within the development pipeline, and allow the company to make clear decisions about progressing new ideas at the right moment.

The AIM process defines the rules to be followed by innovation project teams. The development pipeline is divided into five stages, each containing parallel and coordinated activities designed to refine the definitions of customer needs and develop technological solutions. Each stage ends with a gate, a decision point where a project is reviewed by senior managers who have authority to ensure that it progresses quickly or is discontinued. A project moves to the next stage when these gatekeepers decide that it is technically and economically likely to meet customer needs, as well as Coloplast's financial, quality and environmental impact standards.

One example of a Coloplast innovation involved the development of three alternative bags for patients with ileostomies (where the small intestine is diverted through an opening in the abdomen). The AIM process enabled a clear understanding of user needs to be initially translated into ideas by a task force that included stoma care nurses and patients. These were turned into prototypes which could be developed and tested with users. Technical development of filter and output systems was initiated in June 1997. This was followed by formal clinical trials and test marketing in November 1999, with introduction into the healthcare market from 2000 onwards. AIM is said to have helped ensure faster and more systematic conversion of the initial idea into the final product, enabling extensive learning along the way through the close interaction between the company and users and specialists.

While AIM was regarded as very useful, there was concern that the process did not cope well with good ideas that may eventually lead to innovative products, but were insufficiently structured or too radical to be pursued — ideas entering the AIM process were generally regarded as unlikely to fail. The routines used to manage the AIM process therefore needed to be redesigned and more flexibility injected into the stage-gate method to incorporate a

(Continued)

INNOVATION IN ACTION 4.2   (*Continued*)

greater capacity for failure. Coloplast subsequently set up an 'external R&D' unit to handle open innovation activities such as technology scouting, relationships with external innovators, and in-licensing and out-licensing of innovations. A key process step now involves translating these externally sourced innovations into the Coloplast context and understanding how they can be best aligned with the company's targets and capabilities.

Another change, introduced in 2007, is the From Innovation to Accelerated Global Roll-Out (FIGARO) product launch strategy. This is designed to further reduce overall product development times by accelerating the phases of market analysis, business concept and business case development, and more closely aligning processes for R&D, marketing and operations, and sales.

Sources: Bessant *et al.* (2004), Foss *et al.* (2012), Tidd and Bessant (2014).

---

obtaining pre-market approval can be a complicated process. How much clinical and technical data is required, and consequently the time taken for approval to be granted, is based on a three-tier risk classification system (see Box 4.9).

Mirroring the drug industry, the approval process for medical devices has grown more complicated and expensive, especially in the USA. From the early 2000s, the FDA increasingly required large-scale clinical trials during the pre-market phase due to heightened concerns over product safety and demands for increased scrutiny after recalls of faulty medical devices. It is now said to take US firms over four times as long as European firms to secure approval for innovative products — 54 months from first communication with the FDA to approval, compared to 11 months in Europe (Kruger and Kruger, 2012).

Although the speedier regulatory process may now act in favour of European medical device companies, especially smaller and more innovative ones, they still face significant challenges in the product development pathway. Small companies often lack the relevant disciplines or skills needed to engage with financial partners, regulators or customers, and are too small to fund any trials that are needed for safety or evidence purposes. The generally fragmented nature of the medical devices sector also makes co-operation harder and more costly. Collaboration

---

Box 4.9   BACKGROUND: Risk classification for medical devices

- Class I includes low risk products for which general controls are sufficient to ensure safe and effective use.
- Class II products carry a moderate risk and require additional information to establish appropriate controls.
- High risk (class III) products are defined by the FDA as those which support human life and are of substantial importance in preventing impairment, or those which present potential risk of injury or illness. These include coronary stents, defibrillators, and tissue grafts.

---

between SMEs and universities can be problematic for a host of reasons — a lack of clarity over ownership of IP resulting from collaborative research activity, differences in accounting for the costs of research, and different time horizons, with academic researchers often starting research without necessarily knowing what the endpoint is or when it will be reached.

In fact, adoption — as we will see in the next chapter — is often a far larger problem for medical device companies than the challenges of product development. In the UK, the routes available to the industry for commercialising new products and ensuring they are adopted are widely seen as unreliable (BIS, 2012a), although various policy and other initiatives have begun to focus attention away from supporting the 'push' of new technologies into the health system towards a more 'pull' orientated, needs-driven approach (see below, p. 147).

The role of users in developing healthcare innovations — lead user, user-led and open innovation

We saw in Chapter 2 how 'need pull' can be a powerful trigger for innovation, but this does not mean that end-users are passive recipients of products supplied by innovators. As Joe Tidd and John Bessant

(2014) describe it, the frustrations of users with existing solutions may lead them to experiment and create early versions of what eventually become mainstream innovations.

Throughout history the development of new medical devices has been closely associated with user-innovators. These are often surgeons who see a need for a new product or the possibility of improving an existing one, and then try to develop a solution (Kirkup, 2006). Not only do they represent an important source of new ideas, and sometimes the initial development work, they also often lead the innovation process as originators, developers, entrepreneurs and marketers (Lettl, 2005; Lettl *et al.*, 2006; Metcalfe *et al.*, 2005; Metcalfe and Pickstone, 2006; Storey *et al.*, 2011). This role stems from the particular characteristics of healthcare — a combination of inventive and innovative personalities who work in high-pressure, problem-orientated contexts and organisations where there may be a lack of suitable competences and resources (Lettl, 2005). One study concluded that in the USA almost 20% of about 26,000 medical device patents had been developed by physicians (Chatterji *et al.*, 2008); another found that 22% of surgical equipment was developed by surgeons (Lüthje, 2003; Von Hippel, 2005). Sometimes the basic idea for new medical devices comes from an individual who has no connection to basic or clinical research. For example, the idea and initial model for a device to drain the build-up of cerebrospinal fluid in individuals with hydrocephalus came from the parent of an affected child (Baru *et al.*, 2001). While the development of novel healthcare technology spans all the innovation models, it is important to look in more detail at the lead user and open innovation forms because of their significance in the health technology sector, especially medical devices.

> ➜ *Supplier-centred, technology-push models, lead user and open innovation are described in Chapter 2*

While the user-innovator model has resulted in medical advances, it is not without problems. Doctors or other end-users initiating new ideas often need to augment their innovation with other technical and business skills. A common model is for a doctor to get together with engineers from a local university to develop a prototype before turning to a medical devices manufacturer. The challenge is to ensure that partners are introduced at the right time in the innovation journey. User-innovators may be reluctant to relinquish control of their

---

Box 4.10 CONCEPTS: Healthcare professionals as lead users

Healthcare professionals can also be important lead users in the development of healthcare technologies because of their ability to define problems and then specify or provide input into new solutions (Lüthje and Herstatt, 2004; Hinsch *et al.*, 2014). When it comes to the development and adoption of complex healthcare products — for example, medical and scientific instruments or IT systems — lead users are usually critical for the co-development, testing and early adoption of new products.

---

innovation projects when additional skills need to be brought in, slowing or impeding commercialisation and adoption. Or the perspective of doctors may be narrow, resulting in an imperfect understanding of the health system's procurement and adoption processes, and over-estimation of the size and ease of access to the market. Too narrow a perspective may also mean that an innovation developed by a clinician to address a particular problem may not be accepted by other clinicians, even in the same specialism. In a detailed study of innovations emanating from within the UK's National Health Service (NHS), Clive Savory and Joyce Fortune (2013) found that origins in a clinician-led, user-innovator model did not appear to make adoption any easier. This was partly due to the blurred boundaries between NHS-developed and commercially-developed technologies, which made it difficult to show that the origins of the innovation made a difference. Under certain circumstances, development within the NHS could help smooth the path to adoption, but sometimes it constrained adoption. This occurred when an innovation was narrowly focused, perhaps because individual inventor held a particular perspective on the purpose of the innovation or its possible uses. In contrast, Savory and Fortune suggest that the more market-oriented approach of commercial developers sometimes ensures that the scope of a particular innovation is broadened to attract as wide a market as possible.

The role of user-innovators in healthcare means that there has also been interest in what the concept of open innovation means for the development of new medical technology. Open innovation is seen by some firms in both the drug and medical devices industries as a way of increasing the volume, velocity and value of innovation processes. This is partly a response to the rising cost and declining productivity of traditional approaches to R&D and partly because of the perception that the really interesting innovations are being developed by small entrepreneurial firms, individuals or in universities.

Open innovation in the medical devices sector

The characteristics of the medical devices sector — strict regulations, a product development process that is time- and cost-consuming, the predominance of small firms — all mean that companies increasingly seek to collaborate with external partners when developing innovative new products. In a study of collaborative networks amongst Dutch medical device companies, Pullen *et al.* (2012) show that the most successful companies displayed what they describe as a 'business-like' approach towards collaboration — objective, focused and relatively closed — compared to lower performing companies, which tended to work informally with partners in a network. Nevertheless, the fluid and informal models found within the open innovation paradigm have been heralded as an essential part of the armoury of health technology companies, whether they are sourcing new ideas or they are seeking collaborators to help with the research process itself.

There are some high profile examples of open innovation in the medical devices industry such as GE's 'Ultrasound Innovation Circle', launched in 2012. This is an open innovation initiative to accelerate ultrasound research, incentivising independent researchers by giving them access to GE's technological and human resources. Suitable ideas are brought into the company's own development process, with research partnerships managed by GE's licensing department (Hollmer, 2012). Various open innovation networking platforms are also beginning to emerge. One example is e-Zassi,[2] which aims to help innovators connect and collaborate, and navigate what it describes as a 'fractured medical device ecosystem'.[3]

---

[2] http://www.e-zassi.com/connect/index.html

[3] http://medsider.com/interviews/how-to-facilitate-open-innovation-in-the-medical-device-space-interview-with-peter-von-dyck/

The reality, however, is that in the medical devices sector open innovation has yet to become embedded in everyday practice. Surveys have suggested that while an open innovation culture is slowly emerging — in the sense that there is at least a recognition of the need to incorporate a more outward-facing culture into new product development approaches — medical device manufacturers are only taking measured steps in this direction. In a study by PA Consulting, most respondents aspired to the type of open innovation programme adopted by Procter & Gamble, but very few had an open innovation strategy or action plans in place (Buntz, 2010).

Research by PwC (2013) on innovation trends amongst medical technology companies identified that only a third of companies in the survey had co-created innovative products and services with customers in the past and only 22% of innovative products and services had been developed jointly with external partners. Nevertheless, open innovation was regarded as one of the top two approaches that will generate the most growth in the future — 33% of respondents saw design thinking as the leading growth driver, followed by open innovation (28%), incubators (19%) and corporate venturing (8%). One of the major challenges for the medical technology industry was found to be a lack of collaboration with patients. The report explains how this hampers the introduction more open innovation models as a source of new ideas. It also impacts on the sales process, since healthcare providers and insurers increasingly rely not only on the clinical value of devices or drugs but on broader sources of evidence, including patient satisfaction scores, when they measure the overall per- formance of an innovation. Employing experts with wider health industry experience is one strategy adopted by medical technology companies, but the report concludes is that they also need to look increasingly to external partners to help widen the funnel of potentially commercial ideas flowing into the company.

"Out of all health industry players, medtech companies arguably have had the least insight into patient outcomes and satisfaction. Their business-to-business relationships did not create a burning need to master patient or consumer understanding." (PwC, 2013)

Open innovation in the pharmaceutical industry

To what extent is open innovation possible in the pharmaceutical sector? Creating new drugs requires huge resources to be deployed within a highly regimented development pipeline. There is growing consensus that the task has become too costly and complex for a pharmaceutical firm to handle on its own. The idea of users experimenting and coming up with new drugs (and freely revealing their IP) seems rather extreme. Yet the research productivity crisis of the pharmaceutical industry, described above (p. 105), has prompted it to look at open innovation as one of a range of new innovation models.

In the 1990s, collaborations between research organisations such as universities and the pharmaceutical and biotechnology companies usually took the form of a linear, transactional model: each player was largely confined to a specific role, handing over the output of its activities to the next player in an arms-length manner. Pharmaceutical companies turned research into patented candidate drugs for development and the successful products were eventually marketed to healthcare providers. The latter are described by Pigott *et al.* (2014) as 'passive recipients of what the industry chose to develop and launch.' The system is essentially a closed one: discoveries are patented at an early stage and there is limited interaction between different parties or a wider range of stakeholders. But this model

---

Box 4.11   BACKGROUND: Open innovation initiatives in the pharmaceutical industry

Eli Lilly — InnoCentive Initiative, engaging with external researchers in a hypothesis-driven approach to early drug discovery, providing access to Eli Lilly research tools and data.

Pfizer — Partnerships with 20 academic institutions, emphasising the importance of collaborative rather than transactional relationships.

Astra Zeneca — Open innovation platform to help identify and establish collaborations with partners across all stages of drug discovery, including exchange of compounds, technology and/or knowledge.

GSK — Extensive use of open innovation as part of its competitive strategy, so that around half the company's product pipeline is now the result of open innovation.

contains some fundamental inefficiencies. A large number of research groups and pharmaceutical companies might all be pursuing the same prospective drug target, wasting resources. And a failure to integrate payers and patients into the drug discovery process at an early stage could result in costly late-stage failures because the resulting drug proves to be too expensive or patients fail to adhere to a complicated medication regimen. The traditional closed model in the pharmaceutical industry therefore increasingly failed to deliver, reflected in the falling productivity of R&D in the pharmaceutical industry.

In response, not only have large pharmaceutical companies tried to change their internal organisational structures to try to act more like small, flexible and innovative biotech companies, but they now recognise that a more open architecture for R&D may be helpful. Managing at least part of the innovation process may be easier when it is located 'outside the corporate walls were it can thrive unencumbered' (Pfeffer, 2012). A broad spectrum of innovation models — including forms of open innovation — is becoming common in the pharmaceutical industry (Gassmann *et al.*, 2010). These are not mutually exclusive; larger drug companies have several business areas with different innovation models — some diseases follow more open innovation approaches, others involve acquisition of biotech companies focused on particular targets, and others take the form of more traditional in-house models. Figure 4.2 summarises where different pharmaceutical companies sit in relation to their innovation management approach (focusing on internal or external resources)

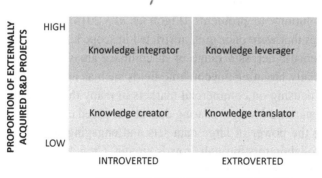

Figure 4.2. New types of pharmaceutical industry innovation model.
Source: Schumacher *et al.* (2013).

and the proportion of externally acquired R&D projects compared to internally generated knowledge:

- 'Knowledge creators' follow the traditional pharmaceutical industry model, relying predominantly on creating new ideas and managing their further development internally.
- 'Knowledge integrators' license or acquire most of their R&D pipeline — drug candidates, technologies and research knowledge — from external sources and apply their in-house expertise to develop them further.
- 'Knowledge translators' generate new ideas internally but then out-source the project portfolio to external collaborators and partners to manage R&D efficiently.
- Companies practising 'knowledge leverage' both acquire externally generated innovation and use a combination of internal and external resources to develop projects further. In Schumacher *et al.*'s (2013) analysis, Shire was the only company falling into this category, with an innovation model that combines open collaboration and corporate venturing with outside partners, and resembles a research foundation. For example, Shire has worked with the Fondazione Telethon, an Italian biomedical charitable foundation, to fund a rare diseases R&D partnership with the Telethon Institute of Genetics and Medicine (TIGEM).

As well as the range of different types of open innovation and other research relationship that exist, the goals being pursued vary. These include the creation of new products, development of tools and models, construction of information databases, and initiatives to access the skills and crowd-sourced solutions to problems (Pigott *et al.*, 2014). Industry-academic partnerships that were once quite restricted in scope have therefore become more systematic across a range of disciplinary areas (Kleyn and Kitney, 2007), initially targeting uneconomic fields such as neglected diseases but now also focusing on commercial markets in many therapy areas.

A recent trend involves sharing data at a reduced cost or free of charge, harnessing the power of large data sets and engaging with a much wider group of collaborators through crowdsourcing. Crowdsourcing is generally described as an online community that brings together inventors and innovators in open forums. A challenge is posted on the Internet and anyone is able to provide a solution. Solutions can be transparent or confidential. Probably the first example of crowdsourcing in drug discovery was initiated by Eli Lilly. This has evolved into InnoCentive,[4] with over 200,000 supporters. Through InnoCentive, the Global Alliance for TB Drug Development was able to accelerate the manufacturing process of PA-824, a new treatment to drastically reduce the time to cure TB. An example of an open source platforms is the Open Pharmacological Space (Ecker and Williams-Jones, 2012). Box 4.12 shows other examples.

Box 4.12   BACKGROUND: Some crowdsourcing initiatives in the biopharma sector

- Lilly's Phenotypic Drug Discovery, a mechanism for researchers' compounds to be tested against a range of assays.[5]
- Bayer Healthcare — funding early stage projects via Grants4Targets.[6]
- Rare diseases initiatives such as Telethon Institute of Genetics and Medicine (TIGEM) — Shire has invested $22m into a rare diseases R&D partnership.[7]
- WIPO Re:Search, a consortium of pharmaceutical and biotechnology concentrating on tropical disease targets.[8]
- GSK has published data on 47 leads for malaria and made a commitment for disclosure of lead structures for tuberculosis.[9]
- The MRC-AstraZeneca collaboration on Alzheimer's, cancer and rare disease research.[10]
- Pfizer is collaborating with academic medical centres through their Centre for Therapeutic Innovation.[11]
- PatientsLikeMe members raise funding for clinical trials that meet the needs of their own special needs.[12]

Source: Judd (2013).

---

[4] http://www.innocentive.com
[5] http:// www.pd2.lilly.com
[6] http://www.grants4targets.com
[7] http://www.genengnews.com/gen-news-highlights/shire-puts-22m-into-rare-diseases-r-d-partnership/81247532
[8] http://www.wipo.int/research/en
[9] http://www.nature.com/news/data-sharing-aids-the-fight-againstmalaria-1.10018
[10] http://www.astrazeneca.com/Media/Press-releases/Article/20121131–astrazeneca-MRC-collaboration-disease-research
[11] http://www.pfizer.com/research/rd_works/centers_for_therapeutic_innovation.jsp
[12] https://www.patientslikeme.com/research/team

Moves towards crowdsourcing and other collaborative models have been prompted by the shift towards more intelligent, targeted approaches to drug development (Box 4.6). The research model is all about early-stage collaboration to tackle the huge volume of data and increase the chances of discovering the factors underlying a condition or disease, before a pharmaceutical company starts designing a drug.

Transparency Life Sciences (TLS)[13] is said to be the world's first drug development company completely based on open innovation. Its ethos is to involve all stakeholders — patients, doctors, regulators, researchers — in drug discovery in areas of unmet need, by collectively generating ideas and designing clinical trials. It seeks to lower the cost of trials by reducing the face-to-face involvement of trial participants in site visits through data obtained by telemonitoring. The portfolio of possible products consists of clinical-stage compounds that have the potential to be repurposed, drawn from other pharmaceutical companies and universities. Value is created by licensing IP and creating co-development deals and joint ventures.

Another feature of open innovation in the pharmaceutical industry is the physical co-location researchers. Both AstraZeneca and GlaxoSmithKline (GSK) have forged open innovation initiatives spanning health research charities, academic researchers and other biopharma companies, which involve scientists sharing laboratories (see Box 4.1).

In the UK, GSK and the Wellcome Trust have established a biomedical open innovation campus, the Stevenage BioScience Catalyst (SBC). This combines an incubator and an accelerator facility with business support services on the same site, providing a 'safe haven' for early-stage companies and networking opportunities. The premise

"The more accessible you make yourself to great science by being porous, by encouraging people to flow through your building and by having people in your building, the easier it is for our scientists to have those informal interactions and therefore start new things ... We're saying, 'you know what? We don't mind if you're in our labs. We really want to work together.' That makes us a much more attractive collaborator and it means we give as much as we take. That's really important." Mene Pangalos, AstraZeneca's head of innovative medicines (cited in Roland, 2014)

---

[13] http://transparencyls.com/

is that building an incubator next to a major pharmaceutical company facilitates engagement and leads to new business opportunities. The Wellcome Trust aims to promote translational research through early academic–industrial engagement. Also supporting the initiative are the UK's Technology Strategy Board and the Department of Business Innovation and Skills, keen to boost local economic development.

There have been concerns about the use of crowdsourcing from the perspective of IP protection (Foreman, 2014). The transparency inherent in crowdsourcing means there is the potential risk that an outside observer could file for a patent before the inventor does or that a patent's commercial value could be diluted unintentionally. This is less likely to be the case with open innovation models involving an organised and trusted platform led by a major pharmaceutical company. These provide inventors with evaluation of their idea and product development support but without the risk of their idea being stolen or personal capital lost.

Still at the fringes of open innovation in drug development is the concept of 'biohacking'. This is essentially a 'DIY biology' movement which aims to democratise biological engineering, making the necessary tools and resources available to non-professionals.[14,15] Roche announced in 2015 that it was spending EUR 200,000 to support an open access 'big data' research programme on the epidemiology of cancer at La Paillasse, a biohacking space in Paris. Roche have no specific business objectives and have explained that:

'As part of an open approach, and contrary to conventional methods in epidemiology, we are not asking scientific questions initially. So we don't know what we will get. It is therefore difficult to know what comes next.' (Raynal, 2015)

Government support for creating healthcare technology innovation — the case of the UK's NHS

In the UK and elsewhere, healthcare technology development is seen as an important part of the economy, so there is concern to make the

---

[14] http://www.wired.com/2011/08/mf_diylab/all/
[15] http://www.wired.co.uk/news/archive/2012-12/12/biohacking-europe

process as effective as possible. The peculiar features of healthcare as a market for medical technology mean that governments often play an active part in shaping the innovation process to ensure that new technologies are successfully developed and commercialised. Intervention occurs across all stages of the innovation pipeline, from basic research, through technology development and trialling, to adoption and diffusion.

The UK medical device market is one of the largest in the world, yet until recently, relatively little attention was paid to its features and needs (Prime Faraday Partnership, 2003). The majority of companies are SMEs — 58% have 10 or fewer staff and over 90% have fewer than 50 (BERR, 2008). Medical technology firms in the UK face a range of problems bringing innovative technologies to the market. These revolve especially around access to the right kind of finance at the right time and the difficulties in readily selling to their home market's biggest purchaser, the NHS.

An anti-innovation culture?

There is a widespread belief that the organisational culture of the NHS undervalues innovation — there is little expectation on staff to engage in innovation activities and there are few financial or other incentives for them to do so. There are also many other factors that impede innovation, both in relation to the adoption of new technologies developed by the medical devices industry and also to the internal generation of innovations within the NHS:

- The structural and cultural characteristics of the NHS. These include its functionally-based organisational structure, comprising professional hierarchies and departmental and financial silos (Rushmer *et al.*, 2004). These lead to a 'not invented here' mentality, as well as impacting on the economics of innovation.

➔ *Chapter 3 discusses the peculiarities of healthcare for innovation*

- The power, functional specialisation and autonomy of clinicians, which means that innovation is potentially limited by the views of individuals (Worthington, 2004), although these attributes can also stimulate user-driven innovation, as described above, p. 134.

- The day-to-day operational demands of delivering a consistent health service mean that innovation projects are given little time or priority.
- The pace of change and frequency of reorganisation within the NHS ensure that a degree of 'innovation fatigue' inevitably sets in.

In recent years, great efforts have been made to create a more innovative NHS. This has occurred in two ways. First, by supporting the generation and commercialisation of innovations developed internally, by trying to capture and protect IP produced within the NHS and exploiting it through licensing or the creation of spin-off companies. Second, by putting in place mechanisms to improve adoption, and supporting a culture of process re-design and continuous improvement, to ensure that innovations and recognised best practice are shared throughout the service. We discuss the ways in which governments have

---

Box 4.13   BACKGROUND: How innovation is defined in the NHS

In the late 2000s, there was mounting concern over the lack of innovation in the NHS and the impact of this on health system performance. The Darzi report (Department of Health, 2008) envisaged higher quality and innovation being driven partly by staff being committed to self-improvement. A subsequent report (Department of Health, 2011) argued:

- 'Innovation has to be more than a simple improvement in performance, and to achieve its maximum added value to the NHS it needs to be replicable — and replicated — across similar settings ...'
- 'So innovation is as much about applying an idea, service or product in a new context, or in a new organisation, as it is about creating something entirely new. Copying is good.'

The Carruthers report (Department of Health, 2011) defines innovation as 'an idea, service or product, new to the NHS or applied in a way that is new to the NHS, which significantly improves the quality of health and care wherever it is applied'. Compare this to the classification of innovations in Chapter 2.

supported the adoption and spread of innovation in the NHS the next chapter — here we concentrate on the mechanisms for promoting a strong medical technology sector.

Bridging the funding gaps

Given the importance of the medical technology sector to the national economy, it is not surprising that an important part of government industrial and health policy involves supporting innovations created in the UK through their journey from initial idea to the market.

As we saw in Chapter 2, the innovation 'pipeline' is conventionally regarded as a series of stages embracing invention, evaluation, adoption and diffusion. It is now accepted that these are neither discrete nor linear — the innovation process is messy, with feedback and adaptation occurring between different stages. For many new healthcare innovations the journey from initial concept to adoption and diffusion does not take the form of a neat pathway. This is particularly the case for products that also involve a degree of organisational or service change, as is common in healthcare.

One of the major problems for medical device innovators and manufacturers is the availability of appropriate financial support at different stages in the innovation pathway. This problem is not unique to the UK — across Europe the mechanisms for seed funding and early-stage financing are seen as inadequate and an impediment for start-ups to reach critical mass. The problem seems more acute in the UK, though, where a report from the European Commission (European Commission, 2009; NESTA, 2009) found that 19% of SMEs (not specifically medical technology ones) saw limited access to finance as a constraint — the corresponding figures for SMEs from Finland was 7% and 9% for those from Denmark. Of course this implies that most UK SMEs did not struggle to gain access to finance (NESTA, 2009), although the trend in the late 2000s was that access was becoming harder (BIS, 2012b).

Typically new innovations progress through different stages of a funding 'escalator' (Figure 4.3) as the technology and the business develop and capital requirements change. However, for UK medical devices firms a

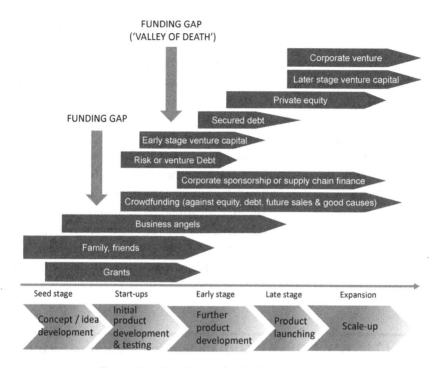

Figure 4.3.   Funding sources by innovation stages.

smooth transition through these stages seems to be the exception rather than the rule (see Case study 4.1 on the development of the Peezy Midstream device). One widely recognised problem is the existence of different 'funding gaps' in relation to equity and growth capital. These largely occur around the mid stages of the innovation pipeline.

The initial R&D phase may be financially supported by government bodies or research funders, but a gap occurs when the feasibility of a prospective new technology needs to be proven in sufficiently large trials prior to further development, testing and launch. This is often known as 'the valley of death'. Its presence means medical technology SMEs may have periods of limited or no revenue. This makes start-ups a higher risk, which either drives away investors or means they require the SMEs to have follow-on finance in place before making an investment. There may also be a gap later on in the innovation process, when finance for scalable commercial development is needed, assuming the innovation has progressed sufficiently for there to be a compelling business case. Limited data on potential revenue makes investors risk averse, leading them to favour larger deals with more established medical technology companies.

A growing range of funding sources is becoming available at different stages in the innovation process, from seed capital provided by angel investors, friends and family through various forms of venture capital funding to initial public offerings and secondary offerings. Venture capital funding tends to be concentrated in certain industry sectors, including biotech and some parts of medtech. Crowdfunding and other peer-to-peer funding models are also emerging as a link between investors and innovators. There are different models, but essentially they require innovators to pitch their ideas to a crowdfunding platform and then — supported by the platform — generate a funding campaign.

Box 4.14   BACKGROUND: Rationalising the infrastructure for technology innovation in France and Denmark

Responding to concern about the fragmentation of its existing system for supporting developers of new technology, France has been renewing its innovation infrastructure. This includes establishing larger regional technology transfer organisations and putting in place new mechanisms for supporting proof-of-concept and prototyping. In 2012, new 'technology acceleration' companies were established (*Sociétés d'Accélération du Transfert de Technologie*, SATT), backed by a EUR 1 billion national loan. Some of the activities of the SATTs are targeted at the creation of innovative medical technologies, financing proof of concept for promising new technologies to help them reach a sufficient level of development to move towards commercialisation. A SATT acts as a single point of contact in a region, with the expertise to manage patents, licenses and industrial contracts. Before the creation of a SATT, in Alsace there were six different *valorisation de la recherche* (research commercialisation organisations). Following establishment of the *Conectus*

(Continued)

Box 4.14   (*Continued*)

Alsace SATT, the length of time needed to agree licenses fell from 9–12 months to 2–3 months (LIF/Vasco Advisers, 2013).

Denmark has also sought to strengthen its national technology innovation strategy. Like France, a multitude of organisations and funding mechanisms for supporting innovation had emerged over the years and the system had become too complex, with many overlapping services. There was also concern about the lack of strategic investment in innovation funding (Crasemann *et al.*, 2012). A new Danish innovation strategy has been put in place, which includes combining the activities of three different national bodies into a single council for strategic research, innovation and advanced technology, with its own innovation investment fund. A 'market maturation' (*Markedsmodningsfonden*) fund has also been established to help SMEs tackle barriers in the technology commercialisation process.

Sources: Crasemann *et al.* (2012); LIF/Vasco Advisers (2013).

In the UK, a range of mechanisms has been put in place to support medical technologies through the different stages of the innovation journey (we return to this is more detail in Chapter 5). Like other European countries (see Box 4.14), there are now many overlapping organisations and funding programmes, from the Research Councils providing funding for basic research to organisations such as Academic Health Science Networks (AHSNs) designed to support adoption and diffusion. The healthcare innovation landscape is comprehensively mapped, but in terms of public funding, by far the largest proportion still goes to the research stage (Barlow and Burn, 2008), partly bolstered by tax credits for allowable research activities (HMRC, 2012). Venture capital funds such as the UK Future Technologies Fund have also been established to support innovative technology-based SMEs, using public and private money to target all development stages. There is still criticism, however, that support is incomplete, especially around the 'valley of death'. This has been the target of the Small Business Research Initiative, but the available finance remains relatively small.

Case Study 4.1   Peezy Midstream

Forte Medical is a small start-up company which develops low-tech, low-cost specimen collection systems. The first product, the Peezy Midstream, began life in 2001. Despite its simplicity, performance and low cost, it is only now beginning to be more widely adopted. The case study illustrates the difficulties faced by small companies bringing new medical technologies to market, the way different funding sources are used at different stages, and the importance of securing both clinical evidence and credible economic evidence.

Background

Analysis of urine samples can be as clinically important as blood testing, but sampling standards are not as stringent. Current hit-and-miss collection methods result in urine specimens contaminated by mixed growth. Of the 65 million samples collected by the UK's NHS each year, 15–30% show mixed growth, and need to be re-tested at a cost up to GBP 52 million. There is also emerging evidence that a lack of diligence in basic urine specimen collection may lead to the over-prescribing of broad spectrum antibiotics, especially in out-of-hours health services, where prescribing may take place before urine analysis confirms the targeted antibiotic required. As Giovanna Forte, CEO of Forte Medical, describes it,

> *'Urine analysis is a vital diagnostic tool in many clinical areas, but puzzlingly it seems to be seen as a second-rate citizen. Hit-and-miss collection is unacceptable. Sending a contaminated urine specimen to the lab is like asking a detective to solve a crime by looking through a dirty window.'*

Not only do existing collection methods fail to meet the UK's standards for microbiology investigation of urine, for individuals they are inconvenient and potentially unhygienic, with wet bottles, wet hands and the spread of urine across clinical settings. Despite developing a simple solution for these problems, Forte Medical's journey to bring this to market has proved hard and long.

Peezy Midstream is a simple funnel and a universal container. These fit with the commonly used 30 ml universal container and the 10 ml primary tube that fits directly into laboratory analysers. But despite its simplicity, performance and low cost, the product has taken over a decade to become accepted.

(Continued)

Case Study 4.1   (*Continued*)

A long history of development

In 2001, Dr. Vincent Forte, a general practitioner, concluded that conventional approaches to collection resulted in unreliable analysis, diagnosis and treatment in female patients with unresolved urinary tract infection. He listened to complaints about collection methods, invented the Female Freedom Funnel and obtained patent protection. The following year, the device was a winner at the Medical Futures Awards. Supported by his sister Giovanna, they conducted market research, explored business partnerships and began design development. This was initially financed with personal funds; Vincent from savings and Giovanna through the PR business she ran at the time.

By 2006, after researching various technical options, including flushable eco materials, GBP 150,000 seed funding was secured, half from the London Development Agency Early Growth Fund and half through angel investors. Additional investment in kind came from their initial manufacturing partner, who took shares in the business in return for supporting research, development and prototype tooling. This allowed proof of concept trials to begin. In 2008–2009, the first prototypes were manufactured and trialled. The team developed a quality assurance programme and submitted it for certification, before registration with the MHRA (the UK's medicines and healthcare products regulatory authority). A major challenge was persuading the MHRA that the early proof of concept trials were not of a clinical nature; a lesson learned was that no clinical trials could take place without prior approval from the regulatory body. The quality assurance work included satisfying a testing and certification body that the product complied with a number of quality standards.

A second investment round raised further finance from existing shareholders and new angel investors, allowing work to be carried out on the specification of product materials and the manufacturing process. Production began in 2009. Despite support from leading clinicians at the Norfolk and Norwich Hospital NHS Trust, a proposed clinical trial proved too costly for the company to support. They turned to less formal evaluations at a number of settings such as different hospital ante-natal departments. However, data from these evaluations were not collected in a sufficiently rigorous way.

Parallel to evaluation work, a marketing and sale campaigns began, helped in 2009 by an Innovative Health and Social Care Technology award from the NHS Health & Social Care Awards. This was followed by Best

(Continued)

Case Study 4.1   (*Continued*)

Industrial Product and Best of Show accolades from the design industry bible, Design Week. The following year consisted of sales visits to nurses in urology and ante-natal departments across the UK, to encourage trials and evaluations to feed into design improvements. A third investment round raised more finance from existing investors and new business angels.

By 2012, manufacturing had been refined to create a single injection mould and reduce costs. Steps were also taken to further protect Peezy Midstream's IP and it was listed in the UK's Drug Tariff. More finance was obtained from a new syndicate of private investors and existing shareholders who continued to support the business. At this time, Forte Medical completed an NHS Supply Chain tender for urology products and secured a place in the NHS Catalogue, making it easier for frontline staff to order Peezy Midstream. Unfortunately this did not help sales, and sales personnel were engaged to continue UK-wide visits.

After completing design iterations that incorporated improvements based on suggestions by frontline nurses and patients who tried the Peezy, a new version of the product was released in 2013. A detailed evaluation from the urology department at Pennine NHS Acute Hospitals Trust was peer reviewed and presented at the Société International d'Urologie 2013 and World Congress of Endourology 2013 conferences. Leading urologists who liked the Peezy concept recommended that the company should contact UCL School of Medicine, where a clinical trial was being set up to investigate the most efficient urine collection methods. This trial compared standard techniques with Peezy Midstream and catheter urine collection, in terms of accuracy, efficiency, patient preferences and economic implications of right-first-time urine specimen collection. Results were pending at the time of writing this case study.

Meanwhile, Stanford Medical School in the USA found Forte Medical by way of an internet search for 'accurate urine specimen collection', and contacted the company because they needed to reduce a high contamination rate in their emergency department. This led to a fully randomised clinical trial to compare Peezy with traditional collection methods and pre-collection cleaning with a microbial wipe. This trial has yet to be completed, with full results expected after July 2016.

The fifth funding round was launched in 2013, to support scale-up production and continuing sales and marketing campaigns. At this

(*Continued*)

Case Study 4.1   (*Continued*)

time, the existing R&D partner and manufacturer recommended that a new manufacturer was needed to cope with the volume sales that they began to foresee. In 2014, a novel tooling-for-equity deal with a specialist plastics manufacturer was secured. This also allowed final design improvements to be made, allowing urine to be taken from patient to laboratory analyser with no decanting, this reducing handling and risk of contamination from external sources.

Sales were growing across the UK, with orders from ambulance services, urology and haematology clinics, mental health, maternity services and others via the NHS Supply Chain contract. Two major private hospital groups also adopted Peezy Midstream for accuracy and patient safety reasons. Purchasing by the private sector was less constrained than the NHS market, where 'silo budgeting' (see Chapters 3 and 5) meant that the department purchasing Peezy Midstream — which costs more than other options — would not necessarily receive the benefit of savings due to reduced retesting. At that time, the majority of NHS Trusts also implemented a blanket 'no new products' policy in order to meet government pressure to save money. An additional problem arose with the private laboratories appointed to handle NHS services; these are often paid on volume, which means reduced retesting is unwelcome as it is likely to reduce profits.

In 2014, Forte Medical was approached by a specialist sales company, which subsequently failed to meet the ambitious targets it had set itself. Later that year, Forte Medical regained control of sales and developed a new marketing strategy. This included greater use of social media, and a strategic partnership with a national parenting brand to facilitate an awareness and sales campaign to midwives, community nurses and pregnant women. Forte Medical has also gathered champions and supporters from parts of the health sector. As well the two private hospital chains, this includes the nursing trade union which feels that its members could benefit from Peezy's infection control, patient safety and right-first-time benefits. The focus of Forte Medical is now on specific sectors such as antenatal, elderly care and paediatric medicine, and the promotion of prescription Peezy for patient populations that need very accurate urine testing, such as pregnant women. A sales partnership in the USA has also been established.

To improve the prospects for adoption within the NHS, Forte Medical has appointed a health economist to explore the potential savings to the NHS. This

(*Continued*)

Case Study 4.1 *(Continued)*

work is now being translated into an economics marketing and media campaign, which will be bolstered by the results from the UCL and Stanford university trials. The company has also appointed senior sales executives to deal directly with NHS finance and procurement directors, where an awareness of cross-budget savings is more likely to be in evidence. Meanwhile, feedback from the market is helping the company to identify new unmet urine sampling and other specimen collection needs; new products are now being developed for EN2 prostate cancer, cervical cancer and bladder cancer urine tests, as well as stool sampling for bowel and colon cancer.

Key lessons

The Peezy Midstream case demonstrates how the development and marketing of a seemingly simple and low cost medical technology innovation can require patience, persistence and a flexible approach to funding.

- Since 2001, **different funding sources have been used at different stages**. These range from a mixture of personal funds and grants, to angel investors and other private investors across five separate funding rounds. Each round has unlocked the ability of the company to conduct the activities needed to progress through the innovation pipeline. In addition, support has come from manufacturing partners in the form of shares in the business in return for supporting R&D and prototype tooling, and a tooling-for-equity deal with a specialist manufacturer to allow final design improvements to be made. Forte Medical feels that it has learned that it should never overestimate sales forecasts and underestimate funding requirements.
- The importance of securing early **clinical trial evidence**, as well as a clear understanding of **customer and patient benefits**, is another lesson learnt by Forte Medical.
- Over time gathering **credible economic evidence**, in the form of tangible cost savings for different stakeholders, also became very important. And evaluation was not a once-off activity — it needed to be carried out in a variety of contexts and continue as the product evolved. Funding had to be raised for evaluation, including hiring a health economist. Engaging with world-leading university partners unlocked the possibility of conducting detailed trials.

(Continued)

Case Study 4.1 (*Continued*)

- Forte Medical learnt lessons about the **sales process**. It was important to identify individuals who could champion the Peezy in their organisations and more widely, for example through medical conferences. Once initial sales had been made, maintaining regular customer communication to gather their feedback on the product and establish regular sales was essential.
- Finally, the development of Peezy Midstream shows how continuous design development, drawing on customer feedback, requires both regular funding at different stages and an **awareness of when to secure protection of IP** — in this case after the initial invention and once the manufacturing process had been refined.

Questions

- Should Forte Medical consider focusing its attention on a market outside the UK, where there are more private sector healthcare providers and the market is less complex? What would be the pros and cons of such a strategy?
- Do you think further government support would have helped speed up the development of the Peezy Midstream? What might be an effective type of support in this case, and at what stage in the development process would it be most useful?
- How could Forte Medical tackle the problem of silo thinking in the NHS? What kind of arguments might be most convincing to persuade purchasers to adopt their product?

Source: Case study prepared in collaboration with Giovanna Forte, CEO, Forte Medical.

Towards an open and user-led innovation model within the NHS

Since the late 1990s, interest in improving technology transfer from public sector research institutes into healthcare practice, along with finding ways of exploiting IP generated within the NHS has gradually increased. The NHS's potential role as an active partner in 'pulling' innovation from the health technology sector has been increasingly emphasised (Baker, 1999; Department of Health, 2002; HITF, 2004). NHS innovation hubs, modelled on commercial and university technology transfer offices, were set up to assist the transfer of technology developed within the NHS to wider markets. The extent to which these have been successful in capturing and exploiting IP generated within the NHS is, however, uncertain (Savory and Fortune, 2013). This may partly be due to difficulties in translating a commercial technology-transfer model to the NHS culture (Savory, 2006).

Broadly, the government policies and initiatives put in place over the last decade or so have begun to view the NHS as part of a wider innovation system in which interrelated factors affect both the creation and adoption of health technologies. There is recognition that adoption by NHS organisations does not take place in isolation from other activities in the innovation system, so effective strategies to facilitate adoption need to consider the relationships between different activities (Savory and Fortune, 2013). Of particular importance are the links between assessment of clinical need, promotion of research and dissemination of its findings, support for the creation of appropriate innovative technologies, and improving the NHS capabilities to get them adopted.

It is here that open and user-led innovation perspectives potentially offer valuable lessons (Savory and Fortune, 2013). A key challenge is to ensure that knowledge is effectively transferred between the different organisations involved in the healthcare technology innovation system — NHS organisations and staff as lead users and developers, patients, companies developing new technological solutions, researchers and funders. This leads Savory and Fortune (2013) to propose an extension of what is known as the 'triple-helix' model of technology transfer (Etzkowitz and Leydesdorff, 2000), which emphasises the relationship between universities, government and industry. They argue that innovation in health technologies often occurs on the periphery between formal research organisations, industry and NHS organisations. In contrast to examples of open innovation where commercial technology manufacturers maintain a degree of power over the trajectory and focus of the innovation, examples from the NHS show how its staff were able to maintain influence and act as clinical champions and opinion leaders. The triple-helix model therefore needs to embrace a more user-led perspective to capture the innovation processes characteristic of medical technology (see Arnkil *et al.*,

2010 for a discussion of a 'quadruple helix' model embracing a continuum of user involvement). The fourth strand of the revised model is, therefore, the healthcare system itself. Such a refinement, Savory and Fortune argue could represent a useful basis for understanding the various transfers of knowledge that result in the creation and adoption of new technology in the NHS. This would also help to build the 'absorptive capacity' of the NHS to adopt innovations.

Chapter summary

- Many companies producing innovative drugs or medical devices go through the same practices of technology and innovation management as companies in other industries: stage-gate decision-making, balancing their portfolios of potential new products according to likelihood of success, deciding how much R&D to conduct in-house compared to contracting out, and so on.
- But there are also characteristic features of technological innovation processes in the healthcare sector compared to other sectors.
- The development of new health technologies brings together universities and other R&D organisations, drug and device manufacturers, funders and governments and regulatory institutions, and end-users in national, regional and sectoral innovation systems.
- While there are some similarities between the pharmaceutical and medical devices sectors, the former is subject to a much more structured and highly regulated development process.
- For both the development of many health technology innovations can be very time-consuming and costly, because of the amount of scientific and engineering content and regulatory process.
- Development of medical devices is often user-driven, for example by clinicians who have identified a particular need that has not been fulfilled. Innovation may take place within an open innovation network or within a wider network of knowledge and resources.
- Government support may be needed to address the 'translation gap' between research and implementation, and support innovations at different stages in the technology development process.

Questions for discussion

1. Why do companies often find it hard to bringing new healthcare products to market? Provide examples to illustrate your answer.
2. What are the key stages in the development and commercialisation of healthcare technologies? Describe the activities typically take place at each stage in the innovation process for a new drug and a new medical device.
3. Describe the 'stage-gate' approach to the development of new products. Are there differences in the way this model is applied between medical devices and new drugs? What alternative models are used by innovators?
4. Recalling the lessons from Chapter 2 on new product development and the need to balance experimentation and risk management, and referring to Innovation in Action 4.2:

   - What were the pros and cons of adopting a standardised stage-gate approach to new product development? To what extent do you think this potentially compromised Coloplast's internal creativity?
   - What challenges do you think Coloplast might face in selecting externally sourced ideas for further development?

5. To what extent do you think the innovation efforts of the pharmaceutical and medical device industries are stalling? Why? What are these industries doing to overcome its innovation productivity challenges?
6. In what ways are open- and user-driven innovation advantageous to the medical device and pharmaceutical/biopharma companies? Describe the potential benefits and challenges for companies adopting this type of approach.
7. How important are healthcare practitioners in medical technology innovation?
8. Discuss how pharmaceutical companies tackle the technological and market uncertainties associated with the development of new drugs.

9. Why do developers of new medical devices often resort to personal networks, friends and family, and crowd funding at certain stages in the innovation process? What other options are available?

10. Select an example of a medical technology start-up and outline the problems they faced regarding funding. How did they overcome these problems?

11. What is the cash flow gap that small companies developing medical devices often face and why is it called the 'valley of death'?

12. Why should governments provide assistance to innovators in healthcare? Choose an example of an initiative, describe its purpose and evaluate how effective it is.

Selected further reading

Burns L, Nicholson S, Wolkowski J (2012) Pharmaceutical strategy and the evolving role of merger and acquisition. In Burns L. (ed.), *The Business of Healthcare Innovation*. 2nd Edition. Cambridge: Cambridge University Press.

Chesbrough H (2006) *Open Business Models: How to Thrive in the New Innovation Landscape*. Boston: Harvard Business School Press.

IMS (2012) *IMS Market Prognosis International 2012–2016*. IMS Health.

Lindqvist G, Sölvell O (2011) Organising clusters for innovation: lessons from city regions in Europe. CLUSNET final report.

Metcalfe J, James A, Mina A (2005) Emergent innovation systems and the delivery of clinical services: The case of intra-ocular lens. *Research Policy* 34(9): 1283–1304.

Northrup J, Tarasova M, Kalowski L (2012) The pharmaceutical sector: Rebooted and reinvigorated. In Burns L. (ed.), *The Business of Healthcare Innovation*. 2nd Edition. Cambridge: Cambridge University Press.

Savory C, Fortune J (2013) *NHS adoption of NHS-developed technologies*. Final report, NIHR Service Delivery and Organisation programme.

Von Hippel E (2005) *Democratizing Innovation*. Cambridge: MIT Press.

INNOVATION PROCESSES PART 2 — IMPLEMENTING AND SUSTAINING INNOVATION IN HEALTHCARE ORGANISATIONS

05

THIS CHAPTER WILL HELP YOU TO:

- Understand the reasons why innovation adoption in healthcare requires careful consideration of the wider context and the nature of the innovation itself.
- Explain what role benefits evidence plays in adoption decision and why its collection is hard for many healthcare innovations.
- Understand why governments use financial approaches to incentivise healthcare organisations to adopt innovations.

In the last chapter, we explored the challenges faced by innovators trying to create and bring new healthcare technology to the market. In Chapter 5, we turn to the perspective of healthcare organisations trying to adopt and embed innovations into their everyday practice. We also discuss mechanisms put in place by government policy makers to stimulate innovative behaviour in healthcare providers. We pick up an issue introduced previously, the question of evidence for the benefits of innovations and the way this enables or constrains their adoption. As we have argued, an innovation is more likely to be adopted when it has perceived benefits, we can try it out and observe its impact, it is compatible with the organisation or health system that is adopting it, and it is not so complex that it cannot easily be replicated. But many healthcare innovations are complex and involve a mix of technological, organisational and service delivery change, so despite good evidence for their benefits, potential adopters view them cautiously.

There are two case studies in the chapter. The 'Columba project' (Case study 5.1) illustrates the difficulties in implementing and scaling-up a complex innovation, which combines new technology with changes to the health and social care service delivery model. These difficulties were a result of the need to engage widely across the care system and the changing goals of the project, as different stakeholders responded to emerging health policy needs. Case study 5.2 looks at the use of financial incentives to stimulate healthcare providers to adopt haemodialysis in patients' own homes. Different types of incentive were tried out in England's National Health Service, with varying results. One problem was that local healthcare providers lacked an understanding of their costs of delivering dialysis. This meant they were unable to clearly see what they were gaining from the financial incentives.

Mini Case 5.1 describes the development of polio vaccine in the 1950s. The story is one of a medical community being given the confidence to use a new product because technology trials delivered unambiguous feedback about its benefit. Mini Case 5.2 illustrates how a similarly clear and evidence-based technology was initially slow to take-off, but was given a boost with the publication of guidance from a medical professional body. Mini Case 5.3 looks at the problems of introducing remote care (telehealth and telecare) from the perspective of the manufacturers of the technology, and the way a fragmented and disorganised market impedes adoption.

The received wisdom on the adoption and diffusion of healthcare innovations is that it is a problem — a problem for policy makers, for industry, for healthcare providers and for payers and governments. While there are often pockets of excellence within health systems, where what is recognised as best practice or the latest evidence-based innovation is readily taken up, often these new ideas do not spread further. Sometimes the knowledge about them fails to be transferred because the mechanisms for sharing the information between medical professionals, managers of health organisation or policy makers are imperfect. Or an innovation fails to develop beyond the phase of small-scale trials — even in the local region where the trial is being carried out — because the challenges are felt to be too high compared to the perceived payoff. Perhaps there are insufficient local resources — skills or finance — to expand an innovation trial further. This can happen when the funding committed to a pilot project has come to an end and no-one is prepared to pay for a larger trial or invest in rolling-out the innovation into mainstream healthcare practice — there are echoes here of the 'valley of death' problem for innovative medical products we saw in Chapter 4.

As we describe later, the quality and nature of evidence for the benefits of an innovation can be very important for convincing the sceptics; a perceived lack of evidence is sometimes used as an excuse for inaction. So often it is not the innovative technology itself — at least not its physical or technical attributes — that is the problem. It is the organisational and financial challenges surrounding its adoption that are considerably more important.

What research on adoption from outside healthcare tells us — a recap

Chapter 2 drew on the mainstream body of research to look at the adoption and diffusion of innovative products. We argued that until relatively recently, this research has had some limitations. First, its focus was overwhelmingly on the introduction of new *manufactured products* rather than innovations in *services* or *business models*. Second, the specific innovations studied tended to be *individual* products with *unambiguous* characteristics, in other words an innovation delivering clear and specific benefits, such as the mobile phone, microwave oven or hybrid corn. Third, the explanatory framework has often concentrated on the aggregate effect of *individual* adoption decisions by *independent decision-makers*; situations involving collective or organisational decision-making have been relatively neglected by researchers. Finally, until relatively recently, there was little research on the adoption and diffusion of innovation in the public or non-profit sectors.

Sometimes the conventional models of adoption and diffusion from other industries are applicable in healthcare. This may happen when there is no ambiguity in the innovation itself and the characteristics described by Everett Rogers — trialability, observability and so on — can be clearly seen to influence an individual clinician's decision to adopt it. Or the adoption decision is taken by more or less fully informed individuals who can weigh up the pros and cons and make a decision to adopt, uninfluenced by others factors. The case of polio vaccine is a good example from healthcare. Another example is the adoption and diffusion of lipid emulsions in anaesthesia, which was stimulated by a combination of emerging awareness of the benefits, the introduction of formal guidelines for use and a simple decision-making context (see Innovation in Actions 5.1 and 5.2).

INNOVATION IN ACTION 5.1: When clear innovation attributes help adoption and diffusion — the story of polio vaccine

As Everett Rogers (2003) argued, the perceived attributes of an innovation — its 'relative advantage', 'compatibility', 'trialability', 'observability' and 'complexity' — together influence the speed and extent of adoption. Sometimes in healthcare these attributes are clear and adoption takes place rapidly. Richard Nelson and colleagues describe how sharp, persuasive feedback on the evidence, combined with growing benefits as it was more widely adopted, resulted in the rapid diffusion of polio vaccine (see Chapter 2, Table 2.4, for details of Nelson *et al.*'s explanatory model).

In the late 1940s, there was uncertainty about whether the best approach to vaccinate against polio would be to use a live (weakened) virus or a killed (inactive) virus. The live virus, created by Albert Sabin, would take longer to develop. Past experience of vaccines suggested it could provide longer immunity, but also possibly result in more virulence. The alternative killed vaccine was championed by Jonas Salk. This could be developed faster but there was uncertainty about the length of immunity it provided.

(Continued)

INNOVATION IN ACTION 5.1 *(Continued)*

Development of both technologies began in the early 1950s and by 1952, Salk had created a candidate polio vaccine which showed promising results in monkeys and a small number of humans. In 1954, the vaccine was trialled in 1.8 million children across the USA. The results, presented in 1955, showed clear evidence for the benefits of the vaccine and within days of the announcement the US government licenced production to six vaccine manufacturers. Because the trial's results were so unambiguous and accepted by the bulk of the medical community, use of the vaccine diffused rapidly. Within a decade over half the population had received it. Yet there was still some reluctance to use the Salk vaccine, partly because it required a course of three separate injections to cover each strain of polio. In 1959, Albert Sabin developed a live virus that could be administered orally and protected against all three polio strains. Following a very large trial in the Soviet Union, the vaccine was judged to be as effective as Salk's vaccine. It also conferred immunity faster and was longer-lasting. Soon after the vaccine became available, it was endorsed by the American Medical Association and it spread rapidly through the developed world. By 1968, it was more widely used than the Salk vaccine.

Nelson *et al.* (2004) describe the case of polio vaccine as a story of technology trials generating rapid feedback of efficacy to both the medical community and population of consumers, resulting in growing confidence about its use. This was reinforced by previous experience of the benefits of vaccination more generally. Although there was a false start, with the initial diffusion of what proved to be an inferior technology, the low switching costs from the Salk to the Sabin vaccine meant that there was no problem of 'lock in' to the earlier technology.

Source: Nelson *et al.* (2004).

But healthcare innovations are typically not like this. Adoption and diffusion often takes place in a context that is more ambiguous or complex. This occurs when the attributes of the innovation are less clearcut because they involve elements of technology and organisational change, and the adoption decision is taken by an organisation rather than individuals or is heavily influenced by government objectives. It is

INNOVATION IN ACTION 5.2: The role of guidelines in the adoption of 'lipid rescue'

Lipids are a group of naturally occurring molecules that include fats and fat-soluble vitamins. They can be included in a lipid emulsion for human intravenous use. The possibility of using intravenous lipid emulsion to treat serious overdoses of local anaesthetic drugs was first mooted in 1998. This was followed in 2004 by publication of a suggested treatment regimen for local anaesthetic-induced cardiac arrest in humans, dubbed 'lipid rescue'. While lipid rescue is not superior to orthodox treatments, its successful use in patients suffering this type of cardiac arrest was reported in peer-reviewed journals during 2006–2008. Research suggested that there would be little to lose from administering intravenous lipid and potentially everything to gain if it saved a life. Moreover, lipid emulsions were familiar to anaesthetists and already stocked in most hospital formularies, at minimal cost. Widespread adoption of lipid rescue should therefore be straightforward. In August 2007, the Association of Anaesthetists of Great Britain & Ireland (AAGBI) published guidelines recommending lipid rescue. Picard *et al.* showed that at that time only just over half the relevant hospitals in one region of the UK used lipid rescue. Adoption grew rapidly after the guidelines were published, so that by the time of a survey a few months later only 14% of hospitals reported not having lipid rescue (see figure).

Lipid rescue therefore spread widely and fast — the first published reports of its use in humans appeared in mid-2006; by December 2007 around 80% of hospitals in the survey region had adopted it. However, this was not just due to the publication of evidence and the AAGBI guidelines. The diffusion curve was already on an upward trajectory as knowledge spread. The guidelines merely reinforced what was underway; other factors were at play. In many hospitals, adoption was driven by a single enthusiast acting seemingly almost alone; in others enthusiasts were thwarted by the local drugs and therapeutics committee. Although the hospitals were geographically close and are staffed by doctors with similar training, the adoption of lipid rescue occurred in different ways in different hospitals. In fact, only about a half the hospitals adopting lipid rescue attributed its introduction to the guidelines' publication.

(Continued)

INNOVATION IN ACTION 5.2 *(Continued)*

Uptake of lipid rescue from January 2005 to January 2008 in the hospitals responding to the survey.

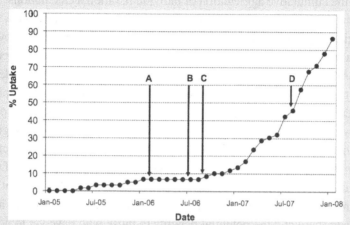

A: February 2006 — Anaesthesia editorial
B: July 2006 — First case report published
C: August 2006 — Second case report published
D: August 2007 — AAGBI Guidelines published

Source: Picard *et al.* (2009).

useful, therefore, to distinguish between different contexts for adoption decision-making:

- decision-making in situations where the *individual* is the main decision-maker, independent of peers,
- decision-making where choices are made jointly with others in a social system and accompanied by peer pressure or formal requirement to conform (*collective*), and
- situations where decisions are taken by a few individuals because of their power, status or expertise (*authoritative*) (Rogers, 2003). The latter is particularly characteristic of healthcare systems.

We also saw in Chapter 2 how the diffusion of an innovation often takes the form of

> → *See Chapter 2 for a discussion on decision-making in an organisational context. See Box 2.10 for a description of the role of information in adoption decision-making*

an S-shaped curve, resulting from its cumulative take-up by a population over time. Decisions to adopt and the resulting impact on diffusion have been studied from several perspectives. Economists typically view the process as the cumulative aggregation of individual, rational calculations. These are influenced by an assessment by adopters of the costs and benefits of the innovation, and made under conditions of limited information. However, this is a rather narrow perspective because it ignores the effects of feedback and learning between individual and organisational actors, or the wider system within which adoption is taking place. As the innovation is deployed, users learn more about its potential or its limitations and either adapt it or feed lessons back to the innovation's developers; this in turn changes the nature of the innovation itself or its pace of adoption. 'Network effects' are another example of feedback within a system altering the pattern of adoption. Here the benefits of adopting an innovation grow as the population of users grows — the more people who own a mobile phone, the greater are the benefits to them and the potential benefits to those who have yet to adopt.

Researchers therefore stress the importance of information, created and shared by actors in a given population or social system. The emphasis is on the way different social systems, with their own values and beliefs, explain the diffusion of an innovation. Actors within these social systems may well have distinct ways of understanding the important features of an innovation, such as its relative advantages, its costs and benefits or its compatibility with the existing organisational or social context — in short, the 'evidence'. Because of this, the most appropriate channels of communication may vary according to the type of innovation and the context.

The role of 'opinion leaders', 'change agents', and learning and communication forms part of this perspective. As we see later, these have been used as part of the process of encouraging adoption and assimilation of healthcare innovations. Opinion leaders carry information across boundaries between groups, operating not from the top but as brokers between groups. They are recognised by peers as competent and trustworthy, and have extended personal networks. As such, they can be critical for the adoption and diffusion of new ideas or products, especially where changes in behaviour or attitudes are involved. We return to the role of knowledge and communications below, p. 202.

The importance of information, feedback and network effects therefore means that it is unrealistic to assume all potential adopters are similar and that the take-up of an innovation necessarily takes place in an obvious S-shaped curve. While such a curve can be observed for many new products, including those in healthcare, the pattern may be erratic, especially in the early phase before the curve takes off. Typically, following the introduction of a new product or service into the market there is a 'pre-diffusion phase' of limited introduction, market testing, trial and error, and adaptation as user needs become clearer (Tidd and Bessant, 2014). The time taken for innovations to be adopted and widely diffused can therefore be long and the rate of adoption irregular. The example of telehealth (see Case study 5.1) — using sensing devices to monitor a patient's vital signs or movement and respond appropriately — shows how long the adoption period can be for a new healthcare technology. Despite many years' development and widespread trialling, telehealth remains in the early stages of adoption, with technology developers complaining about the difficulties of persuading healthcare organisations to take up their innovations. Novel drugs have particular characteristics that may make their adoption difficult. Once successful trials have ended a lengthy period of pre-launch marketing and engagement ensues, prior to adoption, involving input from clinicians and regulators. This in itself may be a difficult process — a doctor and patient must be motivated to use the particular drug innovation and other stakeholders — payers, insurance companies or other gatekeepers — may be involved in the decision to dispense the drug (Northrup *et al.*, 2012).

Innovation adoption and diffusion in healthcare

Throughout the chapters so far, we have alluded to the fact that health-care innovations are often complex, with attributes that make their adoption hard:

- There may be multiple individuals or organisations involved in adoption and implementation decisions, the end-users (i.e. 'consumers' or patients) of the innovation may be far removed from the decision process.

> ➔*Chapter 3 discusses why lessons from mainstream innovation research may need to be adapted when they are applied to healthcare*

- They may be adopting an innovation which is multifaceted, perhaps combining several objectives (e.g. quality *and* safety improvements), or which is less well defined because it embraces elements of service *and* product innovation — a diagnostic test which changes the processes in a care pathway would be an example.
- The impact of the innovation may be felt more widely than just in the adopting organisation. Multiple stakeholders from across primary, secondary and social care may be affected, all with the potential to veto adoption decisions. Decision-makers may be situated in different organisations, the interests of which all need to be aligned. The case of telehealth is a good example, where the investment might be made by a hospital organisation in tandem with the local primary care provider.
- The evidence for benefits may be contested because those people involved in adoption decisions come from different parts of the health and social care systems, have different professional or cultural characteristics, and view what is acceptable evidence in different ways.

Thus the adoption and diffusion of healthcare innovations may not follow a neat S-shaped curve. What might be generally acknowledged as best practice or a clearly evidence-based innovation may well be unevenly adopted across a health system, with many silos where outmoded approaches continue to be used. This can result in significant geographical differences in access to the best care — hence the interest of policy makers in improving the effectiveness of healthcare innovation processes and, in particular, the spread of best practices across the system to reduce variations in healthcare outcomes.

So how have researchers tried to explain the processes of innovation adoption and diffusion in healthcare? The range of perspectives is wide. Researchers have emphasised:

- The attributes of the innovation itself, including its complexity (e.g. Plsek and Greenhalgh, 2001; Denis *et al.*, 2002; Coker *et al.*, 2004; Atun *et al.*, 2007).
- How the innovation is perceived by individual adopters (e.g. Foy *et al.*, 2002; Pierce and Delbecq, 1977).
- The importance of the organisational context, including leadership issues (e.g. Pettigrew *et al.*, 1992; Coker *et al.*, 2003; Atun *et al.*,

2006; Meyer and Goes, 1998), presence of local professional 'silos' in an adopting organisation (Champagne *et al.*, 1991), and wider health system factors (Atun *et al.*, 2005a, 2005b).

- The prevailing cultural norms, beliefs and values of actors and institutions within the adoption system (e.g. Atun *et al.*, 2005c), especially professional groups (e.g. Ferlie *et al.*, 2005).
- The role of peer and expert opinion leaders (e.g. Locock *et al.*, 2001; Fitzgerald *et al.*, 2002) and the impact of social networks (e.g. West *et al.*, 1999).
- The systems and structures that enable organisational learning (e.g. Shortell *et al.*, 1998) and 'absorptive capacity' of adopting organisations (e.g. Barnsley *et al.*, 1998; Ferlie *et al.*, 2001), and the existence of a 'receptive context' (Pettigrew *et al.*, 1992; Dopson *et al.*, 2002).

What lessons can we extract from this wide-ranging literature? (see Box 5.1). Collectively, it reinforces the idea that innovation adoption and diffusion is highly dependent on the interactions between the innovation,

---

Box 5.1 CONCEPTS: The essential research lessons on healthcare innovation adoption

- There is often no *single adoption decision*. A series of decisions are taken to first try out an innovation in a small-scale pilot project, then expand it to a larger scale trial, and only then go mainstream. Hence, we need to study the *adoption and assimilation* of innovation in everyday practice as a continuous activity.
- *Power and politics* potentially play a vital role in shaping adoption processes, with the dominance of the medical profession a significant factor. Sometimes changes in the need for innovative thinking are dictated by changing government policy.
- The characteristics of the *decision-making process* around adoption are important — is it decentralised or centralised, formal or informal, is it mandated by regulation or just recommended by policy?
- Decisions about adoption often take a short-term perspective but the *longer-term dynamics* of implementation are often neglected, especially the impact of an innovation as it ripples across the health system in sometimes unpredictable ways.

the local actors involved, and the wider context. A key message is that far more importance needs to be placed on relationships between different professional and other interest groups than in previous (largely non-healthcare based) research on adoption and diffusion of innovation.

Two important reviews of the literature on the adoption of innovations by health service organisations are those carried out by Greenhalgh *et al.* (2004a, 2004b) and Robert *et al.* (2009). Although the primary focus of both was on the UK's National Health Service (NHS), they represent an important contribution because they systematically summarised the research literature and identified gaps in the knowledge, at least at the time of writing. The reviews echoed concerns about a lack of understanding of technology adoption processes that had been raised within the wider innovation research literature. Especially important were concerns about overly determinist perspectives, which assume that the implementation of technology necessarily leads to readily identifiable consequences. Their conclusion was that the bulk of prior research had failed to recognise the complexity of the innovation adoption process within healthcare and the fact that multiple factors are often at play.

These reports present a conceptual model of innovation adoption and assimilation, which comprises three elements — the innovation, the innovators and the 'user system'. Greenhalgh and her colleagues identify the following as especially important in influencing adoption:

- The *nature of the innovation* itself, i.e. its attributes, components, complexity.
- Its *'inner context'*, i.e. the individuals and their organisational environment directly responsible for adopting the innovation.
- The *'outer context'* of the innovation, i.e. the wider environment into which it is being deployed.
- The *linkages* between all of these.

They argue that none of these exist in isolation; there is a dynamic relationship between them and the health system as a whole. The adoption processes individuals engage in are shaped by the characteristics of the innovation itself, and by the nature, capacity and activities of external factors such as communication and influence. This makes the behaviour of the elements and their relationships unpredictable.

A subsequent study by these researchers (Robert *et al.*, 2009) drew on a wider literature on the role of routines in shaping the practices and behaviour of individuals, groups and organisations and on influencing organisational learning. This is impor-

> ➔*Go to Chapter 2 for more information on the social construction of technology and innovations*

tant because of the way routines influence the nature of work, professional identity and the response of individuals and organisations to the introduction of new technology. Robert *et al.* also considered various models from research on technology adoption using 'structuration theory' (Barley and Tolbert, 1997; De Sanctis and Poole, 1994; Orlikowski, 1992, 2000). This highlights how technology adoption can create and reshape social structures, and how individuals can influence the way technology is introduced into organisations, and sometimes reshape the technology itself. We discuss later in the chapter how this has informed work on the 'normalisation' of innovation within healthcare organisations.

The innovation itself — its characteristics and 'inner context'

The characteristics of the technology associated with an innovation play an important role in the extent to which adoption takes place. Relative advantage, compatibility, complexity, trialability and observability are all potentially important, but these attributes on their own do not fully explain adoption behaviour. Sometimes the particular characteristics of a healthcare innovation are unambiguous. Its benefits and costs, its implications and impact are all obvious — we can 'touch and feel' the benefits of a better scalpel. The innovation may also be relatively 'discrete' — the new scalpel may not require new training or redesign of organisational processes for it to be used straightaway. A novel drug may also have these characteristics. Its benefits are obvious and prescribing and administering it are straightforward, as we saw with polio vaccine. But even in the cases of simple innovations, a wider impact may ripple across the healthcare system as fewer people may need to go to hospital or they can be discharged faster.

What constitutes a 'healthcare innovation' may well be rather opaque, though:

- It may consist of some hard technology but also a lot of soft technology (see Chapter 2), such as new protocols for its use, new service delivery models or organisational changes.
- It may be designed to achieve several objectives simultaneously. For example, the objective of shifting to a single bedroom layout, perhaps an innovation for a specific hospital, may be to tackle infection control, speed patient recovery, and improve patient satisfaction.
- The evidence base for its efficacy may be contested by different stakeholders, there may be no generally agreed criteria for judging its benefits, or the techniques for gathering evidence may be underdeveloped.

Telehealth is an innovation characterised by all these features. It is still often viewed with caution by potential adopters, despite its perceived benefits, an ability to trial it and observe its impact — there have been thousands of published studies on the impact of telehealth — and even when it is compatible with the adopting organisation's systems and values.

One reason for differing perspectives on evidence is that we may not all view or use the same technology or innovation in the same way. As Chapter 2 explained, researchers have argued that a particular technology will be inscribed with ways of working that reflect different values and organisational procedures and processes. This relates partly to the way different types of knowledge — tacit or codified — are embedded and evolve as we learn about the technology as it is used in a specific context. Learning may take place through formal processes, as in the example of minimally invasive cardiac surgery in US hospitals, or it may taker place in a more experiential way, shown in the CT scanner example (see Box 5.2). In the case of innovations in diagnostic tests, the problem for those appraising their

➔ *Chapter 2 outlines the different types of knowledge sometimes used in innovation research*

➔ *Go to Chapter 6 to find out about innovation in diagnostic tests*

Box 5.2 BACKGROUND: Learning and implementing of healthcare technology — the adoption of minimally invasive surgery and CT scanning

Edmondson *et al.* (2001) carried out a qualitative study of teams implementing an innovative technology (minimally invasive cardiac surgery) in 16 US hospitals. They examined the collective learning process taking place among the users of the technology and found that sites where successful implementation occurred underwent a team learning process that was qualitatively different from that experienced on unsuccessful sites. Training simulations involving groups responsible for implementation led to a fuller understanding of the technology's benefits.

Barley (1986) investigated why the introduction of the same technology (the CT scanner) played out differently in two US hospital radiology departments. He argued that adoption was shaped and constrained by the pre-existing social structures of the hospital, in other words people's 'interpretive frames' (how they understood the technology), power and influence, and professional codes of conduct. He concluded that the same technology, introduced in different contexts, will have different impacts because of variations in historical, contextual and social factors. He also argued that causality runs in two directions: technology influences patterns of human activity and technology changes as it is modified through day-to-day activity (cf. Orlikowski 1992).

---

effectiveness is that the same test may be used in different ways or for different purposes. This is compounded by less rigorous criteria for testing diagnostic innovations than new drugs. We return to the way evidence-based medicine and approaches to health technology assessment influence the adoption of innovations below, p. 179.

The 'outer context' for the innovation

While many healthcare innovations involve relatively simple, discrete products — the new type of scalpel — and a single decision-maker, this is often not the case. The innovation itself may require organisational change to ensure that it is embedded within healthcare processes or it may have a significant impact on healthcare organisations outside the adopting organisation. Implementation might involve multiple stakeholders from across the healthcare system, all of whose interests need to be aligned. Decision-making may be subject to complex regulations. The inner and outer contexts of the innovation do not exist in isolation — there is a dynamic relationship between them and the wider health system. Furthermore, this relationship may not behave in a predictable way. Successful and sustainable implementation is likely to require a degree of *compatibility* between the innovation and its wider context at both the organisational and wider care system levels. Compatibility was defined by Rogers (2003) as the 'degree to which an innovation is consistent with the existing values, past experiences and needs of a potential adopter.' A new electronic patient record system would therefore need to be seen by adopters as easy to integrate with existing methods, relatively straightforward to use, not overly demanding to learn, and so on.

Complexity, stakeholders, engagement

One way in which the relationship between the inner and outer context of a healthcare innovation manifests itself is through the range of stakeholders involved and complexity of the innovation. The nature of the innovation — whether it is radical or disruptive, for example — will also make a difference. Writing about the adoption and scaling-up of new types of healthcare intervention, Atun *et al.* (2010) argue that the level of complexity varies according to the number of elements involved — the extent of the technological, organisational and process changes, the range and type of stakeholders involved in adoption decisions, and how many stakeholders are impacted by the innovation; in short the compatibility of the innovation with the existing health system. Also important are its trialability and the observability of its impact, to use Everett Rogers' terms, especially the time taken for cause and effect to manifest themselves. The risks, costs and benefits associated with an innovation may not all be immediately apparent in the context in which it is being implemented, and may evolve over time. The organisations and individuals involved therefore need to find ways to cope with these changes as they arise. The learning process can be costly, both in financial terms and also for patients; in the early days of adoption procedures may be carried out on patients who do not need them and errors may occur, as in the case of laparoscopic cholecystectomy (Denis *et al.*, 2002).

Using a simple model, Rifat Atun and his colleagues group innovative health interventions according to their complexity along one dimension of the model, and various other characteristics (number of episodes of care, number of stakeholders, degree of user engagement) as another dimension (see Figures 5.1a and 5.1b). Vaccination for childhood illnesses, for example, might involve a new technology in a selected client group, administered by a health professional in a single episode of care. The impact of the innovation is therefore readily trialable and observable, its compatibility with the existing health system is probably apparent, along with the perceived benefits or any adverse effects. In contrast, a new integrated maternal and child health programme is considerably more complex, and is potentially much harder to introduce because it involves multiple interrelated and interdependent interventions, delivered over a period of time, and embraces a range of multidisciplinary health workers. Denis *et al.* (2002) suggest that the more the benefits and risks arising from an innovation are aligned with the distribution of interests, values and power of stakeholders in the adoption decision, the more likely a coalition for adoption can be created and the faster the adoption process.

Complexity can also be seen in terms of the number and nature of new technologies used and degree of user engagement needed to achieve improved outcomes. Some interventions comprise a single drug, administered once a year, possibly in a mass treatment programme. These are inherently less complex than interventions, such as an

> ➜ *We look at the implications of these points for implementing and scaling-up innovations later in the chapter*

HIV/AIDS programme, which involve multiple new technologies (e.g. diagnostic tools and new drugs), the introduction of new processes such as treatment guidelines, and different types of health worker (e.g. outreach workers, doctors, nurses, social workers), all engaging at different levels across the health system and with other sectors, such as education. Success of these interventions is likely to require strong stakeholder involvement and user engagement.

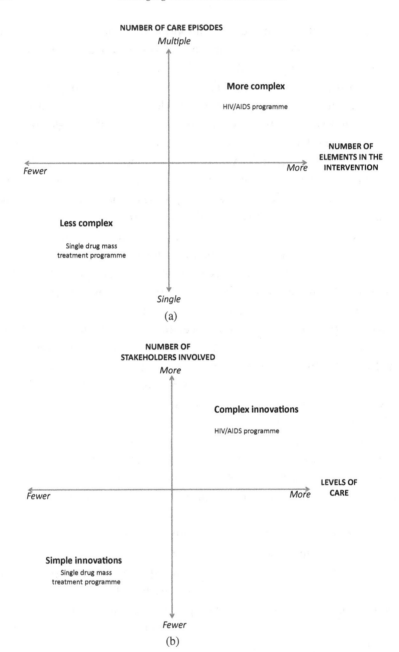

Figure 5.1. *(a) and (b) Understanding the complexity of care.*

Source: Based on Atun *et al.* (2010).

The greater the complexity of the innovation, the greater the likely need for it to be *adapted and modified* to ensure it is compatible with its wider context. Denis *et al.* (2002) show how complex innovations often consist of a 'hard core' of elements — prerequisites for the innovation to work and for successful adoption to take place — and a 'soft' periphery of elements which can be adapted to the local context (cf. Lewis and Seibold, 1993). As they describe it, the boundaries of some innovations are fluid and negotiable. In one example, the introduction of low molecular weight Heparin for deep vein thrombosis, ambiguity in methods of follow-up allowed various non-standard practices to emerge, which helped implementation of the innovation according to the organisation's mix of interests and impacts.

The existence of the soft periphery means, however, that the distribution of benefits and risks for adopters is not necessarily fixed or predictable; a given innovation may be implemented in a variety of ways not fully clarified in the trial stage. This has two implications. First, these types of innovation do not necessarily have a readily replicable adoption and implementation pathway. Second, the more uncertain

> ➔ *The case studies on remote care (5.1) and the Whole System Demonstrators programme (7.2, in Chapter 7) illustrate the problems of gathering evidence on complex innovations that is agreed by all parties.*

the definition of the innovation and ways it can be applied, the more scope there is for controversy over the evidence. Denis *et al.* (2002) discuss how the evidence for the different individual components of 'assertive community treatment' (ACT) for psychiatric patients was not theoretically or empirically clear. This meant there was disagreement over the relative importance of each one and whether or not reliable effects required implementation of the entire package.

Organisational characteristics and innovation adoption

In healthcare, we are more likely to be interested in corporate decisions than the decisions by individual users about the adoption of many types of innovation — whether or not a hospital decides to adopt a new, innovative scanner or whether it decides to embark on a series of radical changes to operational processes is likely to be decided at a corporate level.

Organisations in healthcare are complex entities, so their adoption of innovations is likely to be influenced not only by factors such as the number and nature of key stakeholders — who may have the possibility to veto decisions — and their goals and how powerful they are, but also organisational culture. This is closely associated with an organisation's attitudes towards creativity and the promotion of innovation, as well as its propensity and capabilities towards adoption. Typically, this is seen in terms of a climate conducive to experimentation and risk taking, the presence of staff in pivotal positions who can advocate for an innovation, clear strategic vision and strong leadership.

Glenn Robert and colleagues argue that an important factor which helps to explain why healthcare organisations adopt (or fail to adopt) innovations is their 'organisational antecedents' (Robert *et al.*, 2009). These are the size, maturity, resources, leadership, hierarchies, decision-making approaches and strategic priorities of the organisation, as well as its previous innovation capabilities and experience. Another factor they see as important is 'organisational readiness' to accept an innovation, influenced by many factors, including the pressure for change an organisation faces, the degree of 'fit' (i.e. 'compatibility') with the innovation and its implications, the capacity to evaluate its impact, the levels of support and advocacy that are present, and the availability of dedicated time and resources to support implementation.

The ability to absorb and apply knowledge from outside — an organisation's 'absorptive capacity' — is closely linked to the notion of 'innovation readiness' (Weiner, 2009) and in turn to discussions in healthcare about knowledge translation (Savory, 2009b), the process of turning research into applications for healthcare practice. In the UK, the National Health Service (NHS) has tried to encourage innovative culture within its organisations by putting in place mechanisms to support knowledge sharing across its organisations and capacity building for innovative behaviour.

➔*Approaches to knowledge sharing and capacity building in the NHS are discussed below*

Box 5.3   CONCEPTS: Questions for healthcare organisations seeking to be innovation ready

- What formal structures are needed to support effective decision-making by health professionals, patients and other stakeholders about adopting and assimilating innovations?
- How can organisations ensure they have sufficient absorptive capacity to allow the inward flow of knowledge and skills to support adoption processes?
- How can an organisational climate be created which is supportive of adoption and ensures that it is not inhibited by political, financial, managerial or informational factors?

For an example of a tool designed to help organisations benchmark their readiness for innovation, see the NHS Institute's 'spread and adoption tool' — http://www.institute.nhs.uk/index.php?option=com_spread_and_adoption

---

Healthcare organisations, therefore, face a series of challenges they need to address if they are to become effective in taking-up innovations from outside. Of course, many of the challenges described in Box 5.3 could be applied to any industry or organisation.

Evidence and innovation — too much, too little, too late?

Since the early 1990s, the introduction of evidence-based approaches to medicine and the design of health services has become an integral part of clinical governance, the mechanism for setting standards, improving quality and monitoring health services. The UK has a well-established system for assessing certain medical innovations — largely new drugs and some medical devices and therapies — through the National Institute for Health and Clinical Excellence (NICE) (see Box 5.4). As well as evidence-based medicine, the notion of evidence-based policy has also emerged, with governments seeking to test new policy ideas, including those in health

Box 5.4 BACKGROUND: Evaluating new health technology

Health technology assessment (HTA) is the established process for evaluating the effectiveness of new medical devices and drugs. It is a critical part of the translation of research into clinical practice because unlike the earlier stages of the innovation pathway described in Chapter 4, which are concerned with efficacy and safety, HTA focuses on the economic case for an innovation. It is closely linked to decisions about the business case for a new technology (Rogowski *et al.*, 2008). While its focus is on economics — the potential for cost minimisation, cost benefit, cost effectiveness and cost utility — HTA may also consider wider implications such as ethics or impact on procedures and processes.

Systems for HTA are now used in many countries, but it is argued that there is a lack of consistency between approaches, posing problems for the developers of new technologies (Hutton *et al.*, 2006; Neumann *et al.*, 2010). There is also concern about the application of HTA methodologies which were developed for the assessment of new drugs to a much broader range of technologies, with little or no modification. As well as the problem of assessing benefits such as 'quality of life', some technological innovations may have no direct outcomes affecting the patient because they support other interventions involved in their treatment. New diagnostic tests which make another process more efficient are an example (NICE, 2011).

The use of systematic reviews of the evidence for an innovation has formed an increasingly important element of HTA. While this may make sense in the context of new drugs, in situations where the innovation is less clear cut, what is being measured can vary from trial to trial and a diverse range of assessment approaches may have been employed, making comparison hard. This problem has bedevilled systematic reviews of the evidence for telehealth/ telecare, where one study found that although there were almost 9000 published studies, evidence for various forms of benefit remained unclear (Barlow *et al.*, 2007). Because of this, alternative methods of evaluation are increasingly used for many types of healthcare innovation, especially 'realistic evaluation', developed by Pawson and Tilley (1997) to assess policy interventions and public health initiatives. Here the concern is to identify not only the outcomes but also the factors that lead them to arise in specific contexts.

In the UK, health technology assessments carried out by the National Institute for Health and Clinical Excellence (NICE) are used to provide national

(Continued)

Box 5.4 (*Continued*)

guidance on technology purchasing. The NHS is legally obliged to fund medicines and treatments recommended by NICE. Although the quality and rigour of health technology assessments from NICE are widely praised, only a limited number of innovations are selected for assessment. This means that adoption decisions about new technologies not assessed by NICE are left to local health service organisations, which can result in geographical differences in their availability. Another concern is that NICE economic evaluations are too narrow and do not consider the wider benefits of an innovation to society.

There are now some moves towards the use of wider cost-effectiveness measures in decisions about the adoption of novel or orphan drugs. This can be seen as part of a broader agenda on value-based pricing, where the notion of 'value' considers a range of societal factors, along with the health and quality of life gains for individual patients that form the basis of conventional approaches. Value-based pricing is essentially a method of pricing new medical technologies according to perceived benefits to the patients and the wider society (Persson *et al.*, 2010). It combines the use of wider cost-effectiveness measures with performance-based reimbursement strategies, where development risk of new drugs is shared (discussed later in this chapter, p. 216). The cost-effectiveness measures include the value of lost production, and cost savings to healthcare and other services. By placing a premium on factors that would be ignored under conventional evaluations, adoption may be speeded up. Sweden has used a value-based pricing model with wider cost-effectiveness measures since 2002 (Sussex *et al.*, 2013). There is evidence that this has helped to encourage the development and adoption of innovative drugs, although this may also result from Sweden's use of a 'coverage with evidence development' scheme (Persson, 2012). Italy also uses a value-based pricing approach, in combination with use of wider cost effectiveness measures (Adamski *et al.*, 2010), see p. 217.

and social care, before they are implemented (Walshe and Rundall, 2001; Black, 2001).

Some have suggested these moves represent a shift towards a more scientific and bureaucratic approach to medicine, combining medical knowledge derived from research with standardised rule-based protocols (Harrison, 2002). How far this has actually affected the behaviour of clinicians is an open question. Greenhalgh *et al.* (2004a, 2004b) suggest that in the real world of healthcare, the application of evidence-based medicine is in practice more nuanced than implied by its philosophy — it is applied within a local context with local actors, and this influences the way guidelines about recommended new practices or innovations are adopted. It is clear, however, that 'evidence' is a very important shaper of the adoption and spread of innovation in healthcare. We have touched on this throughout the book so far. Why is evidence so important? The answer relates partly to the way adoption decisions are made in healthcare organisations and partly to the methods used for evaluating innovations.

Adoption decisions in healthcare often involve a range of stakeholders. The evidence used to support the decision needs to be both *sufficient* and *relevant* to all parties. This raises important questions about the basis of that evidence — how is it interpreted and by whom, and how much agreement is there about its epistemological basis? The evidence base for an innovation may need to engage and persuade stakeholders from widely across the care system, including GPs, hospital consultants, nurses and social care workers. All these may have different expectations about what constitutes convincing evidence for an innovation (as well as what constitutes the innovation itself).

At one end of the spectrum, a strictly evidence-based decision-making view of

"(Information needs to be presented) in a format that is easily understood and statistically valid, which appeals to doctors."
(Rogers *et al.*, 2004)

"Saying that clinicians are much more interested in innovation if you show them clinical evidence (is not enough) ... They will think it is a good idea, not that it needs to be adopted."
(Technology supplier, quoted in Barlow *et al.*, 2012)

"There'll be some groups which will be very strong supporters (of an innovation) based on the evidence, others who will just not be. I think it's going to be a mixed bag ... GPs typically have three reactions — enthusiast, sceptics and indifferent."
(Health service manager, quoted in Barlow *et al.*, 2012)

"At the Mayo Clinic, they're very conservative. I adopted it because the Mayo Clinic was doing it ... for me, it's not a scientific article that would get me to change my practice, it's when I hear that another institution in which I have confidence has adopted it. We're a small hospital here — this isn't the place to innovate."
(Denis *et al.*, 2002)

the world would essentially regard adopters as a unified set of rational actors; evidence of clinical and/or cost-effectiveness forms a key part of a single calculated decision whether to adopt an innovation (Denis *et al.*, 2002). Evidence-based decision models generally assume that an innovation is well defined. It can be delineated and its attributes specified in such a way that a randomised controlled trial (RCT), or some other type of formal evaluation, can be conducted and useful data collected. This is then a powerful influence on the decision to adopt, and it is assumed that the innovation will be adopted 'as is', i.e. with no changes to the intervention that was evaluated. In other words, the presence of benefits evidence leads to two alternative states — adoption and non-adoption, or before and after the decision.

But the reality in healthcare is rarely, if ever, like this. The fluid and negotiable boundaries of many innovations, the fact that different actors may imbue a given technology or innovation with differing meanings, the uneven distribution of benefits and risks across the health and social care system adopting the innovation, and

> ➔ *We explore the implications of complexity theory and systems thinking on the implementation of healthcare innovations in Chapter 7*

the idea that innovations and their wider context evolve over time all ensure that adoption isn't necessarily a one-off, all or nothing, event but more like a complex adaptive process.

Implementation and 'normalisation' are not the same as adoption

There is a growing literature on the *implementation* of healthcare innovation and evidence-based practice, including the emergence of 'implementation science', which seeks to understand methods to promote the integration of research findings and evidence into healthcare policy and practice. Implementing and subsequently absorbing a healthcare innovation into everyday practice is seen as a distinct stage of the adoption process. The end point for successful implementation is the integration of an innovation into everyday practice, described by Mair *et al.* (2009) and May *et al.* (2007) as the point when it is 'normalised' (see Box 5.5). This

Box 5.5   CONCEPTS: Normalisation process theory

Normalisation process theory (NPT) is closely associated with the work of Carl May and Tracy Finch (May *et al.*, 2007; May and Finch, 2009; Mair *et al.*, 2009). As described by the Normalisation Process Theory On-line Users' Manual and Toolkit:

'NPT is a sociological toolkit that we can use to understand the dynamics of implementing, embedding, and integrating some new technology or complex intervention. It helps us disassemble the human processes that are at work when we encounter a new set of practices ...' (May *et al.*, 2010).

The theory focuses on the nature of work involved in implementing, embedding and sustaining new practices in particular organisational and social settings. It asks questions about the factors that promote or inhibit these processes and how they can be understood and explained. Normalisation process theory is, therefore, an 'action theory', concerned with explaining what people do to enact a new healthcare intervention, practice or technology, rather than simply their attitudes or beliefs about it. The practices involved in enacting innovations are shaped by four core constructs:

- coherence (how people understand the qualities of the innovation),
- cognitive participation (the work involved in building and sustaining a community of practice around it),
- collective action (the operational work that people do to put in place the innovation) and
- reflexive monitoring (what people do to assess and understand the ways it affects them and others around them).

Normalisation process theory overlaps with the extensive literature on socio-technical systems (STS). Both are concerned with how innovation is produced and stabilised over time in ways that depend on its compatibility with the values and cultural norms of its context, both focus on the practices of users involved in adopting an innovation, and both argue that a technology can have diverse meanings for different people. The differences lie in the perspectives of NPT and the STS literature on predictability — NPT suggests that the trajectory of an innovation can be anticipated within certain limits, assuming we know enough about it and the context for its implementation; STS takes a more contingent view, emphasising the heterogeneity of circumstances and the emergence of processes.

is when the innovation is embedded in everyday work practices and operational processes, and this is sustained. But before this happens, the implementation journey can be slow and hard. Once the decision to adopt has been made — perhaps following a decision to proceed after a successful trial — implementing it may be neither straightforward nor instantaneous. Even when there is senior healthcare management commitment to adopt and implement an innovation — with clear lines of responsibility and accountability, provision of training where needed, good communication between organisational stakeholders, and user-participation (Karsh, 2004) — normalisation can be tortuous. This is a problem both

> ➔ *Scaling-up healthcare innovations is discussed later in this chapter*

in developed countries and in health systems in resource-poor countries, where there is a long history of failed projects to scale-up new healthcare interventions, practices or other innovations, as we discuss below, p. 194.

How formal the approach to implementation needs to be will vary according to factors such as the level of risk associated with implementation, including potential costs, the strength of an innovation's evidence base, and its scale and scope — in short, an innovation's complexity and its consequences for the adopting healthcare organisation or system. Some innovative technologies can be put into service as soon as they have been acquired; others may require an extensive programme of piloting and phased introduction, with implementation treated as a formal process drawing on project management skills and methods. There may also be an overlap between the *development* of an innovation and its *implementation* into practice, where users such as clinicians are also the creators of an innovation. The boundaries can be blurred, for example, when implementation is closely linked to experimentation, prototyping, trialling and incremental improvement of the innovation, all of which take

> ➔ *Chapter 4 explores the role of clinicians as developers of healthcare innovations*

place in the same location, such as a hospital. The development of innovations in hip replacement and intraocular lenses are well-known examples (Metcalfe and Pickston, 2006).

For complex innovations, which comprise many elements or have ramifications for healthcare practices and processes involving multiple stakeholders, healthcare organisations may be more favourably disposed towards innovations that can be piloted or introduced on a trial basis. This helps to reduce the risk and increase the visibility of an innovation's impact, both to local stakeholders who will be affected by it and more generally by contributing to its evidence base. Trials and pilot projects can also provide useful lessons for the best ways of implementing and scaling-up the innovation, and how to integrate it into existing services.

But despite their usefulness, trials and pilot projects often fail to provide good evidence about the likely impact of an innovation once it has become part of mainstream practice. This is because resources — people and funding — are often poured into them; those involved tend to be highly invested in the project and optimistic about its success, not necessarily a good predictor of what happens in the real world (Bate and Robert, 2003; Sanderson, 2002; Maguerez *et al.*, 2001). Small-scale pilot projects therefore have limited usefulness when developing lessons for scaling-up services; issues resolved in pilot projects often fail to translate when attempting to implement the innovation in the real world.

Pilot projects can also become 'closed' to outsiders, such that project teams are unwilling to let go of 'their' project and handover to others. In this way, the creation of small pockets of activity through pilot projects can be divisive, even in areas where there is a tradition of collaboration across different parts of the health and social care systems (Hendy and Barlow, 2012). Hendy and Barlow found that in one example of a telehealth implementation project, rather than being seen as working for the good of the organisation its staff began to be seen by others as working for themselves. Pilot projects, therefore, need to be set up in a way which ensures they can be readily integrated into mainstream health services, providing they are successful in meeting their objectives.

Another problem is that fragmented healthcare systems, coupled with local autonomy, can lead to repeated pilot projects on the same innovation being carried out, yet despite this replication, their findings may never see the light of day. Others are too small or too short-term to deliver *"Pride can also prevent adoption of innovation — 'not invented here' is ... rife in the artificial kingdoms created in the NHS."* (Barratt, 2014) rigorous data on outcomes. Worse, carrying out trials and pilot projects may itself act as a barrier to adoption because they can hold up the mainstream implementation of an innovation. This occurred in the UK with the Whole System Demonstrator programme for telehealth and telecare which included the world's largest RCT of this

> ➔*The Whole System Demonstrator programme is also discussed in the case study in Chapter 7*

type of innovation. It is thought that many NHS trusts and local social services authorities delayed implementing the technology more widely until the research was finished and published, although others believed that the evidence base was sufficiently robust to allow them to move forwards and went ahead anyway (see below, p. 188).

The UK's recent history of 'remote care' — telecare or telehealth — provides lessons on how government policy, evidence gathering and innovation complexity are intertwined, with sometimes unexpected outcomes. There are different variants of remote care, but essentially it involves the use of vital signs or movement sensors to provide an 'electronic security blanket' around patients who are frail and elderly or have a long term health condition. The aim is both preventative (identifying changes in a person's condition and keeping them out of expensive hospital care) and reactive (responding in the event of a crisis).

The UK has been especially prominent in both developing remote care technologies and attempting to bring them into mainstream health and social care practice. In the 1970s and 1980s, it had the world's largest network of 'social alarms', basic fall detectors for elderly people. Since the late 1990s, many UK government reports have emphasised its role in coping with an ageing population and funding has been made available for pump priming its implementation. But both in the UK and elsewhere, the adoption of remote care for elderly people has been much slower than predicted 20 years ago.

The 'Columba project' in the early 2000s was an early example of an attempt to trial and then implement remote care (see Case study 5.1). This shows how stakeholders from across the care system needed to learn and adapt the innovation both during the planning stages and during implementation. The project provided useful lessons on the challenges of designing and implementing remote care in the messy, real world of health and social care services. After many similar trials, attention in the UK began to shift towards the need for gather robust evidence for the benefits of remote care. In 2006, this led the government to fund the largest ever

RCT of remote care, the 'Whole System Demonstrators' (WSD) programme. One of its lessons — apart from useful findings on the impact of the innovation — is that using an RCT for evaluating this type of innovation has a downside. Whilst evidence on the impact and implementation challenges was gathered, the time taken for the trial to be rolled out and evaluated held back investment decisions, as local authorities and health trusts waited for the full evidence to become available (Barlow *et al.*, 2012; Chrysanthaki *et al.*, 2013).

Another lesson of the WSD story is on evidence-based policy making (see above, p. 179), especially the way governments can take limited evidence and make a decision about implementing a new policy or innovation. Box 5.6 shows how early headline findings were reinterpreted by

---

Box 5.6   BACKGROUND: The Whole System Demonstrators programme and evidence-based policy making

Source: With thanks to Stefanie Ettelt and Nicholas Mays (Ettelt *et al.*, 2015).

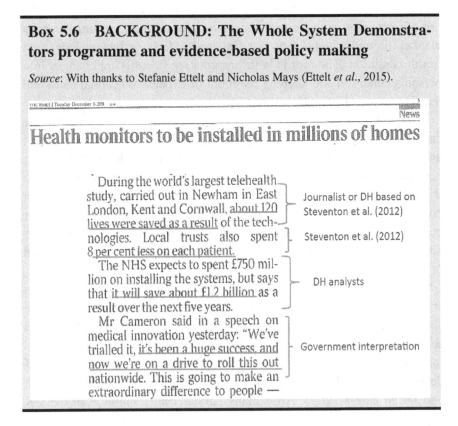

mainstream media and Department of Health analysts, prior to the Prime Minister announcing the launch of a programme to roll out the technology to three million people. This has not, however, been delivered. One of the problems is the perception of health and social care commissioners — responsible for investing in remote care — that evidence base remains ambiguous, despite the WSD programme and numerous other trials.

The story of the WSD shows how hard it is to get the balance right between creating sufficiently robust evidence for the impact of an innovation that is satisfactory to all its stakeholders, but not holding back mainstream implementation or stifling experimentation. For complex innovations, even when there have been many trials, variety in the local context for implementation can mean the evidence may still be ambiguous — findings from a small trial in one area do not automatically tell us what will happen in another or across the wider health system level if the innovation is deployed at scale.

➜ *We discuss the question of piloting innovations and modelling their effects in Chapter 7*

CASE STUDY 5.1 The Columba project to provide intermediate care and telecare in north west Surrey, UK

As a concept, Columba was relatively straightforward. Frail elderly people who had been admitted into hospital and who might otherwise have been discharged straight into residential care would be supported in their own home by a new package of care services, including telecare. By using telecare, the risks associated with independent living would be reduced. The project mixed short-term intensive residential rehabilitation (the service element of the innovation) with telecare (the technology element). The rehabilitation component was to be delivered in a residential care home, where an independent four-bed rehabilitation unit would be built. This was designed to replicate home conditions and familiarise the elderly users with the same telecare systems to be installed in their own homes.

(Continued)

CASE STUDY 5.1   (*Continued*)

Background

When it was first mooted in 1999, there was a considerable R&D activity on 'smart homes' technologies. Companies around the world were developing electronic devices to help control the functions of homes, such as heating, lighting and audio-visual entertainment. Prototype smart homes and demonstration projects had been set up in many countries. As well as creating products for the high end of the domestic market, attention was also being paid to the needs of highly disabled and elderly people. It was argued that if their homes could be made more readily usable, they could achieve greater independence and avoid having to move to institutional care. At the same time, it had become clear that in the UK, the extensive network of social alarms (fall detectors) and local monitoring centres, could be used as a basis for a more advanced telecare network. Around a quarter of the entire global user population of social alarms was said to be in the UK — over 1.5 million people — so the potential to use this to leverage telecare into the social and healthcare systems was evident.

Project objectives and partners

Columba's objective was to reduce the need for residential home admissions by frail elderly people and help tackle the problem of delayed discharges from hospital. It played into a narrative in health and social care policy and practice about the importance of providing people with greater choice over care options and increased independence in their homes. It was also partly motivated by the local social services' objective of reducing the number of residential care beds in the area by 25%. Initial estimates suggested that of the 100 frail elderly people discharged each year from the local acute hospital to a social services-funded residential home, about a quarter would be suitable for the Columba care package.

The project's core partners were the *customer* (the local NHS acute hospital trust), the *suppliers* of telecare and related services (the local community hospital, the social alarm monitoring centre and the equipment manufacturer), and the *funders* (the local social services authority and two NHS primary care trusts).

Project development

In December 1999, a group of senior clinical and social service staff met to discuss the development of older people's services in the local area. Several

(*Continued*)

CASE STUDY 5.1 (*Continued*)

members had knowledge of telecare and formed a project steering group to consider how it might be used. This led to a project proposal in October 2000 to use some local health authority funds, which were available for stimulating the development of remote care. A project manager was appointed in February 2001, and an early task involved bringing together local care teams. As the project manager put it, 'reluctant consent' for Columba had been achieved by summer 2001. The concerns were largely about additional workload and cost.

By October 2001, a revised project plan had been agreed. This proposed recruitment of the first patients by September 2002. Some of the intervening time would involve creating the four-bed rehabilitation unit in the existing residential care home. During the first half of 2002, the service specification and care processes for Columba were created. However, what became clear during this period was that a much larger range of different stakeholders from across the local care system needed to be brought on board to ensure Columba was implemented. A large number of individuals and groups within the core partners had to be engaged in order to develop the service model and ensure it was implemented. These included hospital discharge co-ordinators and care managers, members of the occupational therapy teams from social services and primary care, the managers of the local residential care home, the intermediate care and 'home from hospital' teams, and the community social care team. Representatives of service users, their families and informal carers were also involved. All these became involved in the design of the project on a sequential basis, as it became clear there were gaps in the Columba core team's knowledge about the detail of care pathways for elderly people. This slowed the pace of development.

There were also delays in sanctioning expenditure for upgrading the social alarm system to accommodate telecare sensors. Another problem was that this phase in Columba's development coincided with a major national restructuring of health and social care services, which made it hard to engage stakeholders, who had other concerns. The project manager then left the team in July 2002. Further delays occurred during the autumn when workshops for operational staff were organised. Columba was eventually launched some four months late. However, there were severe problems in identifying and recruiting appropriate patients for the scheme. While these were partly overcome by establishing a dedicated coordinator role to work across the boundaries in the local care system, it took much of 2003 to build local awareness of Columba.

(*Continued*)

CASE STUDY 5.1   (*Continued*)

By April 2004, only 22 people had been through the scheme (after this pilot stage, the project was closed).

The innovation lessons from Columba

The Columba project was developed in the early days of telecare, and there was little experience and knowledge for its protagonist to go on. It did, however, provide useful lessons that showed how designing and operating a complex innovation — involving a hybrid of technological innovation, organisational change and new service delivery models — can be much harder than initially envisaged, not necessarily because of technical problems. Columba demonstrates the way an innovation with seemingly straightforward objectives and using relatively simple technology is heavily influenced by the interactions between the innovation, the local actors involved and the wider context.

Columba was designed from the outset to allow for scaling-up and 'normalisation'. This would be achieved through future organic expansion, after collection of positive evidence from a small-scale trial. However, it was not possible to move to full-scale implementation. This was for several reasons:

- The **organisational and operational complexity** of integrating remote care into the existing care system was poorly understood at the project's inception. What appeared to be a relatively simple concept — adding simple telecare technology to the existing processes for discharging elderly patients from hospital — in fact had a series of unforeseen implications for the roles and responsibilities of the health and social care authorities, and for the distribution of costs and benefits between them.
- As knowledge about the local implications of remote care became clearer during the planning stages, an **increasing range and number of stakeholders** needed to be involved in the project, beyond the initial partners. This led to severe delays in the development and implementation of the trial.
- The project manager, who was based within the primary care organisation, did not have authority across stakeholders from other services — there were many points in the planning and decision-making chain where **others could veto decisions.**
- It became clear as the trial progressed that stakeholders from primary, acute and social care services held **different perceptions of risk** and

(*Continued*)

CASE STUDY 5.1 *(Continued)*

what they saw as convincing evidence for the benefits. This not only meant that some were more sceptical about the project, and hence less engaged, but it also damaged the potential to scale-up the project on completion of the trial.

Problems were also caused by the **fast moving external context** for the Columba project. Local and national health policy priorities and targets were evolving. As the project developed, pressure grew to free hospital beds 'blocked' by elderly patients unable to return home. The overall goal of Columba therefore shifted from one which aimed to enable elderly people to remain generally independent towards one more narrowly designed to address 'bed blocking'. Consequently, the target population changed towards older and frailer patients. This meant that referrals into the scheme were inappropriate for the existing technology and its abilities — they were too old and frail. The change in type of patients not only affected health and social care stakeholders' views of the risks associated with the technology, but changes to the patient population also meant that the evidence collected in the trial on costs and benefits was ambiguous. Modelling work suggested that the timescales over which any financial, clinical or quality of life benefit might be delivered were unclear, making it hard to justify decisions to scale-up the scheme, which was eventually abandoned.

Questions for discussion:

- What type of innovation would you class Columba and why? Refer back to Chapter 2.
- Identify the main barriers to adoption and suggest ways to overcome them from the perspectives of the different stakeholders involved in planning and implementing Columba.
- What strategies might the partners have used to improve the process of implementing the Columba project, and helping to scale it up?

Source: Draws partly on Barlow *et al.* (2006).

Simulation and modelling can help here because it helps us to explore the effectiveness of interventions in this type of situation and improve the basis for decision-making (Barlow and Bayer, 2011).

Scaling-up

'Scaling-up' is a related concept to implementation and normalisation, more rooted in the literature on global health innovation and public health interventions in resource-poor settings. The concept has become the dominant way of understanding pathways for transforming health services in developing countries (Bloom and Ainsworth, 2010). Various frameworks and practical guidance tools for scaling-up have been published and there is a growing literature on the constraints and opportunities associated with it. There is, however, no clear consensus on the operational meaning of the term in healthcare; broadly it can be divided into:

- The agendas of large global non-governmental organisations and other organisations seeking to 'go to scale' through top-down technical activities.
- The process of transforming demonstrably successful small-scale pilot projects or trials into larger programmes.
- Use of grassroots mobilisation, empowerment and collective action to take an intervention to scale.

In the first of these narratives, scaling-up essential refers to 'doing more in a big way', increasing the coverage of externally validated, standardised health interventions or increasing the resources required to expand coverage. Scaling-up is essentially conceived as a technical exercise following a linear trajectory from initial trial to design, implementation plan and their implementation. This requires putting in place the right local conditions and ensuring that the innovation is standardised as much as possible. The approach has been much criticised for imposing a blueprint model that focuses on reproducing interventions with total fidelity to the plan and failing to address the complexities and uncertainties of the local context (Glasgow and Emmons, 2007; Kaplan *et al.*, 2011; USAID, 2010; IHI, 2010).

The second and third narratives are related to the earlier points above about normalisation and implementation, and emphasise scaling-up from trials or pilots to mainstream interventions or programmes. This work has developed partly in response to criticisms of blueprint approaches and the many failures of pilots and trials to grow to scale. Problems that may hamper efforts to scale-up include cost, the institutional setting, differences in values or poor relationships between stakeholders, and a lack of understanding and adaptation to local context. Because of the focus on process, this body of research stresses the importance of context, as well as social and political considerations. Like other research on the implementation of innovation, there is much emphasis on the need to adapt to local realities, preserving the benefits, goals and standards of an intervention, but at the same time ensuring that it is relevant and culturally appropriate to users. Adaptive strategies and learning

> ➔ *We discuss the role of complexity theory in the creation and implementation of healthcare innovations in Chapter 7*

approaches are seen as important, echoing the points made by Denis *et al.* (2002) on the hard core/soft periphery of healthcare innovations, along with close participation of stakeholders to encourage ownership of the initiative.

Writing about two cases of successful scale-up and spread, Lanham *et al.* (2012) draw on lessons from complexity science about self-organisation, the process by which interactions between actors in a system result in the emergence of new patterns of organisation. Briefly, complex systems are characterised by a degree of uncertainty that cannot be reduced by better information, and by nonlinearity in the way the impact of change plays out, so patterns of organisation are unpredictable. This poses challenges for the scale-up of innovative healthcare interventions, which may display trajectories that are difficult to control. Lanham *et al.* argue that designs for scaling-up innovative interventions that rely heavily on the dissemination of information and knowledge amongst stakeholders may be ineffective, and more sensitivity to the interdependencies within a system and capacity among stakeholders for sensemaking — how they understand others' perceptions of the system and its interdependencies — is needed (Box 5.7).

Box 5.7   CONCEPTS: Key features of a complexity science informed scale-up and spread effort

Acknowledge unpredictability

Design

- Allow design to be tailored to local contexts.
- Emphasise discovery in each intervention setting.
- Design for multiple plausible futures.

Implementation

- Encourage stakeholders involved in scale-up and spread to conceptualise surprises as opportunities.
- Encourage them to collectively learn and adapt during interventions.

Recognise self-organisation

Design

- Develop 'good enough' scale-up and spread designs with the expectation that the design will be modified as initial plans are implemented and experience is gained.
- Use focus groups to solicit input into intervention design and implementation.
- Conduct pilot studies to observe local patterns of organising.

Implementation

- Be attentive to existing and developing interdependencies in scale-up and spread settings.
- Facilitate sensemaking.

Facilitate interdependencies

Design

- Acknowledge interdependencies as critical to scale-up and spread success.
- Develop methods to assess the quality and strength of interdependencies.

Implementation

- Reinforce existing relationships when effective.
- Foster new relationships where needed.

(Continued)

Box 5.7 (*Continued*)

Encourage sensemaking

Design

- Encourage focused experimentation.

Implementation

- Encourage participants to ask questions, admit ignorance and deal with paradox.
- Seek out different points of view.
- Provide abundant opportunities for reflection and conversation.

Source: Lanham *et al.* (2012).

Innovation adoption from the perspective of health technology suppliers

What does all this look like from the perspective of the suppliers of technology? Joe Tidd and John Bessant (2014) argue that conventional marketing approaches may use the language of innovation — referring to 'early adopters' and 'majority adopters' for example — and this may be adequate for understanding how to promote many products and services to potential users. However, it does not adequately describe the process by which many innovations are taken-up. Studies from marketing which investigate the factors which affect the success of new products have differed in emphasis, but there is broad consensus about the best criteria for success. These include factors similar to those identified by Everett Rogers: clear product definition and product advantage in the eyes of the customer, and supply-side factors such as assessment of development risks, market and knowledge of user needs, project organisation and resources, proficiency of execution, top management support and presence of champions.

The pre-diffusion phase can be critical but costly for companies selling innovative products. Large-scale diffusion may be preceded by long periods of trial-and-error experimentation. From a management perspective, this is risky. Many companies

> ➔*Chapter 2 discusses the role of lead users in the new product development process and Geoffey Moore's adoption and diffusion 'chasm'*

involved in the creation of new products or services fail before they diffuse widely, a fact of life for small start-up companies. The 'chasms' in
the diffusion process, noted by Moore (1991), reflect this and demonstrate
the importance of a suitable market introduction strategy. This includes
identifying the best potential customers or 'lead users', who can show the
way to subsequent customers. As Tidd and Bessant (2014) put it, introducing a new product is usually a matter of deep pockets and long breath.

Perhaps nowhere is this more the case
than in healthcare. Selling to healthcare
providers such as hospitals or health authorities can be hard, especially when a complex innovative product is involved. Firms
face a host of challenges: a fragmented and
complicated procurement process with
diverse purchasing organisations ranging in
size and experience, a tendency for health-

> ➜ *See the Peezy*
> *Midstream case study in*
> *Chapter 4 for the*
> *difficulties faced by a*
> *small start-up bringing an*
> *innovative product to*
> *market*

care organisations to focus on 'lowest cost' rather than 'best value'
when weighing up the benefits of an innovation, and — in the case of

---

INNOVATION IN ACTION 5.3: **The introduction of remote
care into the UK from the suppliers' perspective**

To ensure an innovative product is successfully and widely adopted, technology suppliers need to provide a business case in terms relevant to an NHS
purchaser from a hospital or other provider organisation. Equally, NHS purchasers need to be clear about their needs and provide suppliers with the right
kind of information. But this idealised picture often fails to be matched by the
reality in the NHS because:

- The devolved nature of the NHS means that companies selling new technologies often face a fragmented market. Individual NHS organisations
  have considerable freedom to determine their own approaches and
  requirements against which they assess technology business cases.
  A business case for a particular technology may satisfy the requirements

(Continued)

INNOVATION IN ACTION 5.3   (*Continued*)

of one NHS trust, but not another. This is confusing for suppliers, who often receive little guidance on how best to meet the requirements.

- To be able to make a clear case for investment, health authorities need information about outcomes, value for money and the impact on patient experience, but they generally lack the skills and resources to identify and compare different options. On the other hand, companies wishing to sell technological innovations, especially those producing new medical devices, are often small and also lack the skills and resources to do the necessary economic modeling.

The example of remote care (telehealth/telecare) illustrates this well. Despite a long history of technology development and the existence since the 1970s of a basic infrastructure in the form of 'community alarms' — pendants and fall detectors for elderly people — companies in the remote care industry have complained it is hard to make headway within the UK. The 'pre-diffusion phase', described by Tidd and Bessant (2014) has been long and hard.

By the time of the government-funded 'Whole System Demonstrators' programme (see main text), designed to gather the evidence required to stimulate adoption through the world's largest randomised control trial on remote care technology, many suppliers felt that the market was trapped in a vicious circle. Uncertainty about demand led to an unwillingness by the NHS to commit to investment; this meant that suppliers were not keen to invest in further development of their products.

Suppliers were particularly concerned about the fragmentation of the procurement process in the NHS, which they felt made it difficult for them to negotiate and deliver substantial projects. Fragmentation on the demand side meant that health and social care providers did not have strong enough market muscle. Suppliers also felt that NHS organisations generally did not have the organisational capabilities and capacity to act as 'smart purchasers', with a clear understanding of their own needs and consistent approaches for procuring new technology. Maintaining collaborative relationships with purchasers within a fragmented NHS was seen as costly and unrewarding.

But there were also problems on the supply side. First, NHS purchasers were concerned about the immaturity of remote care products; from their point of view the market looked complex and unstable, with a danger of 'technology

(*Continued*)

INNOVATION IN ACTION 5.3   *(Continued)*

lock in' due to equipment interoperability issues. Second, the remote care supply industry was relatively small-scale and fragmented. In 2009, the industry
comprised some 47 companies generating more than GBP 550 million in sales.
The turnover of the UK's largest remote care supplier was only GBP 190m.
No single player had all the capabilities to provide an integrated remote care
service, so partnerships were needed to bring solutions to market, yet it was
hard for firms to identify suitable partners and business models — how the
various components of the remote care value chain fit together and how value
is created and delivered. This related to the ambiguous evidence for the economic benefits of remote care, which made it hard to pin down precisely where
the costs and benefits lay. The difficulties in identifying precisely what savings
arose from remote care — translating reduced numbers of bed days in hospital
or emergency admissions into real savings, bankable by a hospital or primary
care organisation for example — made it hard for companies producing the
technology to accurately price their products. What is the value of a remote
care system to a social services department or hospital or GP over time? How
much should be charged for the product or service?

Source: Barlow *et al.* (2012).

innovations that impact across different parts of the health system —
problems resulting from costs and benefits falling across different budgetary silos. Compared to the pharmaceutical industry, where the process for
introducing of new drugs is at least more structured and regulated, medical device companies face a landscape in many health systems that can be
hard to navigate, with rather unattractive market opportunities (see
Innovation in Action 5.3). A common complaint is that the cost of sales is
too high, deterring smaller suppliers.

Supporting adoption and spread

Implementing evidence-based practice — whether innovative or not —
in a timely and efficient manner has long challenged governments,
healthcare providers, clinicians and technology suppliers. The lag between
research being conducted and it being taken up and used can be

BOX 5.8   BACKGROUND: Research translation gaps in healthcare

The Cooksey review of innovation in the UK's NHS (Cooksey, 2006) identified the presence of two significant gaps in the translation of health research into NHS practice: translating ideas from basic and clinical research into the development of new products and approaches (the first translation gap), and implementing new products and approaches into clinical practice (the second translation gap). The review found that the funding arrangements for supporting research translation were insufficiently coherent and comprehensive, and did not function well. It identified a range of issues relating to the culture and economics of the NHS that limit research translation, including a conservative approach to new ideas and technologies, lack of standard procurement routes for new technologies, especially those developed by smaller medical technology companies, and a tendency by managers to see innovation primarily as a pressure on costs, without looking at its potential for longer term efficiency gains.

substantial. Some have estimated that the time between new knowledge being discovered until half the population of physicians acts on it is around 15–17 years (Balas and Boren, 2000). This has been called the 'second translational gap' (Cooksey, 2006), the barriers to implementing new products and approaches in healthcare practice. Improving the capability of healthcare organisations to absorb, recreate and make use of knowledge associated with technological and other innovations is therefore the goal (Davis *et al.*, 2003; Savory, 2009b; Savory and Fortune, 2013). Behind this is a concern that the absorptive capacity of healthcare providers to adopt new innovations and practices is limited by a lack of the right quality and quantity of evidence, and the skills and resources needed to interpret it.

Two factors are important here. First, as Maynard (2007) describes it, the *supply* of evidence may be corrupted by poor quality science or weak peer review, and by consultancy firms, patient lobbies and other, not necessarily disinterested, experts. Second, even if the production and quality of evidence is improved, there are problems on the *demand* side for research. Clinicians, politicians, policymakers and other stakeholders are limited in their capacity to evaluate evidence, and the political imperative for swift action can override more careful consideration of objectives, design of evidence-based interventions, piloting and evaluation, and then implementation (or not). A range of other demand-side barriers also prevent healthcare providers from making use of research findings (Savory and Fortune, 2013):

- The values, skills and awareness of research users such as doctors, nurses and managers needed to understand and evaluate research.
- How open the research users and other stakeholders in the organisation are to innovation, and how much power they have to implement it.
- The quality of research that underpins specific innovations and how effectively this is communicated.

In short, how well equipped is the research user to make sense of the innovation and how good is the research evidence for it?

Knowledge management, knowledge mobilisation or knowledge translation?

Efforts are underway in some health systems to find better ways of tackling these demand-side problems. These draw heavily on the interest within mainstream management research in 'knowledge management' (Lavis *et al.*, 2003; Williams and Dickinson, 2010). There are several definitions and other terms are also used such as *knowledge transfer, knowledge translation* and *knowledge mobilisation*. Broadly, the overall concept is about the environment that can best support the creation, sharing and use of knowledge within an organisation

"... a dynamic and iterative process that includes synthesis, dissemination, exchange and ethically sound application of knowledge to improve the health of Canadians, provide more effective health services and products and strengthen the health care system." (CIHR, 2015)

(Turner *et al.*, 2002). A commonly used definition in healthcare is that of the Canadian Institutes of Health Research (CIHR, 2015).

The premise behind 'knowledge translation' is that it is important to improve the ability of healthcare staff and their organisations to make use of new knowledge. The assumption is that knowledge can be translated or exchanged (Berwick, 2002) and that translation can be managed. In reality, knowledge translation is rarely — if ever — a rational and linear process. Many have argued that knowledge is not simply assimilated. Rather it is interpreted within a specific context, shaped by interaction between different parties and the way they negotiate a shared meaning for that knowledge (Greenhalgh *et al.*, 2004a, 2004b). Turning evidence into practice is thus seen not in terms of an individual's response to a specific piece of research or a specific innovation but in terms of the interplay between many factors, including the people involved and the context. In practice, therefore, knowledge translation may be a contested process in which individuals negotiate around the ambiguity of a piece of evidence, reach consensus and act accordingly (Williams, 2007). Partly for this reason, some researchers prefer to use the term 'knowledge mobilisation' in order to convey a broader, looser perspective which does not convey implicit assumptions of 'management' and linearity (Crilly *et al.*, 2013).

The diverse perspectives and variety of situations within healthcare in which knowledge mobilisation (or knowledge translation) take place mean that there is no recommended 'one size fits all' approach (Grimshaw *et al.*, 2004; Haines *et al.*, 2004). But there are mechanisms which can help strengthen the mobilisation and absorption of knowledge. We know that knowledge often 'sticks' at the professional and organisational boundaries within healthcare systems (Ferlie *et al.*, 2010). Research demonstrates that 'boundary bridging' mechanisms in the form of people with the right skills and brokerage abilities are needed to create more fluidity and overcome the stickiness of knowledge (Wenger, 2000). Action to improve the relationships and links between individuals, teams, departments or organisations can help here. In the UK 'Collaborations for Leadership in Applied Health Research and Care' (CLAHRCs) have been set up to help. These are local health system collaborations designed to operationalise innovation and evidence-based best practice. The CLAHRCs have adopted different approaches to knowledge translation and mobilisation. In one, studied over a period of five years from its inception, it was clear that the approach had to be flexible and evolve in response to the

---

INNOVATION IN ACTION 5.4:   The CLAHRCs as learning organisations

As new organisational models for supporting knowledge translation, the CLAHRCs were themselves innovating and learning about the best approaches. Detailed research on one CLAHRC showed how it needed to adopt a flexible approach to knowledge mobilisation as its organisational structure and relationships with the local healthcare community developed. Initially, the CLAHRC's senior management implemented a 'push' model of knowledge translation, driven by top-down leadership and fairly rigid performance management regimes associated with knowledge translation activities. Although this approach helped the management team to develop a technical infrastructure by which to measure knowledge translation activity, it was seen as heavy handed by those responsible for specific innovation projects and healthcare staff more widely. It therefore became necessary to move to a model that promoted shared accountability and built local leadership capacity amongst clinicians. The emphasis shifted to self-reflection and knowledge pull ('what do I need to know?') and the exchange of knowledge and learning between staff. The CLAHRC's senior management team reframed their approach towards one that emphasised the development of clinicians' capacity to lead improvement and accommodate more experiential, collaboratively constructed knowledge. Greater discretion and support was given to clinical leads from local projects, resulting in a more successful knowledge translation model.

Source: Spyridonidis *et al.* (2015).

---

way local health and social care staff engaged with the various knowledge mobilisation activities (see Innovation In Action 5.4).

Much has been written about the types of linkage between individual and organisational actors — strong and formal versus weak and informal — and success in knowledge mobilisation and or translation. Research suggests that strong linkages are more effective for transferring complex knowledge, while weak linkages are more effective for transferring simple forms of knowledge (Hansen, 1999; Henderson and Clark, 1990). Network forms of organisation are potentially better able to accelerate organisational learning and spread knowledge (Ferlie *et al.*, 2010), but knowledge translation remains a problem in healthcare precisely because of the complexity of networks and the presence of multiple linkages and boundaries between stakeholders, networks and silos within the overall health system. There are various forms of knowledge network within healthcare (Currie *et al.*, 2011):

- *Inter-organisational partnerships,* which bring together public, private and third sector organisations and use synergies in resources and expertise, and economies of scale, to deliver mutual benefits.
- *Formal managed networks,* such as those created in cancer care, cardiology and some other specialities to review performance, consider evidence for innovations, communicate knowledge and champion changes in practice.
- *Professional networks,* also based around clinical specialities, which can create the consensus amongst key stakeholders needed for adoption by helping to validate new knowledge associated with innovations. These can act as a forum for members to gain esteem for their work and are able to influence the behaviour of other members (Menchik and Meltzer, 2010), operating as 'shapers and quiet system architects' (Ferlie *et al.*, 2011).

There can be problems, however, in using networks to promote knowledge sharing and stimulate the spread of innovation (Ferlie *et al.*, 2010):

- They can lose focus or become a 'talking shop'.
- They may become dominated by an elite professional group, linked to key opinion formers who advocate for a specific approach and push for adoption of a particular innovation. Conversely, professional networks may resist change and innovation. Strong inwardly looking links within such networks can also inhibit a wider search for knowledge (Henderson and Clark, 1990).
- Insufficient resources or a lack of skilled management can render networks ineffective; networks with looser interpersonal ties may be

maintained for lower cost but their knowledge translation capability is weakened because of infrequent contact.

- The formal constitution of some networks, such as the UK cancer networks, and their role in coordinating clinical services make them more politically accountable than informal networks, with a danger that they can become over-regulated at the expense of energy and creativity (Addicott *et al.*, 2007).

'Communities of practice' are another type of network. These evolve (or are intentionally created) around particular areas of interest and enable

---

Box 5.9   BACKGROUND: 25 years of supporting innovation adoption and spread in the UK's NHS

Since the early 2000s the UK has established a more rigorous and systematic approach to promoting the adoption and diffusion of innovation and best practice in its healthcare system. The policy emphasis has increasingly moved from innovation 'push' – supporting R&D and technology development — towards innovation 'pull' by stimulating demand from health service organisations. Parallel to the Cooksey report (Cooksey, 2006), the *NHS Next Stage Review* reiterated the importance of technological innovation for the NHS and set out aspirations and regional plans for delivering it, including a legal duty on strategic health authorities to promote innovation (Department of Health, 2008). New organisational vehicles for promoting the adoption and diffusion of innovation and research evidence were put in place, notably the fifteen locally-based Academic Health Science Networks (AHSN) and thirteen Collaborations for Leadership in Applied Health Research and Care (CLAHRC). There are also six Academic Health Science Centres, which tackle the earlier stages in the innovation pipeline.

   All these bodies aim to bridge the gap between research and practice, and support the adoption and spread of new approaches to health service delivery. They do this by coordinating stakeholders from across the local healthcare ecosystem, ranging from innovating companies and universities to NHS trusts and other organisations providing healthcare. An important function of the AHSNs and CLAHRCs is to create a pull for innovations by ensuring that the

(Continued)

Box 5.9 (*Continued*)

flow of knowledge is optimised, and a climate for its adoption into practice is created amongst healthcare providers and commissioners.

The AHSNs support knowledge exchange networks to promote the early adoption of innovations, and coordinate a programme to connect key health sector challenges with innovative ideas from industry by funding competitions such as the Small Business Research Initiative. Essentially, AHSNs are integrators that link different parts of the local health ecosystem across traditional boundaries.

The focus of the CLAHRCs is largely on operationalising innovation and new evidence-based practice. These are partnerships between universities and surrounding NHS organisations which seek to improve patient outcomes by addressing the 'second translation gap' identified by the Cooksey report (Box 5.8). Each CLAHRC has a slightly different slant — some are more focused on applied health research and others on the application of improvement science to the delivery of healthcare. An important part of the CLAHRC approach is to include research as part of the remit of key healthcare staff, giving them the necessary time and support and ensuring that they engage with a wide range of stakeholders at different levels (NHS Confederation, 2012; Currie *et al.*, 2013).

After a decade or more of reforms both to the broader structure of the NHS and to the landscape of organisations and initiatives designed to support innovation, there is now a complicated pattern of bodies and funding programmes. These provide support across all the stages of the innovation process, from the various national Research Councils funding basic research to AHSNs and CLAHRCs designed to support adoption and diffusion. The healthcare innovation landscape is therefore comprehensively mapped, but there are complaints that the landscape remains hard to navigate (Barlow, 2015). Not only are there many potential sources of support, over 20 bodies or funding initiatives are in place to support healthcare innovation and the areas in the landscape occupied by AHNSs, CLAHRCs and the AHSCs to some extent overlap. In October 2014, NHS England published a *Five Year Forward View* of the challenges it faces, highlighting the need to improve productivity in the health system. Parallel to this, two further reviews on national healthcare innovation were announced, one of which is aims to ensure that various organisations involved in healthcare innovation have a clear and simple purpose.

Source: Barlow (2015).

their members — who have similar roles or carry out similar work — to share explicit and tacit knowledge (Brown and Duguid, 1991; Wenger, 1998). Unlike managed or professional networks, their looser and more informal structure allows them to reach across professional silos and organisational boundaries. Within healthcare, this is important because ways of creating and validating knowledge differ between professional groups such as GPs, nurses and surgeons, so communities of practice can potentially break down their differences in epistemology (Ferlie *et al.*, 2010).

Incentivising innovation through financial measures — reimbursing the cost of innovation, paying for performance

Simply sharing knowledge about new research and innovations does not mean it will be taken up and used in everyday practice. The economics of healthcare innovation heavily influence the likelihood that

→ *Chapter 3 discusses the unusual features of innovation economics within healthcare*

potential adopters will actually adopt. To recap, we saw how the costs and benefits of an innovation are often disconnected because of organisational fragmentation across the primary, secondary and social care systems. In most developed countries, these are largely financially autonomous with their own budgetary silos. The costs, risks and benefits associated with large-scale and complex innovations may be spread unevenly across the care system and there may be counterintuitive effects, for example where reducing the demand for hospital beds from frail elderly people through innovative approaches such as telecare is offset by an increase in the volume of more expensive elective surgery patients.

Another problem is that it can be a long time before the benefits of some innovations are realised — long after the typical annual budgetary cycle of a healthcare organisation. In time, an innovation might be cost saving to a healthcare provider (or to society as a whole) but the short-term costs associated with its implementation may be high. These are often unfunded by health system payers — a common problem is 'double running', where costs are incurred by the innovative new healthcare service as it is introduced *and* because the existing service cannot be withdrawn immediately.

Many European countries using a diagnosis-related group (DRG)-based payment system use a higher level of reimbursement to overcome the reluctance of healthcare providers to adopt innovative technologies which may be accompanied by higher costs. When Germany introduced an all-embracing DRG system, it was recognised that the emphasis on improving productivity might impede the willingness of healthcare providers to take up new medical devices, drugs or procedures. Different rules apply for the introduction and reimbursement of innovations, depending on the part of the German healthcare system involved. Broadly the system involves acceptance of the application for use of new technologies ('Nu-B' clearance), agreement with the providers of statutory health

---

INNOVATION IN ACTION 5.5: How the reimbursement system for medical procedures can cause problems for healthcare innovation adoption

The way the system for reimbursing healthcare providers works has long been seen as a barrier to the introduction of innovative new approaches in the UK. Many people have argued that it is necessary to change the structure of incentives within the NHS to influence adoption. One problem is that the increased costs that often accompany a healthcare innovation in its initial stages of implementation — perhaps due to the need for training or need to run the old care service model alongside the new one — are not taken into account. Another perceived barrier to innovation is the possibility that introducing an efficiency improving innovation may result in financial problems, for example by reducing reimbursable activity by a hospital or other healthcare provider. However, the lack of accurate costing information for providing a service means that the financial impact of innovations is also often unclear — poor data on costs mean that NHS trusts struggle to identify potential savings, giving them less reason to drop outdated practices and adopt new ones. We look at this in Case study 5.2, on innovation in renal care.

(Continued)

INNOVATION IN ACTION 5.5 (*Continued*)

Various reforms to the reimbursement system in the 2000s introduced adjustments to the tariff for specific procedures to reflect increased costs associated with the implementation of novel approaches. Several forms of financial incentivisation were also introduced to drive quality, safety and efficiency improvements, with the potential knock-on effect of stimulating innovative thinking:

- In the primary care sector, the Quality and Outcomes Framework (QOF) introduced an incentive system paying a proportion of the income of a GP practice.
- In secondary care, the previous system of block contracts was replaced by Payment by Results, an activity-based payment system with tariffs based on the average cost of a group of procedures under current practice.
- The Best Practice Tariff was also introduced to reward providers that increased productivity and quality in selected clinical areas, by paying a higher tariff price.
- The Commissioning for Quality and Innovation (CQUIN) scheme was introduced in 2009. The bodies responsible for local health service planning and purchasing, Clinical Commissioning Groups (CCG), play an active role in developing CQUIN goals for each local healthcare provider. A proportion of the provider's annual income is conditional on reaching agreed targets. Most of these targets are agreed locally by the CCG, but there are also some national and regional targets around safety, effectiveness, patient experience and innovation.

Concerns have been raised over the use of Payment by Results and Best Practice Tariffs, notably over the quality of cost information on which the tariff is based. Evaluation of the success of CQUIN suggest its effects have been mixed. While commissioners and providers have been helped to identify and prioritise local quality improvement needs, the impact on quality has been minimal. Amongst other problems, the short-term nature of the CQUIN goals was found to limit the motivation for hospital trusts to invest in measures to improve performance.

Source: Abma *et al.* (2014).

insurance about additional payments, and then integration of the procedure into the tariff with any supplementary payment.

In the UK, the NHS tariff system rewards providers for increasing productivity and encourages them to exert tighter control over costs. It also gives the Department of Health the opportunity to incentivise innovation by paying a higher tariff price — the Best Practice Tariff (BPT) — when appropriate (see Innovation in Action 5.5). There are BPTs in various clinical areas, including acute stroke care, total hip and knee replacements, and renal care, described in Case study 5.2.

Pay for performance and outcomes based payments

There is a widely held view that the cost-efficient delivery of high quality healthcare can be inhibited by the payment mechanism, because the reimbursement for a failed procedure on a patient can be the same as for a successful one. Interest is growing in outcomes-based approaches to payment ('pay for performance'), tied to the delivery of agreed patient outcomes and other measures of quality, productivity or effectiveness. By focusing attention on these performance measures providers should in turn seek out and adopt evidence-based innovations and best practice, or develop new approaches themselves. Adoption is accelerated because approval for a new technological innovation is not held back until satisfactory evidence is available. Apart from giving patients earlier access to potentially beneficial healthcare technologies, these schemes also change the incentives for manufacturers towards a model that explicitly rewards health outcomes (Garrison *et al.*, 2013; Carlson *et al.*, 2011).

Broadly, pay for performance and outcomes based payments models link targets to the revenues received by health providers, either via a financial reward or a penalty. The argument is that healthcare provider behaviour is likely to be influenced if they believe that a proportion of their income is at stake. This requires all stakeholders in the provider system to be clear about the expectations of payers and commissioners, and how payments are aligned to them. The emergence of 'integrated care', widely seen as a way forward for health systems facing escalating costs and rising demand, has spurred interest in the best methods for incentivising performance improvement in healthcare providers. One of the key features of integrated care is the adoption of payment systems that incorporate financial incentives and risk-reward sharing mechanisms.

Research on the effectiveness of pay for performance incentives suggests that the evidence is inconclusive (Lagarde *et al.*, 2014; Health Affairs, 2012). This is partly because of the diversity in the design of pay for performance models, which makes them hard to compare. Categories of quality measure generally cover:

- *Processes*: Activities that have been demonstrated to contribute to positive health outcomes.
- *Outcomes*: The effects that care has on patients. Increasingly, outcome measures also include cost savings.
- *Patient experience*: Patients' perception of the quality of care they have received.
- *Structure*: Relating to the facilities, personnel and equipment used in treatment.

Use of outcome measures has been controversial because outcomes may be affected by social and clinical factors unrelated to the treatment provided and beyond the provider's control. Nevertheless, in the USA pay for performance has become popular with policy makers and private and payers. The Patient Protection and Affordable Care Act 2010 expanded their use in Medicare and encourages experimentation to determine which pay for performance designs are most effective. One of the best known is the Premier Hospital Quality Incentive Demonstration project which explored how far financial bonuses improve the quality of care provided to Medicare patients with certain long-term conditions.

Social impact bonds (SIB) are another form of pay for performance contract designed to fund the innovative delivery of public services. Various experiments are underway using SIBs to tackle complex social and health problems, such as care for frail older people with multiple long-term conditions, street homelessness and youth offending. In the USA, there has been some use of SIBs in preventive healthcare services (Crowley, 2014; Fairfax-Clay, 2013; Trupin *et al.*, 2014). Social impact bonds involve a contract to fund innovative interventions between public sector commissioners of health and social care or other services, and private or third sector (i.e. voluntary or charity) organisations. Investors cover the upfront costs necessary to set up the interventions, which are

---

Box 5.10 BACKGROUND: Incentivising innovation and change in integrated care programmes

One of the key features of integrated care is the adoption of payment systems that incorporate financial incentives and risk-reward sharing mechanisms to encourage performance improvement and innovative behaviour. There is, however, wide variety in how 'integration' is defined and applied. This makes it hard to compare the impact of underlying processes of different schemes. A common element underpinning integrated care models, however, is the use of a payment system that incorporate financial incentives and some form risk-reward sharing mechanism.

Financial incentives in integrated care have been used to deliver particular goals, such as process and outcome targets, or the adoption of evidence-based innovations or best-practice clinical practice guidelines. Most incentive and payment systems have focused on healthcare providers, but some of them target on health insurers and patients. Schemes focusing on providers include the 'quality and outcomes framework' (QOF) system in the UK (see Innovation In Action Box 5.5), *Gesundes Kinzigtal* (Germany) and Family Health Teams (Ontario, Canada).

Gesundes Kinzigtal is a population-based integrated care system in an area of south west Germany, introduced in 2005. It covers around 20 preventive and health promotion programmes for specific conditions. Local healthcare providers are given additional pay-for-performance payments for services that are considered important for improving the quality of care, but which fall outside normal reimbursement coverage. There is also a profit sharing element based on the degree of performance improvement, along with safeguards against cherry picking the least risky patients for enrollment in the scheme. *Gesundes Kinzigtal's* model is said to have led to benefits including reductions in morbidity and mortality rates, reduced hospital and nursing home admissions, and morbidity-adjusted efficiency gains of 16% of total costs relative to a control group of patients.

(Continued)

Box 5.10   (*Continued*)

In Ontario, Canada, Family Health Teams were set up in 2005 to provide financial incentives to physicians to manage chronic disease. By 2012, of some 200 FHTs, serving 2.8 million patients, had been established. Almost half of these were led by physicians. The model enables primary care providers to collaborate with other specialists, using a funding model which includes bonuses for achieving preventive care targets and payments for extending the range of services provided. The number of people previously without a family doctor who are now enrolled has risen dramatically, although it is unclear to what extent this is due to the introduction of FHTs. There have also been concerns about the cost of the overall programme and the large number of organisational models, each with its own different payment structure.

Source: Draws partly on Bienkowska-Gibbs (2013), Curry and Ham (2010), Llano (2013), Singer *et al.* (2011).

CASE STUDY 5.2   Financial incentives in kidney care

In the UK, different forms of kidney dialysis (apart from acute and paediatric dialysis) have been paid for by a tariff under the Payment by Results scheme. Hospitals receive a higher Best Practice payment for patients who receive in-centre dialysis with an arteriovenous (AV) fistula or graft, compared to those receiving dialysis via a tunnelled vascular catheter, because patients with a fistula or graft are believed to have fewer complications. A hospital reaching a predetermined proportion of patients undergoing in-centre haemodialysis using the preferred approach receives the higher tariff for *all* its in-centre haemodialysis patients.

Subsequently, haemodialysis carried out in patients' own home (home haemodialysis, HHD) was given its own tariff, paid on a per week basis and amounting to the same sum of money as three in-centre dialysis sessions on an AV fistula or graft. This made the weekly income from home haemodialysis and in-centre dialysis on a fistula the same. Since 2010, there have also been several Commissioning for Quality and Innovation (CQUIN) goals (see Innovation in Action 5.5) relating to the locally negotiated proportion of patients on home therapies (both haemodialysis and peritoneal dialysis). Other

(Continued)

CASE STUDY 5.2   (*Continued*)

CQUIN goals in kidney care aim to reduce the time between a patient starting dialysis and being referred for a transplant. The tariff for HHD should function as an incentive for hospitals because it pays the same as the alternative (in-centre haemodialysis) but is regarded as cheaper to deliver; the Best Practice Tariff should function as an incentive because dialysis via an AV fistula or graft pays more and is cheaper than the alternative (dialysis via a catheter); and the CQUIN is an incentive because it gives an additional (relatively small) sum of money when a certain percentage of patients is on a home therapy.

In practice, the effects of the incentives and mechanisms by which they operate are not so clear. Research showed a statistically significantly increase in the percentage of patients on HHD in hospitals after introducing the CQUIN for home therapies. However, some kidney dialysis centres were concerned about the time taken to balance net income from in-centre dialysis and HHD, so they did not see the tariff for HHD as an incentive. There was also concern about the turnover of patients on HHD and its adverse impact on costs, as upfront investment in training and setting up patients is lost when they cease to be on the programme. To overcome the lack of incentive to invest in meeting short-term targets, some commissioners therefore negotiated a multi-year home therapy CQUIN target, with the target percentage increasing each year. More fundamentally, it was unclear to some kidney centres whether the HHD tariff was an incentive or not because they had very limited knowledge of the costs of the different forms of dialysis they offered. In other words, they did not understand the price signals given by the Payment by Results tariff.

The CQUIN targets, on the other hand, were seen as an encouragement to increase the numbers of patients on HHD. Even though the payment is a relatively small portion of income for the kidney unit, it provides an extra, very visible sum of money for the current year. This additional income seemed to outweigh any uncertainty around the costs of HHD. The Best Practice Tariff for vascular access was also seen as a clear incentive because dialysis with an AV fistula or graft attracts the higher tariff and is a cheaper longer-term option for vascular access. However, kidney units were also concerned about possible detrimental effects of the CQUIN model. They might, for example, be 'punished' financially because a few patients rejected HHD or an AV fistula or graft, and some patients may be pressured into getting a fistula because the

(*Continued*)

CASE STUDY 5.2   (*Continued*)

hospital received the higher tariff. These problems can, however, be addressed by ensuring that informed patient choice is an indicator for reaching the CQUIN target.

Questions for discussion:

- What alternative approaches might have been developed to stimulate the adoption of HHD? What are the pros and cons of these?
- Would a 'top-down' mandate to hospitals to deliver more HHD have achieved better results?
- What tensions might hospitals which already offer an in-centre dialysis programme face when seeking to introduce an HHD programme? How might you resolve them?

Source: Abma *et al.* (2014).

delivered by service providers; the commissioner commits to pay rewards if agreed desired outcomes are reached.

Research on the use of SIBs is limited and there is no consensus about their impact and the ease of scaling them up. Nevertheless, their potential to foster innovation has been welcomed by policy makers, commissioners and service providers; these feel that traditional funding streams such as grants or block contracting lead to programmes that are too focused on short-term, narrow, process measures of success. For example, pay for performance arrangements under SIBs are seen as a way of incentivising service providers to pursue interventions designed to promote preventive behaviour via outcomes-based measures of success over longer periods of time.

Pay for performance in access to drugs

Pay for performance has also embraced the pharmaceutical industry through experimentation with schemes that involve 'paying for pills by results' rather than merely 'paying for pills' (Towse *et al.*, 2012). The argument is that healthcare payers want to know that they are getting value for money and other benefits for patients. However, pharmaceutical companies are not prepared to accept prices that do not reflect the value to patients, the healthcare system and the wider economy of their R&D investments in creating innovative drugs. Paying for the *outcomes* delivered by drugs potentially 'squares the circle' — payers know they are getting value; pharmaceutical companies receive a return which incentivises them to continue innovating. This involves striking an agreement between a payer and a pharmaceutical company, where the price level and/or revenue received is related to the future performance of the drug either in a trial or a real-world environment. The implication is that there is a degree of risk-sharing whereby one party in the transaction — the drug company — is sufficiently confident about its claims that it is prepared to accept a reward or penalty depending on the observed performance at some later point. A weakness of pay for performance schemes, however, that is that clear definition of health outcome measures and a mechanism for monitoring patients, along with penalties for non-compliance with the agreement, needs to be agreed and enforced.

Value-based pricing models are now being tried (see Box 5.4). These combine performance-based reimbursement, where the development risk of new drugs is shared, and the use of wider cost-effectiveness measures (Sussex *et al.*, 2013). Value-based pricing models potentially influence the behaviour of pharmaceutical companies in relation to R&D strategies, and there is some evidence from Sweden that they speed up the adoption of novel and orphan drugs (Persson *et al.*, 2010; Persson, 2012).

The use of 'coverage with evidence development' is another tool for sharing the risk of developing and adopting novel drugs and some other technologies. Because there are often uncertainties over the level of evidence available at the time an innovative medical product is introduced, it is hard to determine an appropriate level of reimbursement. Coverage with evidence development provides temporary funding of innovative products whilst additional evidence of their effectiveness in wider populations is generated (Hutton *et al.*, 2007). Healthcare decision makers are therefore able to make available the innovative product in a controlled manner, defining the type and level of evidence required to support wider adoption.

There is wide variety in coverage with evidence development methods (see Box 5.11) and some moves towards harmonisation (Garrison *et al.*, 2013), along with concerns over the design of schemes (Garber

Box 5.11 BACKGROUND: Coverage with evidence development schemes

A number of countries have now adopted coverage with evidence development (CED), systems. Australia launched a scheme for shared risk in pricing (the 'Managed Entry Scheme') in 2011, based on listing drugs at a price justified by the level of existing evidence, pending availability of more conclusive evidence of cost-effectiveness (Wonder *et al.*, 2012; Vitry and Roughead, 2014). Several European countries have adopted CED schemes, although there are differences in how they operate. A study by Martellia and van den Brink (2014) compares France, Germany, and the UK:

- Since 2010, France, has operated a system for conditionally covering the full cost of selected innovative devices, services or interventions which appear promising but for which there is insufficient data on the clinical benefit. The Ministry of Health, rather than manufacturers, initiates the CED process and defines parameters of the specific study, such as numbers of patients involved, conditions of use, funding period, and location of trials. Full financial support is provided for the trial, with no refunds required from manufacturers should the innovation be recommended for coverage by the DRG system.
- Germany introduced a CED scheme in 2012. This was in recognition of the need for a mechanism to support innovation within the DRG system, which was especially focused on improving productivity. Top-up funding for innovative products is available, with approved products subsequently monitored to ensure they are cost-effective. Unlike France, manufacturers initiate the processes, and receive only up to half the costs of evaluation, which they have to refund if the device is finally reimbursed. The German approach also emphasises new diagnostic and therapeutic treatment methods rather than the device itself.
- In the UK, the National Institute for Health and Clinical Excellence (NICE) has, since 1999, used a system for recommending the use of new drugs, procedures or devices within the context of evidence development. This is either on a 'only in research' (OIR) or 'approval with research' (AWR) basis. To speed up decision-making, NICE has also introduced a 'single technology appraisal' (STA) process, designed to appraise a single product with a specific indication. Since STA was introduced, OIR/AWR recommendations have declined.

(Continued)

Box 5.11 (*Continued*)

All three countries specify the nature of the evidence required, but not how studies should be designed. Unlike the German and French systems, however, NICE does not recommend a funding process for the additional research — this can be the responsibility of the manufacturer or a body such as the National Institute for Health Research.

et al., 2014). One issue is the length of time a post-launch trial of an innovative product should be conducted before there is a price review and a decision about coverage. Waiting for the results of a lengthy — perhaps 10 year — post-launch trial would unacceptably delay patient access, and would also be unacceptable to manufacturers. But given that the alternative is to collect scientific data through much more comprehensive and expensive trials in advance of launch, coverage with evidence development does offer a way to handle uncertainty around the expected value of a new drug in routine clinical practice and speed up adoption.

Incentivising innovation through public–private partnership (PPP) models

The use of PPP in healthcare has grown since the 1990s, especially in the provision of healthcare infrastructure. These were initially developed in some countries to renew outdated facilities faster than would be the case under conventional public funding models. They were also seen as a way of ensuring that facilities were adequately maintained over their lifetime (Barlow and Köberle-Gaiser, 2009). More recently, healthcare PPPs have expanded from infrastructure, and sometimes non-clinical services such as maintenance and catering, to embrace clinical services as well. The argument is that 'bundling' together all aspects of delivering healthcare locally means that the interests of the parties involved are more closely aligned. In this way, innovative thinking is encouraged because the risks, costs and benefits of trying out new ideas all fall within the

Box 5.12   BACKGROUND: New forms of PPP to drive performance change and innovation

Finland has experimented with a form of franchising model. Coxa Hospital, in Tampere, involves the consolidation of existing elective orthopaedic services into a new hospital. The PPP initially brought together a private company, the local university hospital, and the local municipalities which are responsible for purchasing healthcare service. Following a restructuring, all shareholders are now from public sector, the local municipalities. The project was developed at a time of concern in Finland about rising demand for joint replacement surgery, suboptimal clinical outcomes and a lack of cost control. Combining specialisation (focusing only joint replacement surgery) with process innovation, especially the introduction of 'lean thinking' in its operational procedures, was expected to help drive up quality and reduce costs.

Coxa comprises a PPP embracing clinical and non-clinical services, and new physical infrastructure, essentially a 'hospital in a hospital'. Radiology, pharmacy and laboratory services, and orthopaedic training are all outsourced to the partner university hospital. There has been innovation in infrastructure design, with Coxa adopting a flexible model — a 'hot floor' (the core clinical activities) plus 'hotel' (accommodation) and 'back offices'. Organisational culture and structure has also seen new thinking, with greater emphasis on rewarding performance and embedding clinicians within the university to encourage research.

The Finnish example involves the delivery of largely hospital-based services via forms of PPP. Another model involves population-wide service provision, in which a private company provides both the hospital services and the primary care for a geographical area from its own facilities. A well-known example is La Ribera, in the Valencia region in Spain. This extends the idea of bundling services beyond the hospital and is innovative in several ways. La Ribera uses a 'capitation' model, in which the regional health authority makes a standard payment for each member of the population in a single local area. The payments are set so that the cost to the public purse is lower than that previously incurred under purely public-sector provision or in other comparable areas. This aims to encourage innovative thinking in how services are delivered. The terms of the contract discourage the consortium from reducing the volume or quality of services provided to its catchment population, since costs incurred by patients travelling outside the concession are charged to La Ribera. There are also disincentive to offering care to non-catchment area patients.

Source: Barlow *et al.* (2013).

same contractual entity, the PPP consortium. There is now a spectrum of different combinations of PPP, determined by the degree to which the various services and facilities are bundled within the contract (Barlow *et al.*, 2013). How risk management, financing and payment mechanisms are structured in PPPs can vary considerably between different models. Well-known examples include the Alzira scheme in Spain and Coxa Hospital in Finland (Box 5.12).

An important influence on the success of a PPP is the way risk is handled. More discipline in the transparency and allocation of risk should in theory reduce financial uncertainty for all parties, potentially benefitting innovative activities. The healthcare provider side of the PPP, which holds the risk arising from changing regulations or policies, or falling demand for healthcare services, should be stimulated into focusing on the flexibility and adaptability of its infrastructure during the initial planning stages of the project. For the supplier side — construction and facilities management companies — the concern is to minimise financial and reputational damage arising from a poorly managed physical asset, or unforeseen inflation in maintenance and operational costs which cannot be recovered. Both sides should therefore be concerned to inject a degree of innovative design and construction thinking into their project in order to cope with the inevitable changes in healthcare services over the duration of the contract. However, in the UK, a pioneer in the use of PPP for healthcare infrastructure, this theory was not borne out in practice, at least in the initial wave of projects (Barlow and Köberle-Gaiser, 2009). Although there was awareness that future changes in demand posed financial risks for hospitals and some concern over the need for adaptability and flexibility in hospital facilities, the drive by government and the NHS to transfer risk as far as possible away from the public sector meant that construction companies and funders were not interested in putting forward innovative — but untried and potentially higher cost — solutions. Moreover, hospitals needed to reduce project costs as much as possible to meet government 'value for money' norms. To minimise project risks, contracts were designed to ensure cost certainty as early as possible in the design process, further reducing the incentive for innovative behaviour.

The jury is still out on the extent to which these PPP models have encouraged innovative thinking or the adoption of innovations from elsewhere, but the publicly reported outcomes suggest the quality and efficiency of services has improved compared to the previous model that was in place. In Coxa Hospital, collectively sharing risk is said to have resulted in significant process and safety improvements, lower infection rates, shorter lengths-of-stay in hospital, and less readmission for revisions of operations (Lehto, 2009). The PPP model has reduced bureaucracy and speeded operational and strategic decision-making. In La Ribera, the healthcare outcomes are said to show impressive results across a range of indicators, including significantly reduced delays in waiting for surgery and MRI/CAT scans, reduced average hospital stays, lower readmission rates, and increased rates of day and outpatient surgery (NHS Confederation, 2011).

Chapter summary

- Innovation adoption is highly dependent on the interactions between the innovation, local actors involved in adoption and diffusion, and the wider context.
- There is often no single adoption decision and adoption and assimilation unfolds over time.
- The linkages and compatibility between the outer and inner contexts of the innovation are often important and the innovation may be adapted for a better fit.
- Innovation investment decisions usually need a business case, backed by evidence for the potential impact. However, this is often hard where healthcare innovations combine organisational, service and technology change.
- The collection and use of evidence for the impact of innovations can be very important in decisions about the adoption of healthcare innovations. There are tensions between evaluation methods that are based on positivist scientific methods and those based on more qualitative approaches.
- The use of RCTs can be problematic when used to generate evidence for what are very complex and hard-to-define innovations.

- Various techniques have been put in place to support the adoption and spread of healthcare innovations. These include approaches to sharing and spreading knowledge, and financial methods for incentivising the take-up of innovations or stimulating innovative behaviour.

Questions for discussion

1. Refer to the Innovation in Action examples 5.1 and 5.2:

- What do these cases tell us about the role played by evidence in stimulating the adoption of these innovations?
- What were the key characteristics of the innovations that helped their introduction?
- Which of the innovation adoption models described in Chapter 2 applies best and why?

2. Why is innovation in healthcare often such a lengthy process?
3. What factors influence the adoption and diffusion of healthcare innovation? Do you think 'implementation' and 'embedding' are more appropriate concepts when investigating uptake and spread of healthcare innovations?
4. The way in which the distribution of benefits and risks map onto the interests and values of the adopting organisation is critical for understanding how healthcare innovations are adopted and spread. Discuss this statement and explain the reasons for your answer.
5. Use the theories of process researchers such as Greenhalgh *et al.* to discuss the reasons why healthcare organisations might resist adopting a healthcare innovation.
6. Do you agree with the view that successful adoption of an innovation in healthcare is the result of the interaction between economic, social and organisational factors?
7. From the perspective of developers of new healthcare technologies, why might innovation be more than just a matter of developing a technologically superior product? What types of capabilities and competencies do technology developers need to be successful?

8. Refer to Innovation in Action 5.3. If you were running a small company developing telehealth technology, how would you go about marketing your products? Should you focus your activity on one or two potential lead users from the NHS? Should you spend more time and effort gathering better evidence for your products?
9. What role does evidence for the potential benefits of a healthcare innovation play in its implementation? Why is it often hard to gather such evidence?
10. Sometimes stakeholders differ in their assessment of the benefits of specific healthcare innovations. Discuss what effects this might have on the adoption of healthcare innovations.
11. Is it possible for those who *develop* new innovations, those who *pay* for them and those who *use* them to ever agree on the meaning of 'value'?
12. Choose three contrasting healthcare innovations and apply the model developed by John Gourville (Chapter 2) to explain their patterns of adoption. What are the advantages and disadvantages of such a model? Explain the reasons for your answer.
13. To what extent do you agree that government support is often needed to address the 'translation gap' between research and implementation?
14. Do governments place too much importance on supporting the development of innovative healthcare technologies compared to their implementation?

Selected further reading

Atun R, de Jongh T, Secci F, Ohiri K, Adeyi O (2010) Integration of targeted health interventions into health systems: A conceptual framework for analysis. *Health Policy and Planning* 25: 104–111.

Barlow J, Bayer S, Curry R (2006) Implementing complex innovations in fluid multi-stakeholder environments: Experiences of 'telecare'. *Technovation* 26: 396–406.

Bloom G, Ainsworth P (2010) Beyond scaling up. Pathways to universal access to health services. STEPS Working Paper 40, University of Sussex, STEPS Centre.

Denis J, Hébert Y, Langley A, Lozeau D, Trottier L (2002) Explaining diffusion patterns for complex health care innovations. *Health Care Management Review* 27: 60–73.

Ferlie E, Fitzgerald L, Wood M, Hawkins C (2005) The nonspread of innovation: The mediating role of professionals. *Academy of Management Journal* 48(1): 117–134.

Greenhalgh T, Robert G, Macfarlane F, Bate P, Kyriakidou O (2004a) Diffusion of innovations in service organizations. Systematic review and recommendations. *Milbank Quarterly* 82: 581–629.

Hendy J, Barlow J (2012) The role of the organizational champion in achieving health system change. *Social Science and Medicine* 74(5): 348–355.

DISRUPTIVE AND FRUGAL INNOVATION IN HEALTHCARE. WE THINK WE NEED IT — BUT WHAT IS IT?

THIS CHAPTER WILL HELP YOU TO:

- Understand what disruptive innovation is.
- Explain why it is regarded as important in healthcare in advanced health systems and in those of low- to middle-income countries.
- Understand the implications of disruptive innovation for the healthcare workforce and organisations.
- Discuss the similarities and differences between disruptive and frugal innovation.
- Understand the challenges in translating frugal innovations into an advanced health system context.

The notion of 'disruptive innovation' has become increasingly common, both in healthcare and more widely across business and government. But it is often misunderstood and the term is used uncritically. We often talk about 'disruptive' innovation and 'radical' innovation interchangeably. And a growing interest in another concept, 'frugal innovation', is muddying the waters. So we need to be more rigorous and analytical about the characteristics of disruptive and frugal innovation.

This chapter discusses what is meant by the concept of disruptive innovation and how it has been applied to healthcare challenges. It is important to make a distinction between its use in the context of advanced high-cost health systems and countries with more rudimentary health systems. In the former, the issues are largely about the use of disruptive innovation to shift healthcare from expensive settings, using a combination of new technologies and new service models. In the latter, the challenge is to increase access to healthcare by an under-served population, and avoid replicating the expensive models of developed countries. Frugal technologies, created especially for this market, are beginning to help achieve this. The chapter also considers two questions which are largely neglected in discussions about disruptive innovation — the impact of disruptive technologies on the built infrastructure for healthcare services and the extent to which low cost, but possible lower functionality, frugal technologies are transferrable to advanced health systems.

Case study 6.1 focuses on the demand for disruptive technology. There has long been discussion about the possibility of field-based brain imaging for people who have had a stroke, to allow faster diagnosis and therapy with thrombolytic drugs if indicated. However, apart from the technical difficulties in creating smaller and cheaper imaging technology, the costs and benefits of introducing such an innovation are less clear. Much depends of the geographical context.

Mini Cases 6.1 and 6.2 update examples of disruptive healthcare innovation first described in the early 2000s. Coronary angioplasty (Mini Case 6.1) shows how changing evidence for the costs of a new healthcare technology can mean that the economic implications are now less clear than originally anticipated. Mini Case 6.2, on the concept of 'retail clinics', illustrates how a disruptive concept triggered a response from competitors, which led to a further evolution of the original concept. Mini Case 6.3 describes the range of new diagnostic technologies that underpin cheaper and faster diagnosis outside conventional hospital settings.

Since it was first introduced in the late 1990s, Clayton Christensen's concept of 'disruptive innovation' has become part of the currency of management and innovation research and practice. The original theory referred primarily to *disruptive technologies* such as the first personal computers. It

"The core prediction of disruption theory has been boiled down and summarized quite efficiently many times. But these summaries have not precluded widespread confusion." (Raynor, 2014)

focused largely on the way they displace seemingly superior technologies in a given market (Christensen, 1997). Over the years, use of the term has steadily broadened, to explain different kinds of innovation in a wide range of sectors. It is often loosely used to embrace any innovation that is seen as somehow 'radical' — perhaps new-to-the-world — and potentially disruptive to existing ways of working.

Some have argued that this broadening devalues the concept and that we need to be much clearer about how we use it. Researchers have pointed out that different kinds of innovation should be treated as distinct phenomena (Markides, 2006; Danneels, 2004). A disruptive technological innovation is a fundamentally different proposition from a disruptive business model, and a disruptive product is not the same as a disruptive service innovation.

> *"A disruptive innovation allows a whole new population of consumers to afford to own and have the skill to use a product or service, whereas historically, the ability to access was limited to people who have a lot of money or a lot of skill."* (Smith, 2007)

They all arise in different ways, they have different competitive effects, they create different kinds of markets, and they require different responses from incumbent firms in the market. Moreover, disruptive and radical innovations are distinct categories, driven by different forces and with differing outcomes. And now — as we will see — the concept of disruptive innovation is beginning to overlap with that of frugal innovation, especially in healthcare, causing further confusion.

Disruptive innovation defined

The original concept of disruptive innovation argues that products have particular trajectories in the way their performance improves as innovating companies introduce new and improved versions. Once introduced, the technology underlying a tablet computer or mobile phone will continue to incrementally improve its quality and performance. But there are two related problems with this. First, these incremental improvements (called by Christensen 'sustaining innovation') often drive consumer prices up rather than down (Christensen *et al.*, 2011). Second, eventually the pace of technological progress usually exceeds the needs of most customers, as companies try to sell ever-better versions of the product to the most demanding segment of the market for higher profit margins. Think of continually improving mobile phones with features that many people don't want or need.

For a short video of Christensen defining disruptive innovation see: http://www. claytonchristensen.com/ key-concepts/

A disruptive innovation brings to the market a more affordable product (or service) that is simpler to use. Because of this,

Another video is at: http://www.innosight.com/ innovation-resources/what-is-disruptive-innovation-chapter1-part2.cfm

it may be taken up by those customers who are not currently in the market because they demand less — all they want is a simpler, cheaper tablet computer or mobile phone. To qualify as a disruptive innovation, the new product or service must enlarge the overall existing market by attracting new customers. The markets created around disruptive innovations therefore comprise different types of customer and have different success factors compared to those within established markets. Boxes 6.1 and 6.2 describe the key attributes of disruptive innovations.

Box 6.1   CONCEPTS: What is an innovation's potential for disruption?

To determine whether an idea has disruptive potential, companies must ask three sets of questions:

1. Does the innovation have the potential for new-market disruption?
   Is there a large population of people who have historically not had the resources to access a product or service for themselves? Can an innovation be developed so that such a population can begin owning and using the product? If so, there is potential for shaping the idea into a new-market disruption.

(Continued)

Box 6.1 *(Continued)*

2. Does the innovation have the potential for low-end disruption? *Are there customers who would be happy with a product with lower (but good enough) performance if they could get it at a lower price? Can an innovation be created that delivers sufficient profit that price? Innovations that enable low-end disruption may also involve process improvements that reduce overhead costs.*

3. Final check
   Is the innovation disruptive to all the significant incumbents in the industry? If it appears to be sustaining to one or more significant players, then the odds will be stacked in that firm's favour, and the entrant is unlikely to win and it is unlikely the innovation will lead to disruption.

Source: Christensen and Raynor (2003).

Box 6.2   CONCEPTS: Catalysts for disruptive innovation

* Not a sustaining technology (so not resulting in price inflation).
* Produced by an organisation autonomous or separate from the incumbents who dominate the market.
* Less expensive than traditional technology.
* Maintains cost-competitiveness over time.
* Enabled by a rapidly evolving technology (and may start-off worse than existing product but improve over time).
* Demonstrated effectiveness in real-world use (perhaps requiring significant trial and error).

Based on: Eggers *et al.* (2013).

It is important to note that the companies creating disruptive innovation are not the same as the ones that invent new products or services. As Markides (2006) puts it, they 'simply redefine what an existing product or service is and how it is provided to the customer … Amazon did not discover bookselling.' Because these products or services do not satisfy the minimum performance level that is valued by customers in the existing market, and they are produced by companies with a different value chain, incumbent firms in the mainstream market have little incentive to respond — they are not interested in reorganising their business to compete for these customers. Over time, though, incumbent companies may be provoked into a response, especially if their markets are displaced because there is such an improvement in the performance of the disruptive product or service that established customers begin to switch. Incumbent firms, used to concentrating on incrementally improving their existing product, are therefore faced with a dilemma. Do you try to compete with the entrants by creating a lower-performance version of your product, in which case you may end up with co-existing and competing products in the same organisation (Markides, 2006)? We can see this in the airline sector in Europe when some longer-established airlines made an explicit decision to target less demanding or first-time flyers in the face of competition from low cost entrants, after years of focusing on higher-value business customers.

The disruptive innovation concept was encapsulated by Christensen in a simple analytical graphic. A version is portrayed below (Figure 6.1). This illustrates the performance trajectories over time that are demanded

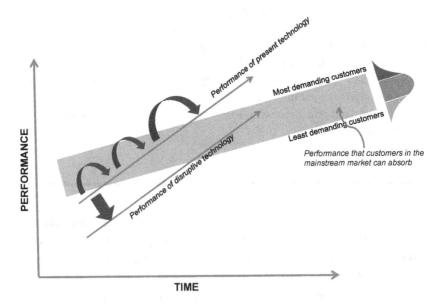

Figure 6.1.   Disruptive innovation — the concept.
Source: Christensen (1997).

by different market segments and catered for by existing and disruptive technologies. It shows that the needs of customers are distributed across the population in some form, perhaps a bell curve showing a small number of high-end, demanding customers and small number of low-end, less demand ones. Customers' needs tend to grow slowly as their expectations change. The application of technological innovation improves a product or service incrementally at a rate that is faster than changing customer needs, leaving behind a segment of potential customers with lower performance expectations. Disruption occurs when a new version of the product or service is created which is more attractive to these potential customers. This brings them into the market and possibly also captures a proportion of existing, mainstream customers. In time, the performance of the new, disruptive product develops its own upward trajectory.

The elision between radical and disruptive innovation was mentioned above. Radical innovations create new-to-the-world products and are also disruptive to producers and consumers, but in a different way from disruptive innovations. Radical innovations introduce new value propositions that fundamentally disturb prevailing markets, undermining the competences of incumbent companies. They are rarely driven by demand, and result instead from a supply-push process originating with technology developers. This may involve a radical shift in the underlying technology, moving the whole performance curve 'to the right'.

> ➔ *Chapter 2 describes different ways of classifying innovations and the links between performance improvement and innovation (Figure 2.6)*

There has been much debate on the concept of disruptive innovation and its validity. Danneels (2004) and others have raised questions about the relationship between a technology and its 'disruptiveness' and the timing of the disruption event itself:

- Can a particular technology be seen as inherently disruptive or is its disruptiveness simply due to the perspective of the companies subject to it? As Christensen has argued, the internet was disruptive to some firms but sustaining to others, depending on how consistent it was with their business model — it was a sustaining innovation for mail-order retailers but disruptive to department stores.

- At what point does a technology become disruptive? Does this happen when it invades an existing market and displaces incumbent firms and their prior technology? For example, did digital imaging become a disruptive technology when (a) it began to displace photo-processing labs, film manufacturers and camera manufacturers, (b) when photographers substituted film cameras with digital ones, or (c) when the services of photo-processing laboratories were no longer are needed?
- How can we know *ex ante* if a technology will be disruptive (Klenner *et al.*, 2013)? As Doering and Parayre (2000) noted, 'Significant emerging technologies are easily seen after the fact, and companies are then congratulated or castigated for their decisions to pursue them or ignore them. But rarely are the winners clear at the outset. Yet, this is the challenge managers face.'
- Does disruption ultimately depend on the impact of the disruptive technology on the resources or competences of firms by rendering established technologies obsolete and destroying the value of the investment made by incumbents in those technologies (Charitou and Markides, 2003)?

In 2014, an article in the *New Yorker* magazine by Jill Lepore provoked considerable debate and a response from Clayton Christensen (Lepore, 2014). She argued that disruptive innovation theory rests on shaky empirical foundations, accusing Christensen of poor scholarship by using case studies that conform to his theory. Lepore also suggests he misreads history since some of the companies he highlighted as doomed in fact performed well over a longer span of time. Lepore, an historian, concluded that disruptive innovation can only reliably be seen after the fact, echoing the point made above by Doering and Parayre (2000). If we take a longer perspective, many successes that are labelled as disruptive innovation in fact look like the result of something

"The choice of the word 'disruption' was a mistake I made 20 years ago. And I never thought about the word 'disruption' in the English language has so many connotations, that people would then flexibly use an idea, twist it and use it to justify whatever they want to do in the first place." (Clayton Christensen, https://www.youtube.com/watch?v=9ouwUs4QmFQ&feature=youtu.be)

else, while many failures that are initially seen as the result of competition from disruptive innovation simply look like bad management. Christensen has vigorously defended his position (Bennett, 2014), refuting these points and arguing that he has always recognised the theory is not only incomplete but also has gaps. He makes the point that disruption does not mean that incumbent companies are necessarily destroyed — US Steel survived the introduction of mini mills and the 'legacy airlines' are still around, albeit vastly changed in the face of low-cost carriers.

Michael Raynor provides another detailed response to Lepore. He argues that she makes two common errors when she describes disruptive innovation purely in terms of cheaper, lower-performance products eventually invading an entire industry. First, disruptive innovation need not start with these types of product, but with a completely new one, where there is no pre-existing competition and the returns are less attractive either because they are more uncertain or simply smaller in absolute terms — mobile telephony is an example. Second, a successful disruptive innovation does not require an industry and its incumbents to be wholly devoured — although mobile telephony has grown at the expense of fixed line telephony, many incumbent fixed line companies simply embraced the innovation and created their own mobile phone networks.

Perhaps our conclusion should simply be that disruptive innovation is best seen as a guide, a framework for understanding innovation trends in a market and their potential outcomes, rather than as some kind of overarching evolutionary theory. Indeed, this point is made by Christensen himself, who emphasises in his response to Lepore that disruptive innovation is not a theory about survivability.

Disruptive innovation and healthcare

Disruptive innovation has been much discussed in the healthcare context, especially in developed countries with high cost health systems that are now facing major resource limitations. These countries are facing a perfect storm for health and social care budgets, with a rising incidence of chronic disease, coupled with an ageing population, at a time of public expenditure constraints and increasing patient expectations.

We know we need innovation but while there is already plenty of technological innovation in health systems, part of the problem is that this leads to innovation-induced demand and cost inflation. It is because of this that many commentators and academics have argued that healthcare is in desperate need of disruptive innovation to avoid an impending resourcing crisis. Listed in Box 6.3 are just a few of the articles on disruptive innovation published in the *Health Services Journal*, the UK's leading weekly news magazine for the sector.

The argument for disruptive innovation is that countries with advanced health systems need to radically rethink the way they deliver healthcare. Disruptive innovation is

"If we do not fix our healthcare system the US may go the way of General Motors — paying more, getting less and going broke." President Barack Obama when launching the planned health system reforms in 2009. (http://news.bbc.co.uk/1/hi/world/americas/8100605.stm)

→*See Chapter 3 for a discussion about the economics of healthcare innovation*

Box 6.3 BACKGROUND: A range of articles discussing disruptive innovation in the *HSJ* — *Health Services Journal*

How the different types of innovation can inspire change, Steve Fairman, 6 March 2015.

Lessons from India: the role of tech and compassionate clinical leadership, Ajit Abraham, 15 May 2014.

Chief executives designed for the future, David Buchanan, 24 March 2014.

Innovation is the lifeblood of the health service, Nick Golding, 6 November 2013.

Clare Gerada: Disruptive innovation does more harm than good, Clare Gerada, 30 July 2013.

Debunking some myths about disruptive innovation in the NHS, Helen Bevan, 14 May 2012.

(Continued)

Box 6.3 (*Continued*)

This is the kind of disruptive innovation the NHS needs, Chris Ham, 25 November 2011.

HSJ interview: Clayton M Christensen, author of The Innovator's Prescription, Alastair McLellan, 3 November 2011.

The judges' verdict: why the NHS should listen to Christensen, Stephen Dorrell MP, Mike Farrar and Mark Britnell share their thoughts on *The Innovator's Prescription*, 3 November 2011.

Stephen Eames: it's time to embrace disruption, Stephen Eames, 18 March 2011.

Remove the barriers to healthcare innovation, Ali Parsa, 26 August 2010.

about disrupting the axiom that technological innovation is synonymous with increasing costs — introducing new models of care, which use new technologies where appropriate, thinking about how to break down complex processes into elements of care that can be provided by healthcare workers whose skill sets are best matched to the setting, shifting care into cheaper locations, and ultimately ensuring that we all take more responsibility for our own health and wellbeing. One way of describing this transformation is in terms of inverting the 'pyramid of care', as shown in Figure 6.2.

So what might disruptive innovation mean for healthcare? We need to answer this question from the perspective of different types of healthcare system and the challenges they face — first, how to tackle escalating healthcare costs in *high income countries* and second, how to improve access to healthcare in *lower income countries.*

Solutions to the cost crisis in advanced health systems

In an influential paper published in the *Harvard Business Review* in 2000, Clayton Christensen and colleagues applied their notion of disruptive innovation to the challenges in the USA's healthcare sector, described in Box 6.4. According to Christensen *et al.* (2000), healthcare in the US

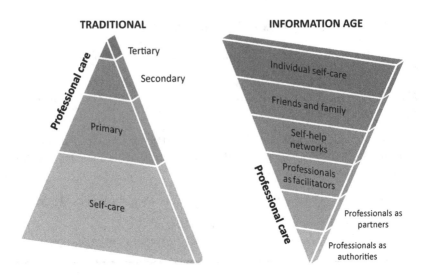

Figure 6.2.   Shift from industrialised to post-industrialised care.

Source: Jennings *et al.* (1997) in NHS Confederation (2008).

Box 6.4   BACKGROUND: The need for disruptive innovation in the US health system

'Make no mistake: the US health care industry is in crisis. Prestigious teaching hospitals lose millions of dollars every year. Health care delivery is convoluted, expensive, and often deeply dissatisfying to consumers. Managed care, which evolved to address some of these problems, seems increasingly to contribute to them — and some of the best managed-care agencies are on the brink of insolvency. We believe that a whole host of disruptive innovations, small and large, could end the crisis — but only if the entrenched powers get out of the way and let market forces play out. If the natural process of disruption is allowed to proceed, we will be able to build a new system that is characterised by lower costs, higher quality, and greater convenience than could ever be achieved under the old system.'

Source: Christensen *et al.* (2000).

needs to 'Invest less money in high end, complex technologies and more in technologies that simplify complex problems'. It is worth spending some time visiting the arguments in this paper. Christensen and his co-authors argue that while there may be a deep crisis in healthcare, history tells us that 'disruptive revolutions' offer ways a systemic transformation might be managed. Creating such a system will therefore involve several steps:

- *The clinician's skill level needs to be matched with the difficulty of the medical problem.*
  Medical problems range from the simple to the complex, with the simplest easily addressed through rule-based diagnosis and treatment. Complex problems, which cannot be solved this way, need to be channelled to clinicians with the right degree of experience and judgement. However, simple problems do not need specialists and can be tackled by primary care physicians or nurse practitioners (or ourselves with suitable support from health information apps and other sources).

- *Invest less money in high-end, complex technologies and more in technologies that simplify complex problems.*
  The development of sustaining — incremental — technological innovations targeted at the most complex problems and used by the most skilled practitioners has undoubtedly been of immense value to our healthcare. But as we saw in Chapter 3, one of the problems for health systems is the cost inflation associated with the adoption of such innovations. Christensen *et al.* argue that rather than focusing on complex solutions for complex problems, research and development needs to concentrate on simplification, enabling the healthcare professional to do things in lower-cost and more convenient settings. One of the examples of disruptive innovation described in Christensen *et al.*'s paper is the case of coronary angioplasty (see Mini Case 6.1).

- *New organisations will be needed to do the disrupting of the out-moded institutions of healthcare.*
  This does not mean that the familiar institutions in a healthcare system will be replaced by new ones offering new business

---

Box 6.5 BACKGROUND: Tools for growing disruptive innovation in the public sector

- Level the playing field: enable the disruptive innovation to gain ground by removing the subsidies and contracts that have allowed incumbents to dominate a market space.
- Change laws: some disruptive innovations may require legal and regulatory changes before they can exist and/or thrive in a given market.
- Phase-out the existing programme: once it becomes clear that a disruptive innovation is positioned for success, funding can be phased out from the current dominant approach to allow for the innovation's further growth, expansion, and development in the market.
- Partnerships: public–private partnerships may help to scale the innovation.

Source: Eggers *et al.* (2013).

---

models — hospitals will always be needed to provide intensive and critical care. Rather, the care of medical disorders that primarily involve a single system in the body should migrate to more focused care providers. This could enable higher quality care to be delivered with less 'complexity-driven overhead', although in practice the net impact would depend on the extent to which the cost of complex procedures gets redistributed over simpler procedures within the particular financial model operating in a healthcare system. Christensen *et al.* suggest that if history is any guide, only the creation of *new* institutions delivering the majority of care will achieve the necessary transformation — a tortuous reform of *existing* healthcare institutions designed for other purposes will not be enough. One view on reforms that might help is outlined in Box 6.5.

- *The inertia of regulation needs to be overcome.*
  Attempts to use regulation to stave off disruptive attacks by new players are common in many industries; for example US car manufacturers relied on import quotas for as long as possible to keep Japanese manufacturers at bay and currently, taxi drivers in various cities around the world have vociferously protested against the entry of Uber into their

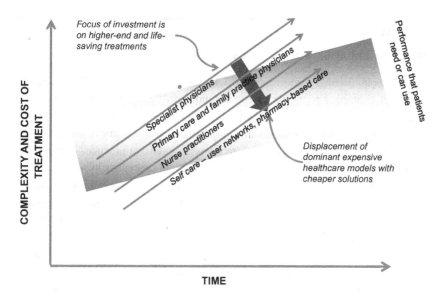

Figure 6.3.   Disruptive innovation concept applied to advanced health systems.
Source: Christensen *et al.* (2000).

markets. The entrenched professions and institutions in healthcare are highly protected by regulation. For example, physician bodies in many parts of the world have resisted the transfer of prescribing rights to nurses, although this has been shown to be very useful. In the USA, the *status quo* has been preserved by strong links between healthcare institutions, federal and state regulators, and insurance companies.

The approach in healthcare is summed up in a simple variant on Christensen *et al.*'s original graphical representation of disruptive innovation — Figure 6.3. This shows how we need to shift advanced healthcare systems towards a model where specialists continue to concentrate on the most complex and serious cases, while less highly qualified and relatively inexpensive healthcare professionals, such as nurse practitioners, take on more complex roles than they are currently allowed to do. But even at the upper end of the treatment complexity and cost spectrum, technological innovation has created new procedures that have allowed cardiologists to treat patients who previously would have needed the services of open-heart surgeons (see Innovation in Action 6.1).

INNOVATION IN ACTION 6.1: Coronary angioplasty — a move to cheaper, simpler healthcare?

Percutaneous coronary intervention (PCI) (formerly known as balloon angioplasty) is a coronary revascularisation technique used in the treatment of ischaemic heart disease. Before product innovations in balloon tip catheters and stents led to the introduction of PCI, another approach, coronary artery bypass grafting (CABG), was used. This is a far more resource intensive practice, requiring a technologically sophisticated surgical team, multiple specialists in several disciplines, and long periods of recovery in hospital and at home. PCI, on the other hand, involves non-surgical widening of the coronary artery using a balloon catheter to dilate the artery from within. A metallic stent, which may be either bare metal or drug-eluting, is usually placed in the artery after dilatation. This far simpler technique enables less expensive or specialised practitioners to treat more people with ischaemic heart disease in lower cost settings, i.e. not in advanced heart hospitals. PCI has spawned a new generation of clinical professionals, interventional cardiologists and radiologists, whose procedures require fewer days of inpatient hospitalisation and result in more rapid recovery.

Christensen *et al.* (2000) describe how PCI was initially used for only the easiest cases and was much less effective than surgery. Because of all the things it and its practitioners could not do, experts were sceptical about the procedure. But over time, in classic disruptive innovation style, the procedure improved. Sustaining technological innovations and the increasing skill and experience of practitioners meant that PCI began to supplant CABG in many cases, and it can now be performed in stand-alone cardiac care centres, not burdened with the high overheads of large hospitals.

While this can clearly be seen as an example of disruptive innovation in healthcare, the economics of PCI are in fact less straightforward than implied in Christensen *et al.*'s paper. Its success has generated high demand, which may have led to greater overall healthcare costs than if it had not been introduced: the 'market' has been extended as more patients can be treated than previously (see Chapter 3, p. 83). And over a five-year period, there may be evidence that medical treatment alone is more cost effective than CABG, and CABG is more cost-effective than PCI (D'Oliveira Vieira *et al.*, 2012). Nevertheless, Christensen *et al.*'s point is well-made — by enabling less expensive practitioners to treat ischaemic heart disease in less costly settings, PCI has disrupted the conventional treatment model without compromising quality.

Sources: Christensen *et al.* (2000), D'Oliveira Vieira *et al.* (2012).

What do disruptive innovations in advanced health systems look like?

The quote to the right sums up the typical perspective on disruptive innovation. By using a range of new technological and business model innovations, the 21st century challenges of healthcare systems in developed countries can be tackled. The reality is rather more nuanced, as we will see.

In the UK, the NHS Confederation (2008) published a report on the potential disruptive innovations which are most likely to have a significant impact on the way health services will evolve over a 10–15 year time horizon, drawing on the views of a range of experts inside and outside the NHS. The report's position was that healthcare needs to leapfrog from a 'pre-industrial', craft-based model to become a post-industrial personal service. Part of this process

"The enabling disruptive technologies and business models that can help drive down health care costs are fairly well understood. Retail clinics, telemedicine, single organ hospitals, surgical robots, medical tourism, and personalized medicine are just a few of the disruptive health care models that hold tremendous promise for breaking traditional price and performance trade-offs in this sector. Virtual patient visits, for example, can cut costs by one-fourth."
(Eggers *et al.*, 2013)

could involve new entrants offering potentially disruptive services in new settings. The report argued that disruptive innovations are likely to appear from unexpected directions and from outside the mainstream (see Box 6.6).

The experts discussed a number of technological innovations. One area where they agreed considerable disruption was possible is diagnostics. The trend toward decreasing equipment costs and size, dramatic improvements in image quality, and reductions in the use of ionising radiation received by patients are all broadening the availability of imaging. The experts also identified similar opportunities in other forms of diagnostics. The use of novel small-scale analytical technology — the 'lab on a chip' — and synthetic biology are behind moves towards adoption of a wide range of 'point-of-care tests' (POCT) (see Box 6.7). These can be conducted in the patient's home, at the hospital bedside or in the GP surgery, and provide more rapid diagnosis or decision-making. We describe this trend in more detail below.

Box 6.6 BACKGROUND: The NHS Confederation's perspective on disruptive innovation in healthcare

'People have often talked about the need to industrialise healthcare. This would be a mistake. The interaction of patient with an individual who is entirely focused on their needs does not fit well the industrial paradigm. Healthcare needs to leapfrog from a pre-industrial approach to a post-industrial personal service providing care, support and knowledge, along with the personal interaction that makes it special. Key to this is for organisations to become very adept at generating and handling information, expert at knowledge management and open to new ways of patients, the public and staff using technology. This opens up the potential for new market entrants providing very different services in new settings — web, phone and retail settings would all expand as delivery mechanisms. This has potential to create a fundamental shift in the relationship between patients and the system.'

Source: NHS Confederation (2008).

Box 6.7 BACKGROUND: Several technology innovation trends are reshaping diagnostics and imaging

- Imaging technologies: smaller-scale equipment allowing localised use, including ultrasound, basic X-ray, bone densitrometry and ECG. Some areas, such as chest X-ray, still require 'big technology' and are unlikely to move to localised use. CT, MRI, and PET scanning are also unlikely to see much movement to localised use in the next 10 years, although small bore MRI will replace some X-ray use.
- Pathologic technologies: analysis of tissue and fluid samples by portable equipment. Some interpretation is done locally (i.e. by the device) and some sent to an interpretation service.
- Physiological diagnostics: better ways of monitoring vital signs through telehealth.

But the NHS Confederation report also raised two questions. First, they were cautious about claims that new diagnostic technology will replace existing approaches rather than adding to them. In other words, expanding the market — in classic disruptive innovation terms — and potentially increasing overall costs to the healthcare system. Second, as the report put it, developing novel forms of diagnostics and imaging 'will be pointless if the rest of the system is not redesigned to respond.' A key area for attention is the creation of new pathways to support the delivery of healthcare in the wider community as far as possible, with only the more specialised elements, access to multi-specialist teams and high technology equipment provided in centralised locations. The report suggested that three forces are coming together to facilitate this:

- People increasingly want access to a wider range of higher quality healthcare services closer to where they live and work — they are less willing to travel to where it suits the system to provide them.
- This demand is being reinforced by consistent policy statements in the UK and elsewhere about the need to take services out of larger hospitals and provide them in the community. For large hospitals, decentralising services to satellite settings has the potential advantage of helping to reduce expensive fixed costs, while at the same time maintaining a revenue flow from the treatment of patients. The trend towards concentration of certain specialist services coupled with decentralisation of follow-up treatment has happened in stroke care, with acute care provided in specialist centres and rehabilitation provided locally. Community provision of cancer care is also increasing, with follow-on chemotherapy being delivered in local settings or the home.
- The introduction of progressively less invasive clinical treatments and diagnostic procedures described above mean that doctors do not need to work in specialist settings. It is increasingly safe and acceptable for diagnostic tests and some acute clinical treatments to be delivered outside large hospitals, even in mobile facilities. The digitalisation of pathology and imaging means that patients do not need to travel to hospitals for the majority of their diagnostic tests, which can be administered locally and the results read and interpreted anywhere.

We are already beginning to see the impact of this technology, with the decentralisation of patient access to some diagnostic services and centralisation of processing, analysis and interpretation. Together, these trends are beginning to reshape the organisational and physical infrastructure for health services in developed countries' health systems.

Point of care testing and imaging — a technological driver of disruptive innovation?

The goal of diagnostics innovation is to improve convenience for patients and clinicians, and deliver high predictability in results within time limits — to combine the convenience of single visits (or access to care closer to home) and same-day results, with high quality interpretation. Point-of-care testing or imaging is a way of delivering the result of a medical test closer to the point in the care pathway where and when clinical decisions are made. For example, diagnosis of heart failure can be hampered by limited access to timely ECG, considered the gold standard of diagnosis. Raised levels of natriuretic peptides have been shown to be a sensitive indicator of heart failure in untreated patients and a predictor of the prognosis for patients with coronary artery disease. In the UK, NICE guidance recommends testing natriuretic peptides in combination with clinical assessment and ECG to rule out heart failure and prioritise those who need urgent ECG. This is driving research into the possibility of a POCT for brain natriuretic peptides.

There are essentially three different types of POCT: they can be used for patient triage, as a replacement for existing tests, or as an addition to existing tests (Bossuyt, 2006). Some types of POCT can be seen as disruptive innovations because they potentially replace high cost, high functionality laboratory testing equipment operated by skilled laboratory technicians, with simpler and cheaper equipment used by nurses, healthcare assistants, paramedics and doctors (see Innovation in Action 6.2), or by patients themselves. Although the quality typically improves over time, POCT may initially provide slightly reduced functionality. However, doctors may be prepared to trade-off slightly less accurate results against improved convenience and speedier decisions. This represents a disruptive innovation in relation to skills required of diagnostics staff and the infrastructure required for a diagnostics service, since POCT enables tests to be conducted outside conventional healthcare settings.

INNOVATION IN ACTION 6.2:   iKnife — disruption in the operating theatre and pathology lab?

iKnife is a diagnostic tool to enable surgeons to rapidly identify whether tissue that is been removed from a patient during an operation is cancerous or not. The surgeon normally takes out the tumour and a surrounding margin of healthy tissue. Because it is often impossible to identify cancerous cells by the naked eye, the tissue is sent to a pathology laboratory for examination while the patient remains under general anaesthetic. This could take up to two hours for results to be available. The iKnife aims to provide this information much faster, and possibly within minutes. In doing so, it represents a disruptive innovation for pathology laboratories.

iKnife uses previous developed technologies that are combined together to create a new concept. These are electrosurgery and mass spectrometry, the analysis of chemicals that are present in a sample. Both these technologies date back many years — electrosurgery was developed in the 1920s and mass spectrometers were developed in the early 20th century. Electrosurgery knives use an electrical current to rapidly heat tissue, cutting through it while minimising blood loss. As this happens, tissue is vaporised, creating smoke that is normally sucked away by extraction systems. The inventor of the iKnife, Dr Zoltan Takats of Imperial College London, realised that this smoke would be a rich source of biological information if an electrosurgical knife was connected to a mass spectrometer. Different cells produce different types of metabolites in different concentrations, revealing information about the state of that tissue. The iKnife works by matching its readings during surgery to a growing reference library of the characteristics of thousands of cancerous and non-cancerous tissues to determine what type of tissue is being cut. The results can be provided in less than three seconds. The tissue type identified by the iKnife in 91 different tests matched the post-operative diagnosis based on traditional methods. Further trials are planned to see whether giving surgeons real time access to the iKnife's analysis can improve patients' outcomes. Other potential applications of the iKnife include the identification of tissue with inadequate blood supply or types of bacteria present in the tissue.

Source: http://www3.imperial.ac.uk/newsandeventspggrp/imperialcollege/newssummary/news_17-7-2013-17-17-32#comments

For the health system, POCT potentially reduces the number of steps in the care pathway (although it may increase steps if the outcome is to send patients for more invasive or expensive tests). It improves process efficiency through speed of delivery of results, and the effectiveness of clinical decision-making because there is an immediacy of dialogue between the patient and healthcare professional. However, there are important economic considerations related to the increasing ease of diagnostic testing and imaging and the effects of this on overall healthcare budgets. As we saw in Chapter 3, technological innovation in healthcare can increase costs because it grows capacity and allows 'more healthcare' to be delivered — hitherto untreatable patients can be treated, previously undiagnosed problems are picked up and so on. One concern is therefore that POCT extends the range of patients who can be tested, increasing demand overall (e.g. Frey, 2010). Demand on health services is also shifting because new POCT markets are emerging in the form of a general public increasingly prepared to purchase self-testing devices for cholesterol, blood glucose, pregnancy and HIV (Box 6.8). While self-testing has the potential to take some demand from formal healthcare

---

Box 6.8   BACKGROUND: 'Test at home, treat online'

QuickCheck Health, has produced a 'retail clinic in a box', an over-the-counter device for home testing. This is all about home diagnostics, supported by a virtual online visit by someone who can interpret the test for you — a 'test at home, treat online' approach. The company has now created 17 rapid tests. The initial market is the USA and the target price for the home test is USD 15 with an optional USD 35 online clinic visit, shared between the provider and QuickCheck. The applicability of these solutions as disruptive innovations for developed healthcare systems is considerable. QuickCheck Health is targeting *streptococcus* throat infection in the USA, where 40 million *streptococcus* tests — 80% of which prove negative — are carried out annually at huge cost. In the UK, Babylon Health offers a 'GP in your pocket' with unlimited online consultations for a subscription of GBP 10 a month. A wide range of tests can be ordered online with the test kits delivered to the customer's home. In early 2016, Babylon Health raised USD 25 million in funding, the highest so far for a digital health venture in Europe.

services, at least a proportion of people conducting their own tests may subsequently seek a second opinion for reassurance or a follow-up consultation from a doctor or nurse. The possible escalation in costs arising from greater use of diagnostics is therefore a concern, but the issues are not straightforward. A key cost benefit question is what are the best outcome measures — how do we weigh up convenience, safety, quality and cost? The answer to this depends on very much on the circumstance and context for using POCT, described in Table 6.1.

Diagnostics procedures can sometimes shift their location to a less expensive context in the community without the introduction of technological innovation, but there are limits to the extent to which a procedure can be widely diffused into community settings. In the case of endoscopy, a minimum amount of equipment and space is needed, along with critical mass in terms of patient numbers. Mobile community endoscopy units are an option, providing equipment can be decontaminated after use. Critical mass remains a constraining factor on distributing the procedure across the community, but mobile units can be found in some east Asian countries where the incidence of gastric cancer is higher than Europe. The experience of community endoscopy in France ended when new regulations on decontamination and increased costs led to units closing. Until a different approach emerges, driven by development of new biomarkers and POCT technology, endoscopy is likely to remain a hospital-based procedure.

In general, though, the future trend in diagnostics is pointing towards far more tests conducted outside hospitals, as technological innovations support changes in practices and new service models. As well as POCT, cheaper, more portable ultrasound is an area where the technology is evolving fast and driving changes in practice. Other important technological enablers of new approaches to diagnostics include machine interpretation of results using carefully designed protocols, along with follow-up remote consultation by experts via telemedicine. The latter may already be leading to a changing relationship between GPs and specialists — through their involvement in regular remote consultations with experts, GPs may improve their knowledge in particular fields of medicine and their ability to manage a higher degree of complexity in their patients (MacFarlane *et al.*, 2006; Cravo Oliveira *et al.*, 2015). Other potential

Table 6.1. The economic implications of point-of-care testing.

Largely cost increasing	Unclear — depends on the context	Largely cost reducing
How those administering the tests are reimbursed may be important.	*Different types of test will have different productivity and efficiency implications for the rest of health services.*	When coupled with better decision-support systems, the introduction of POCT could help to identify when further testing or imaging is appropriate, so addressing concerns about the economic impact of increased demand.
Reimbursement per test may encourage inappropriate use or overuse, which can be mitigated by ensuring payment is only made when the test is performed according to clinical guidelines.	Does improved access to tests increase convenience and improve productivity in other areas, perhaps through reducing hospital length of stay due to rapid access to test results? The financial impact depends in part on whether finance for POCT comes from the same purse that sees the financial benefits.	It could also aid disease prediction and population risk stratification, eventually taking some demand out of the overall health system.
	There may be financial implications in shifting from the old diagnostics model to a new one.	
	An important consideration is the cost of decommissioning the old approach, including the impact on the existing workforce or previous capital investment in pathology laboratories.	
	The prevalence of the disease or condition will influence the configuration of infrastructure needed for testing, i.e. whether tests carried out in a GP surgery, a specialised diagnostics centre or by the patient him or herself (see section on the implications of disruptive innovation for healthcare infrastructure and Box 6.10).	

The overall incidence of a medical condition and speed of its progression will affect the way overall demand arises from introduction of a POCT.

Demand may be influenced by whether the test is for monitoring people who have already been diagnosed with the condition or for *de novo* screening, designed to identify or rule-out particular conditions in symptomatic patients. The latter may pick up large numbers of hitherto undiagnosed cases, resulting in increased treatment costs while the former may result in better disease management and reduced interactions with the health system.

changes in GP practice include more pre-testing before patients go to outpatients so all the key decisions are made at that point, and bundling together tests and consultations in 'one-stop shops'. Although some feel these are more expensive for healthcare providers, the benefits to the patient and for the wider economy are greater because patients spend less time off work. The latter is one factor behind the introduction of 'retail clinics' in the USA, one of Christensen *et al.*'s original examples. The story of what happened to MinuteClinic demonstrates how a disruptive innovation can itself be disrupted (see Innovation in Action 6.3).

Technological drivers of disruptive innovation — does the concept hold for the drug industry?

We have described how technological innovation in medical devices, especially point-of-care-testing, has a potentially disruptive effect on healthcare services. But does the concept of disruptive innovation hold within the pharmaceutical sector. Do the features discussed earlier in the chapter still apply when it comes to drug development?

In the longer term, the development of new drugs targeting complex conditions and co-morbidities could disrupt parts of the healthcare system such as the location and nature of services. For example, drugs that stave off the onset of chronic conditions like type II diabetes might have a significant impact on primary and secondary care in terms of the kinds of health service these patients need and on costs across the overall health system. Of course, this depends on the cost of the drugs compared to alternative approaches to treatment and care. A more immediate question is whether we can see the rise in use of generic drugs as a form of disruptive innovation. In some ways, generics display some of the attributes of disruptive innovation:

- They are certainly cheaper than brand alternatives, and therefore potentially expand the market, although they are not a 'simpler' or only 'good enough' product.
- Generic drugs attack branded drugs that come off patent through lower prices. In these respects, then, they meet Christensen and

INNOVATION IN ACTION 6.3: The story of retail clinics in the USA

What made MinuteClinic disruptive was its business model. Nurse practitioners diagnose and treat the routine conditions that make up the bulk of primary care in locations that are convenient for people's lifestyle, like a kiosk in a retail store. MinuteClinic visits were said to be 30% to 50% cheaper than a visit to a primary care clinic, with very high user satisfaction. The model spread to those US states where nurse practitioners were allowed to write prescriptions for generic drugs that could then be obtained from the same store. As a new business model, however, retail clinics represented a threat to traditional healthcare providers, simultaneously taking away higher-volume, lower-complexity transactions and also helping to reveal the real costs of the more complicated and expensive low-volume transactions which were previously cross-subsidised (Eggers *et al.*, 2013). Subsequently, MinuteClinic was itself disrupted. The story is described by Ron Hammerle, of Florida-based Health Resources Ltd., which works with retail and employer-based clinics to connect them via telemedicine systems with medical centres:

'When Clayton Christensen first anticipated that retail clinics would be disruptive to the established healthcare industry, their business model was potentially disruptive. What has subsequently happened, however, is a prime example of how potentially disruptive movements can be sidetracked. After acquiring MinuteClinic and laying the foundation for taking retail clinics national, CVS Caremark chose to make deals with hospitals, which could easily afford to rent, open and operate such clinics without making money on the front end or facing real disruption. Retail clinics were a loss leader to hospitals in exchange for large, downstream revenues, and slightly-enhanced market share for the retailer's pharmacy. After CVS surprised Walgreens with acquisitions of MinuteClinic and Caremark, Walgreens responded:

1. They doubled the number of their clinics (to 700) in less than two years, thwarted AMA opposition, leapfrogged ahead of CVS in numbers of clinics and totally changed the retail clinic model by setting up employer-based clinics, below the political radar, providing a broader range of services and making profits upfront.

(Continued)

INNOVATION IN ACTION 6.3:   (*Continued*)

2. They began upgrading the design, product mix and customer experience in their clinics, becoming more professional and moving closer to becoming a regular consumer destination, although still lacking what supermarket-based clinics could offer.
3. Walgreens went global with the Alliance Boots acquisition, laying the groundwork — and beating Walmart — for a potential, global supply and service chain.

In the USA, however, Walgreens made peace with hospitals, in exchange for permission to pick up medication management before in-patients ever left the hospital. Walmart, Target, Kroger and Safeway have all stumbled with retail clinics, despite having a core business (with food) that sits at the fulcrum of managing, preventing and treating the three biggest chronic diseases in the world. So, who is left as potential disruptors? "StealthCare" companies with the size and market cloud of Walmart, Amazon, Google and Apple, to challenge big, status quo, players with technologies, market-based purchasing and global sourcing, and less than a handful of telehealth players. It remains to be seen if "disruptive innovation" can come from giants instead of ants.'

CVS is now keen to develop telehealth services and combine these with MinuteClinic, so customers can be provided with direct access to online consultations with a doctor. As well as the need to continue innovating the MinuteClinic offer, the move is driven by CVS' expectation of increased demand because of the Affordable Care Act, the ageing population and a projected physician shortage, as well as the need to replace a USD 2 billion revenue hole following its decision to stop the sale of cigarettes (Rupp, 2015).

Sources: Cusano (2014), Eggers *et al.* (2013) and other sources.

Raynor's criteria for disruption (Box 6.1). They have the potential for new-market and low-end disruption, at least in some parts of the world. But they are not a new technology or service. They are simply free of the burden of the sunk cost of R&D of the original inventors or owners of the IP. Nor are they necessarily disruptive to incumbent drug companies. While there are a growing number of generics and biosimilars producers, there is no reason why incumbent drug firms should not cut their costs in an aggressive way. Novartis, GSK, Merck and Sanofi are all examples of incumbents who have successfully switched part of their business to the production and marketing of generic drugs (Markides, 2012).

* A feature of the original disruptive innovation concept is the emergence of incremental/sustaining innovation in the disrupting technology, something that can now be seen in the generic industry's moves towards 'super-generics'. These are added-value generics, new therapeutic entities or hybrids which offer improvements to the formulation of the original product or its method of delivery. Thus the generics industry is itself becoming a generator of innovation, using new technology platforms to produce new innovative products, and seeking to achieve competitive advantages over their rivals.

The growth in the development and consumption of generic drugs is undeniably a very important factor behind the evolution of the global biopharma sector. Whether it can be described as a disruptive innovation is a moot point.

Disruption and healthcare infrastructure

The impact of technological innovation is having a disruptive effect on the overall landscape of healthcare built infrastructure — the distribution of different types of building and facilities required to deliver healthcare. Clayton Christensen and colleagues' *Harvard Business School* paper alluded to the way new models of healthcare delivery, including those initiated by disruptive innovation, were beginning to impact on where healthcare is delivered (Christensen *et al.*, 2000). They explained how patients who once occupied hospital beds can now be treated in different environments, such as more focused care centres and outpatient clinics, GP surgeries or in their own homes. This was captured in the graphic shown in Figure 6.4. Teaching hospitals, as Christensen *et al.* describe it, 'incur great costs to develop the ability to treat difficult, intractable illnesses at the high end. In the process, they

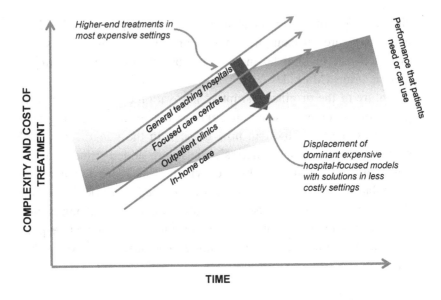

Figure 6.4.   Disruptive innovation impact on healthcare institutions.
Source: Christensen *et al.* (2000).

have come to overserve the needs of the much larger population of patients whose disorders are becoming more and more routine'.

However, the interaction between healthcare services, technologies and built infrastructure is complex. Changes in one element can lead to unpredictable or highly lagged effects on the others. The mix of evolving demographic, social, policy and technological factors is certainly beginning to reshape the future healthcare built environment in the UK, USA and other countries, but the picture is not quite as straightforward as a simple decentralisation of services from high cost teaching hospitals into the community. As well the effects of technological innovation, other trends are at play. Parallel to a movement towards decentralisation, *centralisation* is also taking place. This is both stripping out straightforward elective work such as knee replacement surgery into

→*Coxa Hospital, described in Chapter 5 and Box 5.12 is an example of the concentration of surgery into specialised centres in a developed health system. We discuss Indian examples later in this chapter*

efficient specialised centres and at the same time concentrating more complex procedures in leading teaching hospitals. These include services like stroke, trauma, transplant and highly specialist surgery such as children's heart surgery, where there is evidence for a causal link between the volume and clinical outcomes. This is because there are clinical benefits in concentrating services in locations which carry out a sufficient volume of procedures for team and individual learning to occur and quality of care to improve (Spurgeon *et al.*, 2010). For other conditions, however, the size threshold for quality improvement can be low (Glanville *et al.*, 2010) or there is no clear causal link. In these cases, other factors can be equally important, such as ratios of nurses to patients (Friese *et al.*, 2008) and the capacity to provide 24/7 junior and senior medical cover, hospital system resources (Bellal *et al.*, 2009) or compliance with guidelines and degree of knowledge transfer (Schell *et al.*, 2008).

When considering how to reconfigure services, healthcare planners and managers find themselves faced with the task of trying to optimise across four interlinked elements: quality and safety, cost, access, and workforce. This is challenging because of the complex trade-offs and inter-dependencies that exist between these elements:

- How should we balance centralisation of services driven by technological innovation and policy considerations, with the ability of patients to easily access highly trained professionals and the most up-to-date diagnostic and other technologies?
- What is the trade-off between clinical quality and financial gains achievable through the concentration of services and the social costs to those who are more distantly located or elderly and poorer?

Having to travel long distances may be impractical or costly, and for some life-threatening conditions delay is linked to poorer patient outcomes (Nicholl *et al.*, 2007). However, the timing of the start of appropriate treatment is critical, so innovations in paramedic care, supported by technology such as telemedicine, or faster access to specialists once at the hospital can potentially mitigate this risk (Spurgeon *et al.*, 2010), as shown in the example of stroke care (see Case study 6.1).

CASE STUDY 6.1 Innovating to improve emergency stroke care

Acute ischaemic stroke accounts around 85–90% of all strokes. The risk of disability arising from an ischaemic stroke can be improved in some patients by intravenous administration of tissue plasminogen activator (tPA) to dissolve blood clots, a process also known as thrombolysis. This enables faster treatment and rehabilitation, which not only reduces the suffering of affected patients but also leads to lower healthcare and rehabilitation costs. However, there is a risk of potentially fatal secondary bleeding in the brain if tPA is given to patients with a haemorrhagic — rather than ischaemic — stroke. The type of stroke is determined by a brain scan. The window for administering tPA is 4.5 hours from onset of symptoms. The need for rapid intervention, coupled with the risk of wrongly administering tPA, means the stakes are high.

 Although tPA is the recommended treatment for acute stroke, thrombolysis rates are still low in many countries. A lack of timely access to CT or MRI equipment is a potentially significant factor influencing thrombolysis rates. An important question is where scanning equipment is located. Scanners sufficient for imaging in the acute phase are very expensive, especially when the costs of radiologists to interpret the scans and technicians to maintain the equipment are factored in. Scanning facilities are, therefore, located in larger hospitals or specialist stroke centres. Several different models exist for geographically distributing stroke services, each with pros and cons:

- Patients having a stroke are taken to the nearest hospital but stroke services may be coordinated on a regional basis. If travelling times are short, this can result in faster treatment. However, the quality of care received depends on the availability of stroke specialists and CT scanners, beds in the stroke unit, and out-of-hours cover available at the particular hospital at the time of the stroke.
- Patients may be taken to a specialist stroke centre for the acute phase, after which treatment and rehabilitation is given in a local general hospital or rehabilitation centre. In this model, travelling times might be too high for tPA to be administered in time, depending on where the stroke took place in relation to the hospital.

(Continued)

CASE STUDY 6.1 (*Continued*)

- Acute treatment is provided in the nearest general hospital, linked by telemedicine to a specialist stroke centre, which provides expert advice on the administration of tPA. Issues in this model include the availability of a CT scanner and out-of-hours cover in the local hospital, as well how to meet the needs of patients who require specialist care which cannot be delivered in the general hospital, even with telemedicine back-up.

So even where stroke centres are the norm and the principle that stroke is an emergency is well-established — as in the USA — there may still be problems over accessibility to scanners and thus timely and appropriate thrombolysis. Disruptive technological innovation to help tackle these problems this is possible:

- Work is going on to find ways of improving access to cheaper, but effective, scanning technology. The challenge is to enable a scan to be performed by a paramedic instead of a hospital radiology department and at the same time ensure that that performance is good enough for decision-making. A Swedish company, Medfield Diagnostics AB, is conducting trials of a portable microwave imaging device that facilitates diagnosis of stroke by differentiating bleeding patterns in the brain. In principle, field administration of thrombolytic drugs could also be possible. Thrombolysis can now be given to patients with myocardial infarction in a pre-hospital setting, providing no contraindications are present — previously this could only take place in an emergency department with a cardiologist present. Both these technological innovations can be seen as disruptive to existing models of acute stroke care, moving part of the care away from highest cost facilities and unbundling the tasks in the care pathway so that non-physician healthcare workers can accomplish some of them. As such, they have consequences for the workforce, especially for radiology and paramedics and for the regulatory requirements surrounding the administration of tPA. They also have possible implications for payment and reimbursement across different parts of health systems — who pays for which part of the care process and where do the benefits fall?

(*Continued*)

CASE STUDY 6.1   *(Continued)*

- Another area for technological innovation is mechanical clot retrieval after administration of thrombolysis. This shows potential to improve the chances of good outcomes in some patients if it is performed within six hours of stroke onset. If this novel treatment becomes mainstream for suitable patients, the benefits of streamlining and speeding up the pathways to thrombolysis would also increase, because the time window for bringing a patient to hospital is extended and more patients would be eligible for thrombolysis.

While these technological innovations offer potential benefits in acute stroke care, organisational changes could also make a significant difference. A study in Scotland modelled the potential effects of different organisational innovations to improve acute stroke care (Uzun Jacobson *et al.*, 2015). Given the geography of the country, meeting current guidelines for administering thrombolysis within 4.5 hours of the onset of stroke can be hard where the closest hospital with 24/7 availability of thrombolysis is distant.

By analysing the 2010 Scottish Stroke Care Audit data, covering almost all admitted stroke patients in Scotland, the researchers found that only a quarter of ischaemic stroke patients reached hospital within four hours of onset. Given further delays — perhaps up to 30 minutes — once patients arrive at hospital, those arriving after four hours are unlikely to be eligible for thrombolysis. It was also clear that there was considerable variation between hospitals in the speed and prioritisation of scans for stroke patients.

To address these problems, various organisational changes could be adopted. Patients could be transported to the nearest 24/7 hospital offering thrombolysis, or measures such as moving the physical location of CT scanners in relation to the emergency department could be taken to speed up scanning in hospitals offering tPA. The researchers compared two different scenarios with the current (base) case:

- In one — felt by local experts to be achievable — it was assumed that every hospital installs telemedicine to access a stroke specialist 24/7, who can review symptoms, interpret scans and recommend thrombolysis if appropriate. Hospitals also implement measures to speed up scanning so that they achieve the *average* performance of all 24/7 hospitals. This is achieved by introducing clear and fast protocols to carry out scans. Under

(Continued)

CASE STUDY 6.1 *(Continued)*

this scenario around 25% more patients would be thrombolysed relative to the current position.

- The second scenario assumed that all hospitals achieved the speed of the current *best* performing Scottish hospital in managing the arrival to scan process, as well as having 24/7 thrombolysis provision. This represented an upper limit on how far the thrombolysis rate could be improved by optimising hospital processes. Compared to the first scenario, 50% more patients would be thrombolysed. Almost twice as many patients would be thrombolysed compared to the base case. However, it was recognised that achieving such a streamlined process was likely to be more ambitious than can realistically be achieved, given available resources, and the expedited scanning/expansion of telemedicine scenario was more achievable.

What this case shows is that a wide range of technological and organisational innovations could be developed to improve access to thrombolysis. There is no single 'magic bullet'. As well as the disruptive technology described above, which remains in development, other organisational options could deliver significant improvements to the current situation. These are the kind of decisions health policy makers and health service managers need to make, juggling them with demands of patients and the public, and against a backdrop of changing performance of the underlying technologies.

Question for discussion:

- 'Given the increasing burden placed by stroke on society, we should not miss the opportunities to embrace the emerging technological innovations in the diagnosis and treatment of stroke'. Imagine you have to prepare a report advising a minister of health about the restructuring stroke care services in the medium term (5–10 years). What would your advice be?
- Think about the workforce consequences of the innovations described in the case study, for example for radiology, paramedics and clinicians. What about the possible impact on the system of payment and reimbursement for stroke procedures, and who gains and who loses? What might be the implications for healthcare organisations, such as where to locate new field based solutions?

Sources: Draws partly on Uzun Jacobson *et al.* (2015) and work carried out with Stan Finkelstein, Henry Feldman and Steffen Bayer.

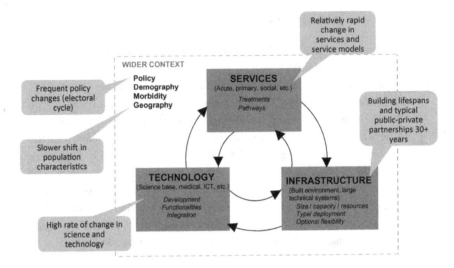

Figure 6.5.   Key elements and dynamics of the healthcare infrastructure system.
Source: Barlow and Köberle-Gaiser (2009).

Forming a backdrop to these challenges are the complex relationships resulting from different cycle times for changes in the technologies, infrastructure and services associated with healthcare. These range from long lasting built infrastructure (i.e. typically 30–50 years), through a more rapidly changing policy context, to frequently changing technologies (see Figure 6.5). The reconfiguration of health services — and ensuing impact on the healthcare infrastructure — is likely to accelerate as remote monitoring technologies (telecare or telehealth) and new diagnostic and imaging tools become embedded as part of health systems. But how this plays out will depend very much on the specific circumstances of a country's health system. In the UK, it is the local general hospitals, rather than large teaching hospitals, that are experiencing the greatest pressure to change. The diversion of services into community settings presents an opportunity to rethink how best to create more responsive and accessible services. But it also raises questions about the future of local general hospitals. These lie directly on a fault line arising from the general reconfiguration of services from acute to community settings, on the one hand, and the centralisation of emergency and specialist services on the other hand (see Figure 6.6). The impact can be seen in the changing number and type of hospital beds in the UK (Box 6.9).

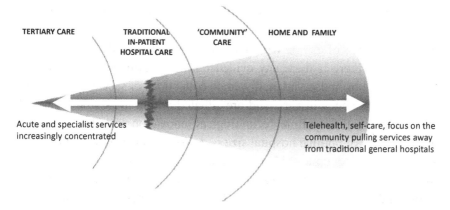

Figure 6.6. An emerging fault-line in the healthcare infrastructure system?

Box 6.9   BACKGROUND: Changing hospital bed numbers in the UK

In the UK, the shift of services out of acute hospitals has been played out over many years, with a significant impact on the role and character of the acute and general hospital. Since its inception in 1948, the number NHS acute hospitals has fallen by 85% and the number of sites where highly specialist care is delivered has fallen even further. During this time the average size of a hospital grew from 68 beds to just over 400 (Imison, 2011). General acute care was delivered in around 200 hospitals in 2011. The trend has been particularly marked since the late 1980s — the total number of general and acute hospital beds for specialties (excluding day beds) fell from 300,000 (1987–1988) to 136,000 (2013–2014) in the NHS in England. During this time, the number of day beds grew from 2,000 to almost 12,000 by 2013–2014 (1). This has partly been driven by the fact that most routine surgery is now undertaken as day surgery. The mean length of stay in hospital fell from 7.9 days (2002/2003) to 5.3 days (2011/2012), with the median length of stay now one day [2].

[1] http://www.england.nhs.uk/statistics/statistical-work-areas/bed-availability-and-occupancy/bed-data-overnight/

[2] http://www.nuffieldtrust.org.uk/data-and-charts/length-stay-hospital-england

Source: Imison (2011).

So how far might these trends take us — what might the future local general hospital look like? There is no one size fits all model for such a hospital in terms of its role within a local care system or design characteristics, nor is there is there any evidence on the optimal size of hospital services — 'hospitals' contain disparate collections of services, each with their own efficiency drivers, and are situated within a specific local and national context. Over time, technological innovation will also impact on any estimates of optimal hospital size — a study published in 1998, which suggested the economic evidence for closing small hospitals was poor, but the merger of some services could improve quality and save money (Normand, 1998), might well come to different conclusions if published today.

While the detailed prescription for a future local general hospital may not be possible, we can still identify broad areas where technological innovation in care services can be combined around local hospital services. There is a clear role for the general hospital as a facility for local, more accessible health services including certain diagnostics and imaging, minor injuries treatment and day case procedures (Box 6.10). These

---

Box 6.10 CONCEPTS: Designing the infrastructure for point-of-care-testing (POCT)

Broadly, low risk and high-volume procedures should be delivered as close to the patient as economically reasonable. The more there is at stake and the smaller the number of patients that need testing at any given time, the more the service should be concentrated geographically and/or conducted by specialists. In some cases, multiple diagnostic skills may be needed, such as diabetes, where eye and blood tests, and examination of feet all form part of the diagnostic process. These considerations imply a move from single task-oriented practitioners to diagnostic experts located in some form of community hub — perhaps a local general hospital — providing interpretation and advice. In other cases, however, the skill is 'in the device', meaning that the healthcare professional — doctor, nurse or other practitioner — can make the diagnosis without recourse to interpretation by diagnostics experts. Or the test may be so simple that the individual patient and their home or place of work is the hub, since self-testing and diagnosis is possible.

hospitals could also represent an important node in the bundle of services designed to enable older people to remain in their own homes. A large proportion of admissions to residential and nursing homes are direct from hospital. With recuperation and rehabilitation, suitable links with social care and adequate availability and funding, many older people could regain enough of their mobility and daily living skills to return home. There is, therefore, a role for the smaller hospital as a rehabilitation facility where older people's long-term care needs can be properly assessed and appropriate packages of telehealth and telecare introduced. This type of model is already well established in some areas. In Northern Ireland, a major transformation programme involving organisational, infrastructure and technological redesign has put in been put in place (see Innovation in Action 6.4).

The other area where infrastructure needs to adapt to healthcare trends is the home itself. This is becoming part of the healthcare infrastructure as hospitals begin to experiment with ideas of 'virtual wards' and telecare/telehealth potentially allow frailer elderly people to live at home, when previously they might have moved into residential care. An early example for a virtual hospital ward was set-up in 2006 by Croydon, a London borough. Around 2,600 patients with a long-term condition and two or more emergency admissions per year were identified and a ward with 100 'virtual beds' (i.e. at patients' homes) was established. The ward processes and staff were similar to those in an acute hospital, with a team which included GPs. Local hospitals, GPs and NHS Direct (the national NHS telephone advice and triage system) were all made aware of patients in the system. 'Beds' in the virtual ward were allocated to patients with the highest risk of admission; if they exceeded a given risk level, they were admitted to the 'real', physical hospital. Evidence of the benefits was mixed. One review comparing the Croydon and two other virtual ward examples with a control group of patient found no evidence of reductions in emergency admissions, ambulatory care admissions or hospital costs; there was however a slight reduction in elective admissions and outpatient attendances, possibly due to greater co-ordination of care (Lewis *et al.*, 2013).

The shift of care from hospitals and other formal settings is beginning to challenge preconceived notions of what type of housing provision is appropriate for people's varying care needs. Remote care can reduce the

---

INNOVATION IN ACTION 6.4:   Northern Ireland's care transformation programme

Northern Ireland has a population of approximately 1.8 million, of whom about 500,000 live in the Belfast area. To tackle the problems of rising demand and constrained resources, the government decided to start a radical transformation programme, taking advantage of emerging technologies such as telehealth and new diagnostics (Northern Ireland Health and Social Care Board, 2011).

It was especially important to rationalise the hospital sector, where 20 hospitals were providing acute services for a relatively small population. Over time, there was a graduated process of closing acute services in some hospitals. Others were reconfigured as community hospitals, and there are some new community hospitals. There are also two teaching hospitals. Northern Ireland is therefore moving towards a system of local health and wellbeing centres, which are vertically integrated with regional acute and community hospitals, and which deliver horizontally integrated health and social services.

From the outset, technology was seen as a key enabler. Northern Ireland already provided an extensive telemedicine and telehealth service. The number of users was set to grow tenfold over a five-year period. Organisational change was essential. As well as the replacement of 20 NHS trusts by five new trusts, the CEOs were given new responsibilities for delivering the full range of hospital, community and mental health services within their locality. To help facilitate fully integrated care between the various care services, 17 networked teams (integrated care partnerships) were established, based around localities with around 100,000 people and 25–30 GP practices. These are collaborative networks bringing together doctors, nurses, pharmacists, social workers, hospital specialists, other healthcare professionals and the voluntary and community sectors, as well as service users and carers.

Inevitably, problems were encountered in implementing the programme. As well as the problems of funding the transition to the new model of care and difficulties of sharing records across the acute, community and primary care sectors, the organisational cultures of the health and social care systems posed challenges. Changing old working cultures, redesigning roles, facilitating integration between professional groups and staff development required considerable effort. Some hospital staff were reluctant to do more of their work outside

(Continued)

INNOVATION IN ACTION 6.4: *(Continued)*

the hospital setting and possibly lose some of the collegiate feeling. Some GPs were unwilling to take on more extensive roles and continued to see themselves as independent operators. These challenges were tackled by using pilots to show what could be done, appointing clinical champions, and nurturing GP leaders who were willing to seize the new opportunities. Extensive public consultation was also needed to allay the fears of local residents about downgrading their local hospital.

Source: With thanks to Professor John Cole, former Deputy Permanent Secretary, Department of Health Social Services and Public Safety, Northern Ireland.

demand for residential home accommodation as people's care needs change or at least delay the point at which they have to move from their home (Barlow *et al.*, 2007; Barlow and Venables, 2004). The mainstream housing stock will, therefore, become an increasingly significant part of the care system, but it needs to be fit for purpose. Measures to improve the physical quality of the mainstream housing stock such as improvements to disabled access or thermal efficiency will need to become part of the care package, posing questions about the cost of upgrading and adapting the housing stock and whose budget this comes out of.

Access to healthcare in lower income countries — disruptive or frugal innovation?

The introduction of disruptive innovation within the complex and high cost health systems of advanced economies is very much about doing more for less — coping with the escalating demands of an ageing population at a time of increasingly constrained financial resources. Viewed from the perspective of lower income countries, the challenges are more about delivering affordable healthcare to as many people as possible, and in some cases providing the poorest people with the most basic services and infrastructure. In doing so, is it possible to avoid replicating, the high cost hospital-centric models of developed countries? Can we leapfrog

20th century approaches to create wholly new models? And do disruptive innovations developed for a more resource-poor context offer lessons for healthcare provision in developed countries?

The healthcare challenges of lower income countries are well known and do not need to be discussed in detail here. The previous UN Millennium Development Goals, and the new Sustainable Development Goals, include the dominant health problems faced by low-income countries, as well

> ➜ *See Chapter 1 for details of the major global health challenges requiring innovative thinking*

as various social and environmental challenges with health implications such as climate change and urbanisation. So where does the disruptive innovation concept fit into this landscape? Part of this agenda is about tackling health problems by increasing access to healthcare resources and infrastructure in an affordable and effective way. Figure 6.7 redraws the Christensen *et al.* (2000) description of disruptive innovation in a developed health system and translates it to a developing health system context.

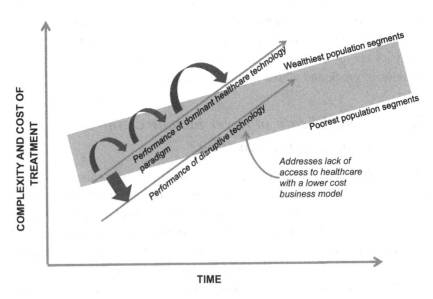

Figure 6.7.   Disruptive innovation concept applied to resource-poor health systems.

This shows that the wealthiest population groups already have good access, often to world-class facilities and care. The performance of this part of the health system improves slowly over time, driven by the same trends in technological innovation found in developed countries, with people treated in high quality hospitals. But bringing the rest of the population into the system requires new thinking — disruptive innovation — to address the lack of access to healthcare for poorer populations (Petrick and Juntiwasarakij, 2011). This may not deliver the same performance standards as the best healthcare services, but it is still regarded as good enough to provide an adequate level of care, certainly when the alternative may be rudimentary at best.

The task of creating innovative low cost healthcare business models for developing health systems was tackled by Prahalad (2006). He starts by asking the question 'what should healthcare innovation deliver in developing countries?' He uses the concept of an innovation 'sandbox', a play pit in which to experiment with different business models for healthcare delivery. Around the edges of the sandbox is a set of constraints which influence the way in which we experiment with new business models. Nothing about these constraints is fixed, however, and a different set might be more appropriate in another context. In the case of Indian healthcare, Prahalad argues that new business models must deliver a set of goals:

- They must result in a product/service of world-class quality.
- High performance level: they must result in a significant price reduction compared to equivalent in a developed economy.
- They must be scalable: produced, marketable and usable in many locales and circumstances.
- Universal access: they must be affordable at the bottom of the socio-economic pyramid.

Within these constraints, there is much scope for innovative thinking in healthcare business models, described in Table 6.2. Using examples of healthcare delivery from India, Prahalad outlines a number of areas where business model innovations have been applied to radically improve the

Table 6.2. The scope for innovative thinking.

Innovation area	Features
Specialisation	Optimise resources, build expertise, build a brand
Pricing	Cost ceiling drives process innovation
Capital intensity	Only purchase relevant equipment, pay higher fixed costs to reduce variable costs
Leverage talent	Focus on skills rather than credentials
Workflow	Process design is critical
Customer acquisition	Volume needed to drive down costs/patient
Values and organisational culture	Deeply held values, direction, motivation

Source: Prahalad (2006).

delivery of health services. He describes examples of innovative health-care business models which fulfil the goals within the constraints he sets, notably the specialist hospitals NH (Narayana Health) and Aravind (see Innovation in Action 6.6), and a cheaper, simpler version of an existing technology, Jaipur Foot. Also particularly important, but not discussed in Prahalad (2006) is the development of cheap POCT and diagnostics, where there is much effort going into creating appropriate technologies for local markets. The Diagnostics For All, CD4 and GE cases are all examples (see Innovation in Action 6.5).

We can see how these innovations meet several of the features required to address the healthcare needs of developing countries: access has been extended, costs have been dramatically reduced, yet results are reliable and quality of care has been maintained. Operationally the focus is on using local skills rather than emphasising professional medical credentials. The innovations are potentially scalable to a wide range of settings. In many ways, these examples can be seen as analogous to disruptive innovations in advanced health systems — in disruptive innovation terms, they provide 'low end disruption'.

In recent years, though, the picture has become somewhat confused with the introduction of the concept of 'frugal innovation'. This refers to innovations that are designed to be inexpensive, robust and easy to use, and which concentrate on meeting the needs of poor consumers in resource-constrained situations. We discuss frugal innovation below.

INNOVATION IN ACTION 6.5: Delivering affordable access to diagnostics

Many companies, large and small, are trying to create cheaper, simpler diagnostics and imaging technology. Some of this technology is designed specifically to improve access to diagnostics in health systems which lack the resources to purchase or deploy equipment found in developed countries' health systems. Some of this technology is designed and produced locally, and is now beginning to be adopted as a disruptive innovation in high cost health systems. As innovations, these examples include both scientifically advanced novel devices, such as Diagnosis For All's POCT technology, and more modular innovations (see Chapter 2), which take an established product and rethink its design concept and make use of readily available existing technology to create a new architecture (MAC 400).

User-led open innovation for HIV-AIDS testing — the CD4 initiative

An individual's CD4 cell count is an indicator of when to start antiretroviral therapy for HIV/AIDS and is current practice in high-income countries where access to diagnostic services is widespread. In low-income countries, HIV/AIDS care is often decentralised to rural clinics, but these frequently lack diagnostic infrastructure, so patients must either attend clinics at larger hospitals in person or send their blood samples. This results in delays and attendance at hospitals can be costly or inconvenient for patients. A large proportion of patients do not return to receive their test results and many results are lost. Specifications for the POCT were established after consultation with healthcare workers in resource-poor countries. An explicit aim of the CD4 Initiative was to develop a new frugal technology rather than trying to modify technology used in high-income settings by simply making it smaller and more portable. Following an open call for proposals, Zyomyx developed a simple simple point-of-care CD4 test that provides results for treatment decisions within 10 minutes, using a fingerprick of blood and without electronic instrumentation, at a cost of less than USD 2 per test.

Sources: Zachariah *et al.* (2011) and Imperial College London. CD4 Initiative.[1]

(Continued)

---

[1] http://www3.imperial.ac.uk/cd4

INNOVATION IN ACTION 6.5:   (*Continued*)

Low cost portable scanning devices

By 2000, GE was a major player in developed countries in the markets for obstetrics, cardiology and general radiology but its performance in lower income countries was deteriorating because its premium high tech and high cost products were far too expensive. The threat of companies from China, India and elsewhere competing on a 'new price performance paradigm' (Immelt *et al.*, 2009), as well as obligations under US healthcare reform to reduce the cost of medical devices, led GE to create 'local growth teams' (LGT) in India and China to develop new products to meet local needs, and exploit local opportunities.

Through these teams working under its Healthymagination programme, GE has developed technologies for use in lower income countries which cost a fraction of equivalent in developed health systems. The challenge for the LGT in India was to create a portable and affordable ECG machine. In doing so, the team became one of the most high profile examples of a company practising a frugal innovation approach to product development. The MAC 400 uses the same analysis software as high-end ECG models but costs a fifth of the price. To keep costs down, the Indian Railways ticket printing system was incorporated. GE also teamed up with Astra Zeneca to provide training on the equipment, using Astra Zeneca's own network.

Another area where there has been considerable technological development is lower cost smartphone-sized imaging devices in ultrasound, designed both for developing countries as well as GP and community health settings in developed health systems. Several devices are now available, weighing a few hundred grams and costing around USD 8,000 compared to at least USD 25,000 for a conventional machine. MobiSante's MobiUS system was the first mobile phone-based ultrasound device. The large global medical device companies have also developed similar products, such as Siemens' Acuson P10 pocket ultrasound device, Philips India's Visiq and GE Healthcare's Vscan. Portable ultrasound now comprise a significant global product line for GE, not just in developing countries. The product has been adopted in advanced health systems in Germany, Finland and elsewhere, where its size and portability mean that it can be deployed in the field or in accident and emergency departments. In India and China, however,

(*Continued*)

INNOVATION IN ACTION 6.5: *(Continued)*

ultrasound use is regulated because it can be used to determine the sex of the foetus and to selectively abort female foetuses (GE/BLIHR, 2009).

Sources: Various, including World Health Innovations Summit, Washington DC, 4–7 April 2011, and Walters (2015).

A not-for-profit company delivering affordable point-of-care diagnostics for developing countries — Diagnostics For All

The starting point for Diagnosis For All (DFA) was the premise that paper is cheap and ubiquitous, so if a diagnostics test can be embedded onto a piece of paper you can dramatically reduce costs. Based on technology developed at Harvard University, DFA has created a platform for simple, portable, low-cost, and easy-to-dispose diagnostic tools. The technology was launched for widespread use in 2013. Through innovation in wax printing and micro-fluidics technology, DFA can produce postage stamp sized tests with the positive and negative controls embedded in the test. The cost per test has been reduced to below USD 0.10 compared to some conventional tests costing USD 4. Biological samples are applied to the paper test, where the sample is channelled to the assay zone, which quickly changes colour. Minimal training is required — the results are easily read by comparing the colour change with a reference scale printed on the device. The completed test can then be easily disposed of by burning. The cost and ease of use mean the technology is highly scalable. A device the size of a typical household printer can print 200 tests in a minute. All the guidance notes are in the packaging for the test or can be included on a mobile phone. A growing range of tests is being developed, including liver function, at-risk pregnancy, nucleic acid detection, and child nutrition. However, the market is not just for healthcare — tests are being created for water, food and crop quality and disease. By drastically cheapening and simplifying the testing process, DFA is enabling much greater access to diagnostics for poor populations.

Sources: World Health Innovations Summit, Washington DC, 4–7 April 2011, Fulmer (2012).[2]

---

[2] http://www.dfa.org/about-dfa/our-technology.php

New business models are just as important as technology

Creating appropriate technologies for local settings is much needed, but Prahalad (2006) argues that new ways of thinking about healthcare business models are just as important as technological innovation. Some countries have become fertile environments for trying out new low cost models of care, which typically combine novel technology, organisational and funding elements. In Mexico, a number of such innovations have been created and scaled-up, such as MedicallHome. This provides affordable telephone-based primary care to a million households for a monthly fee of USD 5, partnering with affiliated providers if further care is needed (Britnell, 2015). But much of the attention has been on India, where there has been widespread experimentation with new healthcare business models. The specialist hospitals, such as NH (Narayana Health) heart hospitals and Aravind Eyecare (see Innovation in Action 6.6), are two of the most

---

INNOVATION IN ACTION 6.6:   India's specialist hospitals for cardiac and eyecare

India's Narayana Health (NH) chain of heart hospitals is one of the most widely reported healthcare models to have emerged from developing health systems. An example of a highly specialised hospital, NH has combined innovation on multiple fronts to provide of affordable cardiac care for low income people. In doing so, it has become one of world's largest providers of cardiac care. NH's innovation model involves specialisation and high volumes, achieved through process and supply chain innovation, and a financial model that uses cross subsidy from higher income patients and cheap health insurance to provide care for poor people. Outreach to rural areas is achieved by using telemedicine and mobile laboratories. The combination of high volumes of work, innovative management practices and donations has meant that around 60% of treatments are free or subsidised. Costs of surgery are disputed — see main text and Box 6.14 — but claims range from a thirtieth of comparable US providers (Prahalad, 2006) to slightly under half that of the UK's NHS (Shetty, 2011).

(Continued)

INNOVATION IN ACTION 6.6:   (*Continued*)

Another well-known example is Aravind Eyecare. This also combines multiple innovations and specialisation. Aravind has become the world's largest provider of cataract surgery. The innovation model is similar to that of NH, involving process and supply innovation to deliver highly lean workflow, local lens and suture manufacture, and outreach through telemedicine to attract the rural poor, and subsidies to ensure that around 60% of patients are treated free, while the remainder pays a small charge. Again, cost comparisons with cataract surgery in developed countries are subject to disagreement (see main text and Box 6.14), but one estimate suggests costs are one fiftieth of comparable US providers (Prahalad, 2006).

famous examples. These have been widely reported in both the academic and mainstream media as lessons for high cost hospital models in developed countries. Both involve changes in clinical and surgical processes, task shifting (i.e. delegation of tasks, where appropriate, to less specialized health workers) and use of cheaper technology to dramatically drive down costs, while maintaining or even improving quality compared to developed countries. The idea is not new, nor did it originate in the Indian hospital sector — lessons from Shouldice Hernia Centre in Canada have informed ideas about hospitals as production lines and date back to 1945.

The business model here is about achieving significant economies of scale by high throughput of patients and process innovation, supported by the application of new technology. Another Indian hospital chain, Apollo Reach Hospitals, has applied a similar model to multi-speciality, rather than specialist, hospitals to deliver high quality healthcare to semi-urban and rural India. This is coupled with a low cost health insurance scheme, financially supported by central and state government, and help with transport costs. Apollo Reach's model is not about specialisation but about standardising protocols to ensure high quality is maintained while also delivering volume throughput to achieve financial economies. Another lesson from Apollo Reach is that while telemedicine links to more remote areas are increasingly important for extending access to healthcare — and are part of the company's business model — there is still an important role for the physical hospital. A significant proportion of the population at the bottom of India's socio-economic pyramid live in large urban areas. Bringing hospitals to this population is just as important as outreach to remoter villages, but design and construction innovation is needed to bring down costs. NH has driven down the cost of hospital construction, building new heart hospitals for USD 6 million instead of USD 60 million, a typical figure for India, by using pre-fabrication and building on a single level.

There is a controversy over the cost comparisons between these Indian examples and hospitals in developed countries. Karnani (2007), Richman *et al.* (2008) and others have argued that for NH the cost savings compared to the USA and other developed countries are exaggerated (Box 6.11). High labour, administrative and insurance costs in the US, and a highly unregulated market in India, make comparisons spurious and the

---

Box 6.11   BACKGROUND: Comparing costs — the case of Aravind

Some have suggested that when adjustments are made for volume of patients treated, Aravind's cataract surgery costs are possibly just 1% of those in the NHS, and with lower post-operative infection rates at Aravind (McKinsey, 2011; Ravilla, 2009; Ravindran *et al.*, 2009). Differences in labour costs only accounted for half the difference (Naran, 2011). Another possible source of the cost variation lies in the type of surgical procedures performed. There are currently two predominant cataract surgery techniques, small incision extra-capsular cataract surgery (SICS) and phacoemulsification. The latter, the normal technique in the UK and other developed health systems, is a far more expensive procedure. It is unclear what proportion of Aravind operations use each approach. It could be argued that since SICS is much a cheaper procedure and after six months there is almost no difference between the outcomes in uncomplicated cases, it should be used more widely. However, it is unlikely that patients in developed health systems would accept this, given the shorter recovery time for phacoemulsification.

What is clear is that the cost of intraocular lens produced by Aravind manufacturing partner, Aurolab, is far below the equivalent in developed

---

(Continued)

Box 6.11 *(Continued)*

countries. Aurolab is able to produce foldable lenses for USD 22 compared to USD 80–100 from multinational companies selling in India (Ibrahim *et al.*, 2007) and USD 150 in Europe and the USA (Rangan and Ravilla, 2007). Savings are not just the result of lower wage levels. Aurolab devised a way to manufacture foldable lenses using existing technology and machinery by hydrating and packing the lens in saline solution (Ibrahim *et al.*, 2007). The lenses have a European Community CE mark, which means they conform to European standards and are therefore comparable in quality to those of other manufacturers (Ravilla, 2011).

efficiency gains shown in India are not necessarily replicable in the USA. However, Petrick and Juntiwasarakij (2011) suggest that this argument is too narrow and it downplays the opportunities that a fresh perspective from India and other developing health systems can bring to the health system problems in developed countries.

Other organisations have created innovative business models where forms of cross-subsidy are used to improve the distribution of drugs, create cheap health insurance or help develop basic healthcare infrastructure (see Innovation in Action 6.7). All these innovations have emerged to increase access to affordable healthcare in parts of the world where health systems are under-resourced. All of them tackle Prahalad's challenges for innovations designed to improve healthcare in lower income countries — they extend access, costs have been dramatically reduced, quality has been maintained, and they are scalable. Their innovation architecture varies considerably, though all display at least some of the seven business model innovation features described in Prahalad's framework. And in disruptive innovation language, they may be 'cheaper' but there is nothing 'simple' about some of these examples, which involve a complex ecosystem of stakeholders:

- Both Aravind and NH combine supply chains of local technology manufacturers and suppliers, research institutes and universities, state and national government, and banks, as well as the knowledge of lean

INNOVATION IN ACTION 6.7:   Novel business models to create affordable healthcare infrastructure

- The *HealthStore Foundation* has set up rural village clinics — Child and Family Wellness Shops — in Kenya, Rwanda, Ghana, Ethiopia, Nigeria and Zambia offering health consultation and distribution of essential drugs using **franchising**, licensing a successful business model for others to use. The premise is that top down models of control find it hard to supervise what goes on at the ground level. Under franchise models like that of the sandwich chain Subway (whose CEO is on the HealthStore board), self-interest protects standards because franchisees want to perform consistently. By combining franchising and standardising healthcare delivery to ensure consistent quality, HealthStore has managed to lower the cost of healthcare to rural populations, address the shortage of pharmacies found in Kenya and elsewhere, and create a model that can be widely replicated.[3]
- *MicroEnsure*'s business model involves **aggregating consumers** who are willing to pay small amounts for healthcare so that collectively they amount to a large market — the so-called 'long tail' of customers. MicroEnsure operates in India, the Philippines, Ghana and Tanzania. Health insurance costs USD 5 per person per year in India, USD 4 in the Philippines and USD 6 in Ghana. The system allows flexible payment options for families of different sizes and those unable to afford to pay the premium in a single lump sum.[4]
- Information is valuable, so **monetising data** from patients — for example selling data to drug companies with appropriate safeguards — and using the revenue to cross subsidise healthcare for the poorest population is another approach. *Arogya Ghar*'s aims to make medical knowledge accessible to rural populations by computerising the protocols for common ailments and preventable diseases, rethinking the best practices and reducing them to simple interactive algorithms, and using the internet to spread knowledge. Revenue to defray the costs of care can be generated by gathering accurate healthcare data for population studies and research, and making critical data available for governments formulating public health policies.[5]

(Continued)

---

[3] http://www.healthstore.org/
[4] http://www.microensure.com/products-health.asp
[5] http://si-usa.org/arogya-ghar/

INNOVATION IN ACTION 6.7: *(Continued)*

- In countries where there is limited or very basic health **infrastructure**, there are ways to tie healthcare development to the provision of water and energy infrastructure. *E Health Point* is a social enterprise which is developing a scalable, self-sustaining model for delivering water, healthcare and other benefits to underserved rural communities. The model, piloted in rural India in a strategic partnership with Proctor & Gamble, combines safe drinking water, access to doctors via telemedicine, on-site diagnostic capability and the provision of medicines via a licensed pharmacy. *E Health Point* is targeting people with an income of USD 2 a day. These are willing to spend a small proportion of their monthly income on water. Once the water supply is established, and revenue is generated, an affordable telemedicine consultation system can be set up. E Health Point has estimated that at least 100 countries could benefit from the model and with USD 4 billion of investment, healthcare and water could be provided to 2 billion people.[6]
- The organisation *Sustainable Innovations* has two schemes which combine innovation in **infrastructure, technology** and **business models**. *Arogya Ghar* (see above) aims to treat common ailments and preventable diseases in rural India at $0.50 per visit cost, via a system of walk-in clinics equipped with self-service kiosks and computerised protocols. As well as providing access to the medical knowledge needed to treat common ailments, the kiosks capture clinical and demographic data. The clinics are built, owned and operated by social entrepreneurs — high school educated people who are trained for 6 to 8 weeks and paid USD 150 a month. It is expected that many will be women who already provide door-to-door healthcare in villages.[7]

Source: Various, including World Health Innovations Summit, Washington DC, 4–7 April 2011.

and other process innovations. Both have sophisticated community outreach programmes involving telemedicine.
- For Aravind access to affordable lenses, predominantly produced in Europe and the USA, represented the largest barrier to improving the quality of surgery. After failed attempts to convince lens producers to

---

[6] http://ehealthpoint.com/
[7] http://si-usa.org/

sell them more cheaply, Aurolab was set up in 1992 with help from the Seva Foundation and Sight Savers International to manufacture lenses (Crisp, 2011). This required regulatory, intellectual property (IP) and financial barriers to be addressed, and suitable distribution models to be established. Aurolab were given *pro bono* legal support to ensure that design and product development did not violate the IP of other lens manufacturers.

- The innovation ecosystem of Healthstore is similarly complex. This brings together Management Sciences for Health (MSH) and the HealthStore Foundation in an alliance under which MSH supplies technical advisory services to the HealthStore, Procter & Gamble distributes its PUR water purifying product through HealthStore's child and family welfare outlets in Kenya, and funding comes from the ExxonMobil Foundation.

Frugal innovation — or disruptive innovation?

The concept 'frugal innovation' has become a hot topic. The term has been predominantly applied to the development of innovative technologies for lower income countries — cheaper, simpler but good enough — but there is also interest in their applicability to developed countries' health systems. A report commissioned by The Lancet explains how greater focus on frugal technology offers 'truly global promise', with novel technologies created in lower-income countries potentially helping to mitigate escalating healthcare costs in high-income ones. Use of the term has been popularised partly by articles in the *Harvard Business Review* (Radjou *et al.*, 2010; Immelt *et al.*, 2009) and *The Economist* (2009, 2011). Consultancies have reported on its benefits and implications for healthcare and other sectors (e.g. PwC, 2011c). Dartmouth College Professor Vijay Govindarajan has written extensively about it

> *"Lessons from a frugal innovator. The rich world's bloated health-care systems can learn from India's entrepreneurs."* (The *Economist*, 16 April 2009.)

> *"First break all the rules. The charms of frugal innovation."* (The *Economist*, 16 April 2010.)

(Govindarajan, 2010; Govindarajan and McCreary, 2010). And there is a website devoted to it, http://www.frugal-innovation.com

But there is no agreed definition of frugal innovation. It blurs with notions of 'reverse innovation' or 'constraint-based innovation'. Essentially the concept means innovation designed to be inexpensive, robust and easy to use, starting from the needs of poor consumers or resource-constrained contexts and working backwards to meet these needs (Govindarajan, 2010; *The Economist*, 2011). Sometimes the use of frugal innovation is restricted to products

> *"Reverse innovation has been described as a process 'under which the organisation starts from the targeted market price for a service and derives an appropriate cost structure for providing that service with appropriate quality'."*
> (Richman *et al.*, 2008:1260).

(Zeschky *et al.*, 2011), sometimes business models and services (Richman *et al.*, 2008), and sometimes both (*The Economist,* 2011; Anand, 2009)

Definitions also include the requirement to be sparse in the use of raw materials and their impact on the environment. Engineers at Santa Clara University, California, have published a list of eight core competencies of frugal innovation in product design (Basu *et al.*, 2013) (see Table 6.3), which are echoed in Charles Leadbeatter's book, *The Frugal Innovator* Leadbeatter, 2014:

• Simple — low cost, easy maintenance, adaptable.
• Social — user-centric and community-driven development.
• Clean — efficient re-use of existing resources and local materials.
• Lean — elimination of supply chain waste.

Well-known frugal technologies meeting these conditions include the Jaipur Foot and neonatal incubators (Innovation in Actions 6.8 and 6.9). There are many examples of technologies specifically designed for the needs of local markets, simpler versions of equipment used in developed health systems. In China, Zhongxing Medical, for instance, has targeted low cost radiography, creating a device that can only do routine chest radiographies, but costs 5% of imported machines. As a result, Zhongxing have captured half the Chinese radiography market (Sehgal *et al.*, 2010).

Table 6.3.   Eight core competencies of frugal innovation.

Competency of frugal innovation	Description
Ruggedisation	The technology is designed with materials that can consistently operate in harsh physical environments
Affordability	The technology is designed to be purchased by very low-income communities, where economic markets are still developing, e.g. distribution and marketing strategies are based on high volume and low unit cost
Simplification	The technology is designed without the added features and functionality that are used to market products in developed countries
Adaptation	Technologies that can be adapted from existing products, e.g. a bicycle-powered dynamo originally used to charge a headlamp is modified to charge mobile phone batteries
Reliance on local materials, manufacturing	The technology can be designed and manufactured without importing equipment or materials
Renewability	Technologies that can be powered by renewable resources
User-centric design	A technology that can be used by semi-literate people, e.g. m-health information technologies that use symbols and colours rather than text
Lightweight	A technology that can be carried by human beings through unreliable transportation systems, e.g. a disaster relief kit that can be carried in a suitcase.

Source: Basu *et al.* (2013).

The involvement of users as co-designers is regarded as one of the essential foundations of frugal innovation (Free, 2004). This can be hard to achieve in resource-poor settings because designs often try to imitate products created in resource-rich countries or are based on perceived rather than expressed needs. Many frugal technology innovations do not originate from the poorest countries (Howitt *et al.*, 2012) — around three-quarters of devices listed in WHO's compendium of technologies that are likely to be suitable for use in low-resource settings came

INNOVATION IN ACTION 6.8: The Jaipur Foot

The Jaipur foot is a rubber prosthetic, designed in India in 1968, for people who have lost their leg and foot below the knee. Unlike advanced prosthetics it can be worn without a shoe, and its flexible design is suitable for walking on uneven surfaces. Founded in 1975, Jaipur Foot now has an annual budget of USD 3.5 million, funded by donations, government support and earned income. It has been adopted across Asia, Africa and South America, and around 400,000 people have been fitted with the foot. The innovation is readily scalable because production costs are low — rubber is locally available and the foot can be mass-produced with commercially available ovens. At 2011-prices the foot cost about USD 45, compared to USD 8,000–12,000 for equivalent prostheses used in high-income countries. However, the Jaipur Foot is distributed for free by a non-profit organisation Bhagwan Mahaveer Viklang Sahayata Samiti, which has grown to become the world's largest provider of prosthetic limbs.

Sources: Kanani (2011), Prahalad (2006, 2010b).

INNOVATION IN ACTION 6.9:   Neonatal incubators

Almost four million infants in low-income countries die annually within a month of birth. Half could survive if they were placed in neonatal incubators. But incubators can cost USD 45,000 each. One approach to providing incubators affordably has been to upgrade obsolete equipment with generic components (Amadi *et al.* 2007, 2010). In a study in Nigeria, performance of recycled incubators over 6 months and for 10 indicators was very similar to modern incubators and better for ease of maintenance. The recycled incubators cost only 20% of modern incubators and maintenance were only costs 25%. At the time of a follow-up study, almost three-quarters of functioning incubators in main Nigerian hospitals were recycled (Amadi *et al.*, 2010).

Another approach is to develop new affordable incubators. The Design that Matters organisation attempted this by taking advantage of car parts, 'an abundant local resource in developing countries' as DtM says. By leveraging

(Continued)

INNOVATION IN ACTION 6.9: (*Continued*)

the existing car industry supply chain and the technical understanding of local car mechanics, a low cost incubator, NeoNurture, was developed. A spin-off from the project was the Embrace baby warmer, a portable and reusable sleeping bag that requires only intermittent access to electricity and costs approximately USD 25. However, despite winning awards, NeoNurture failed to be adopted. While DtM paid attention to the end users of NeoNurture — doctors and nurses in rural areas and families — they had not considered the purchasers of medical equipment, which in developing countries are typically governments. DtM could not find anyone to build their incubator. Design that Matters therefore shifted its attention to designing for manufacture and distribution. It developed a successful collaboration with a medical device manufacturer and a foundation distributing medical technology in southeast Asia to create a device for treating babies born with jaundice, the Firefly. The success of the Firefly project was partly due to close collaboration with partners who have influence in manufacture and distribution. Drawing on these lessons, DtM is has turned its attention back to keeping babies warm, with input from key partners, to create the Otter Warming System.

Sources:
http://www.designthatmatters.org/neonurture
http://www.bizjournals.com/sanjose/stories/2008/04/21/story10.html?b=1208750400^1622061&surround=etf
http://www.notimpossiblenow.com/lives/the-acclaimed-incubator-that-hospitals-never-used-and-what-designers-learned
http://timkastelle.org/blog/2014/12/how-to-design-for-outcomes/

from high-income countries (WHO, 2011). Indeed the greatest drivers of development of frugal technology may well be multinational corporations with operations in major emerging markets such as India and China (Zeschky *et al.*, 2011). From the perspective of these corporations, frugal innovation is a way of expanding their markets by embracing excluded populations, as in the concept of disruptive innovation. As Prahalad (2010a) points out, this means redesigning products and production processes to cut costs to the bone and eliminate all but the most essential features of a product or service to create an affordable product. Some companies see huge potential here — Unilever and Procter & Gamble, for instance, have projected that by 2020, poor people in the developing world may account for around 50% of their global revenues. Companies developing such products must ask themselves questions such as:

• is the problem widely recognised,
• are innovations needed to tackle the problem,
• can tackling it change the industry's economics,
• will addressing it give us a fresh source of competitive advantage and create a big opportunity for us?

Transferability of frugal innovations to developed health systems — what are the limits?

To what extent can high-income countries learn from healthcare innovation in low- to middle-income countries? The interest is in whether developing countries can bring a fresh perspective on healthcare in high cost systems (Wooldridge, 2011; Crisp, 2010; Petrick and Juntiwasarakij, 2011). Innovation at the 'base of the pyramid' is said to breed products that can translate into disruptive technologies and business models in developed markets (Hart, 2005). Research for the World Economic Forum identified 22 innovative healthcare delivery models that help to reduce cost, increase access and increase quality in healthcare, 18 of which originated from low- to middle-income countries (McKinsey, 2011). The Ivey Business School at Western University, Canada, ran a competition to identify innovations created in developing countries that could be applied in Canada, with a CAD 50,000 prize to help finance the winning project. This was a minimal invasive eye pre-screening tool to detect glaucoma, diabetic retinopathy and corneal disease, developed in India (Snowden *et al.*, 2015).

The transfer of technology from developing to developed countries has been described as form of reverse innovation (e.g. Immelt *et al.*, 2009; Govindarajan and Trimble, 2012). Some have argued this implies a flow between regions that is too linear and the reality is much more dynamic — frugal technologies originate in both parts of the world and are shaped and reshaped, as they are tried out in practice in different local contexts (Howitt *et al.*, 2012).

There are certainly examples of medical technologies created in developing countries which are adopted in developed ones. The MAC 400 ECG (see Innovation in Action 6.5) has become popular with German primary care physicians who do not want or need a more expensive high-end machine, rapid diagnostic tests initially developed for resource-poor settings have been taken up in high-income countries, and sometimes new protocols developed in resource-poor settings have become gold standard practice in developed health systems — the Ponseti method for treatment of club foot was first adopted in Malawi because of a shortage of ortho-paedic surgeons, but it delivered better results, while being less intrusive and expensive than surgery, and is now becoming standard practice in high-income countries (Crisp, 2010).

What are the limits to transferability of frugal and disruptive innova-tions from countries such as India to countries with highly developed and expensive health systems? We might reasonably expect that transfer is by no means straightforward, given the complexities of the latter — differ-ences in funding arrangements, the need for integration of innovations into existing organisational models, the legacy infrastructure, the regula-tory environment in developed countries' health systems, and the per-ceived threat to incumbent providers and manufacturers. In contrast, health systems of developing countries are, to some extent 'free of the handicap of an entrenched healthcare system infrastructure that seeks to maintain the *status quo*', as a report by PwC (2011c) puts it, making it potentially easier to develop and try out innovations. The comparative lack of legacy healthcare infrastructure — organisational, regulatory, financial and physical — may reduce some of the barriers to integrating certain innovations into developing countries' health systems, especially where the innovation involves a more complex business model. Simpler funding systems, with a higher predominance of out-of-pocket payments for healthcare (i.e. direct payments by consumers) may also help, because there are not the same payment and reimbursement problems across multiple provider organisations found in more complex health systems. Of course, there are equity issues with out-of-pocket payments and even frugal innovations might be not be affordable to some. Others have argued that the culture and demands for healthcare are different in high- and low-income countries. Nigel Crisp (2010) argues that a mentality amongst poorer populations in India based on 'jugaad' — hacking a make-shift solution, doing more with less (Radjou *et al.*, 2010) — is very different from demands of populations in high-income countries for ever growing amounts of money being spent in healthcare.

Regulation and health technology assessment

An important question which influences transferability is whether there is a sufficiently flexible framework for evaluating and regulating new products with frugal innovation characteristics. One limitation has been the way health technology assessement models work, especially whether they are able to evaluate technologies that are somehow 'inferior' to incumbent technologies.

> *"The National Institutes of Health in the US might as well be called Not Invented Here."*
> (Anonymous interviewee cited in Naran, 2011)

Using a narrow incremental or marginal cost-effectiveness approach to assess whether the benefits of upgrading to a newer and more expensive product outweighs the costs does not serve frugal innovations well. These may be cost reducing but also lower quality compared to incumbent products. Comparisons are not made any easier by the problems of translating

> →*Chapter 5 discusses the role of health technology assessment (HTA) in the adoption of innovations. Table 3.1 in Chapter 3 outlines the possible innovation outcomes and their implications for policy makers and payers.*

efficiency and cost savings achieved in low- to middle-income countries to more highly regulated health systems with high labour and administrative costs, as we have seen (see Box 6.11). More broadly, the ideal for politicians and health service managers is the rare innovation that is both quality improving and cost reducing. The reality is that most healthcare innovations are cost comparable or cost increasing, while quality only improves slightly, if at all. Frugal innovations lie in the politically difficult quality reducing/cost reducing cell in Table 3.1 (Chapter 3), making them hard for regulators to recommend. In the UK NICE guidelines for health technology evaluation have become more flexible, with an increasing emphasis on 'value' rather than cost (Workman, 2014). But despite the calls for disruptive and frugal innovation in the UK to help solve its current health system challenges, there is little in the way of methodology to support its introduction (Hurt, 2014).

Different regulatory environments, especially those relating to patient safety, pose barriers to the transfer of frugal innovation. Under US negligence law healthcare innovations that deviate from a 'community standard' are deemed 'malpractice' (Richman *et al.*, 2008), unlike India, where experimentation is encouraged through trials that measure the trade off between cost and quality (Naran, 2011). Although Aurolab obtained a European CE mark for its intraocular lens, it chose not to compete in the USA where it would have faced the need for approval by the US Food and Drug Administration (FDA) (Naran, 2011). Other entrepreneurs developing frugal technologies have faced problems when trying to break into the US market. Nyxoah, an Israeli company with a cheaper, less invasive and easier to use technology for sleep apnoea than current solutions faced FDA requirements for additional clinical trials, along with high insurance premiums and risk assessments, even though the product already conformed to CE standards. Frugal innovations can, however, enter the USA when multinational companies set up a subsidiary or research and development units in developing countries. GE faced few barriers from regulators because they were regarded as creating 'new demand' and the product is 'significantly equivalent' to other ultrasound scanners that GE produces (Naran, 2011).

Although Aranvind's lens manufacturer Aurolab decided against exporting to the USA, elements of the Aravind model have still been transferred into US clinics. In one clinic, these helped to lower surgical procedure time for cataract surgery from 23 minutes in 1996 to 9 minutes in 2004 (Naran, 2011). Some of the lessons are basic lean production concepts, such as standardising certain processes, ensuring all necessary information is available in advance and booking more complex procedures for the end of the day to avoid possible disruption to routine operations. However, there has also been task shifting at Aravind (as well as NH and other specialised hospital models), which is thought to have reduced costs significantly. This can prove harder to transfer. At Aravind specialist staff deal primarily with diagnosis and surgical procedures and all other tasks have been standardised, enabling less skilled staff to carry out many procedures. Skilled nurses and optometrists provide follow-up care unless there are complications. This would not be permitted in the UK's National Health Service (Naran, 2011). Other aspects of the Aravind model have had to be adapted when it has been transferred to another country. The preparation of patients on a parallel table to where surgeons are operating on another patient (to reduce time between procedures) is forbidden in the USA (Naran, 2011) but the surgery process has still been speeded up in some US hospitals by use of two identical surgeries next door to each other, one for operating and one for preparation.

Chapter summary

- Disruptive innovation is about bringing to a market a much more affordable product or service that is simpler to use, and thus more likely to be taken up by less demanding customers.
- These innovations may start-off with a lower performance than an existing product but improve over time.
- Insurgent companies producing disruptive innovations may invade established markets and displace the incumbent company.
- Disruptive innovations are not incremental, 'sustaining' innovations, so they do not result in price inflation and they maintain their price-competitiveness over time.
- There is great interest in potential disruptive innovations for expensive healthcare systems, which might help to shift care from high-end, complex technologies towards solutions that simplify complex problems.
- The introduction of disruptive innovations has implications for the infrastructure of healthcare — the distribution of hospitals and other facilities.
- In low- to middle-income countries health systems, experimentation and innovation in approaches to healthcare provision is leading to innovations that are helping to increase access to healthcare services
- These often combine technological and business model innovation, with new infrastructure such as telemedicine.

- The notion of 'frugal innovation' overlaps with disruptive innovation, but tends to be applied to new technologies and innovations emanating from resource-poor contexts.
- There are some limits to transferability of these innovations to developed countries' health systems.

Questions for discussion

1. Describe the key characteristics of disruptive innovation, and apply the concept to healthcare.
2. Does disruptive innovation have a role in addressing the challenges faced by health systems in developed countries?
3. Do you agree with the view that the term disruptive innovation is often misunderstood in the healthcare context?
4. Why might established organisations and firms in healthcare do badly from disruptive innovation?
5. Refer to Innovation in Action 6.3 on retail clinics. How effectively does the theory of disruptive innovation explain the retail clinic case study? What would you do to preserve or create strategic advantage if you were running MinuteClinic?
6. CK Prahalad said that 'In order to achieve true innovation in healthcare, it is necessary to set ambitious goals, identify a series of strict constraints and then radically re-examine your assumptions.' Discuss how this idea has been applied to healthcare innovation in India and other countries.
7. To what extent have the constraints faced by healthcare in lower income countries resulted in new business model innovations? Why?
8. What are the similarities and differences between disruptive and frugal innovation?
9. 'Frugal innovation is simply disruptive innovation in a lower income country'. Do you agree or disagree with this statement?
10. Pick two examples of business model innovation in developing health systems. How important are the different areas of innovation that Prahalad outlines? Are they all equally important? Are there any trade-offs between them? Are there other attributes that should be included or substituted?

Selected further reading

Christensen C, Bohmer R, Kenagy J (2000) Will disruptive innovations cure healthcare? *Harvard Business Review* 78(5): 102–112.

Crisp N (2010) *Turning the World Upside Down: The Search for Global Health in the Twenty First Century.* CRC Press.

Govindarajan V, Trimble C (2012) *Reverse Innovation. Create Far from Home, Win Everywhere.* Boston: Harvard Business Review Press.

Howitt P, Darzi A, Yang G-Z, Ashrafian H, Atun R, Barlow J, *et al.* (2012) Technologies for global health. *The Lancet Commissions.* http://dx.doi.org/10.1016/S0140-6736(12)61127-1

Immelt J, Govindarajan V, Trimble C (2009) How GE is disrupting itself. *Harvard Business Review* (October).

Prahalad C (2006) The innovation sandbox. *Strategy + Business* 44 (autumn). http://www.strategy-business.com/article/06306?gko=caeb6

Richman B, Udayakumar K, Mitchell W, Schulman K (2008) Lessons from India in organisational innovation: a tale of two heart hospitals. *Health Affairs* 27(5): 1260–1270.

HEALTHCARE INNOVATION IN A COMPLEX SYSTEM

07

THIS CHAPTER WILL HELP YOU TO:

- Understand why healthcare is often seen as a complex system.
- What complexity theory and systems thinking tell us that can be applied to healthcare.
- What this means for the management of innovation in healthcare from the perspective of companies developing new products and services, healthcare organisations adopting innovations, and those responsible for large-scale transformation programmes in both developed and developing health systems.

If people are to get the care they need and costs are to be kept down everything has to work well as a system. We know that health systems are complex. But we also know that progress in one part of the system sometimes makes things worse in another. There is much talk of a 'whole systems approach' to improvement, sometimes explicitly and often implicitly. Practical interventions and policies are sometimes informed by concepts and lessons from theories about complex adaptive systems. Sometimes introduction of new policies or interventions stimulates a response that ripples across multiple levels in the health system. In this chapter, we explore the impact of complexity on the implementation and consequences of innovation, through examples of initiatives which require both system thinking and also have an impact — not always predictable — across the health system.

The chapter contains three case studies, all illustrating aspects of complexity in healthcare systems and the implications this has for understanding innovation management. All are about whole system change, all describe the need to engage stakeholders from the relevant parts of the health and social care system, and all show the importance of using evidence to bring different stakeholders on board.

Two of the cases are about technology-induced whole system change, one successful and the other less so. Clear goals and top–down direction was a factor behind the success of Sweden's introduction of 'drug utilisation reviews' (DURs), but this was coupled with an awareness that there needed to be flexibility if an innovation that had been developed in the USA was to be introduced into a very different context (Case study 7.3).

The Whole System Demonstrator programme (Case study 7.2) also involved top–down direction, although here it was to ensure that a trial was carried out in a way that delivered the evidence necessary to scale up the innovation in the future. But the rigidities of the trial stifled experimentation and the ability to adapt the innovation to the different local contexts it was being deployed in.

Experimentation was also a feature of the third case study (Case study 7.1), on Scotland's national programme to introduce the four-hour target for hospital accident and emergency departments. This was another top–down initiative. A national team set out actions — often innovative ones for those who were implementing them — but they still allowed a sufficient degree of flexibility for individual health authorities to try out variants of these actions if this was merited by the local context. This programme was initially successful in stimulating the health authorities to meet the four-hour target, but ultimately a lack of ability to coordinate some parts of the local health and social care system meant that progress slipped.

The chapter also includes mini-cases on system-wide healthcare interventions in African countries, illustrating the impact of unintended consequences (Innovation in Action 7.1) and importance of context in influencing success (Innovation in Action 7.2).

What is a complex system and what does this mean for healthcare?

The idea that healthcare needs to be understood as a system — and one that is immensely complex — has been a theme running through this book. We have seen how such complexity often makes it extremely challenging to manage change and innovation, whether from the perspective of a healthcare organisation adopting a new idea, a company trying to bring its new product to market, or a government trying to redesign health services to cope with new demands.

The use of 'complexity theory' has grown increasingly popular in organisational studies, both in research and in management and policy rhetoric (McKelvey, 1999). But although it offers potential to help us capture the exigencies of the real world, applying complexity theory to management or policy has proved hard. A common criticism, made even by its proponents, is that complexity theory is too metaphorical (Anderson, 1999; Paley, 2010). We may be able to show that a firm or organisation exhibits the characteristics and behaviours of complex systems; it is harder to develop practical recommendations to help those who manage them.

The defining characteristics of a system according to complexity theory are described in Box 7.1. Particularly important are the nature of interactions between elements of the system and the potential for the system to adapt and display 'emergence' — the way the interactions over time between the constituent elements of a system make the whole different from the sum of its parts. These characteristics present problems for traditional approaches to management or policy development, which tend to rely on our ability to define a strategy that can be effectively communicated and then deliberately directed towards planned or predictable outcomes.

Complexity theory offers an alternative paradigm and a different approach to planning and managing socio-economic systems, organisational development and the implementation of innovation. It rejects the reductionism of traditional planning and management approaches (Gatrell, 2005) and mechanistic models of organisation (Rowe and Hogarth, 2005). These typically emphasise the attributes of individual variables and their impact on the behaviour of an organisation or socio-economic system.

Box 7.1   CONCEPTS: Complex systems attributes

- Complex systems are open systems.
- They operate under conditions that are far from equilibrium.
- They have histories.
- They comprise many interconnected and interdependent elements.
- Interactions are rich; any element in the system can influence or be influenced by any other.
- Individual elements are typically ignorant of the behaviour of the whole system in which they are embedded.
- Complex systems have structure which spans different scales from the micro to the macro.
- Positive and negative feedback processes may result in counterintuitive behaviour.
- Relationships are frequently nonlinear, i.e. change is disproportionate, small differences in the initial system state lead to large differences later.
- Adaptive agents react to and influence the system and each other through self-organisation.
- Complex systems display emergence — system behaviour emerges from interaction between constituent elements such that the whole is different to the sum of the parts.

'Chaos' and 'complexity' should not be confused. Chaos refers to a situation where nonlinear laws *totally* determine the behaviour of a system. The smallest of errors in the initial system conditions are amplified, resulting in unpredictability. Complexity is all about the emergence of order from the interactions between different system components. These are influenced by simple guiding principles; the idea of 'self-organisation' is a fundamental principle of complex systems.

A complex problem is not necessarily a *complicated* one. the main difference is that with the latter, outcomes can usually be predicted if we know the starting conditions. In a complex system, different outcomes can emerge from the same starting conditions, depending on the way elements in the system interact.

Source: Various, including Cilliers (1998), Maguire *et al.* (2006).

Instead, complexity theory embraces notions of interconnectedness between variables and agents in the system, and the way these impact on the behaviour of the whole system. It is an adaptive view of the world, where agents organise themselves into new relationships and behaviours, rather than a deterministic one in which deliberate strategy and processes of control result in change (see Table 7.1).

Some researchers have sought to demonstrate mathematical evidence of complexity in real world examples. For example, research has shown a power law, rather than a normal, distribution in hospital attendance and waiting list data (Love and Burton, 2005; Papadopoulos *et al.*, 2001). More common, however, is the use of complexity theory to help inform understanding of aspects of organisational change. So with proper engagement ('interconnectedness') and 'simple rules', practitioners organise ('self-organisation') for change ('emergence') around a shared vision (an 'attractor').

Table 7.1. Contrasting paradigms in planning, implementation, and organisational development.

Current paradigm	Complexity paradigm
Reductionist: Behaviour of individual variables can impact on behaviour of the whole.	**Interconnected:** Relationships between agents can impact on behaviour of the whole.
Deterministic: Deliberate strategy and control processes result in reorganisation and change to meet forecast changes in environment.	**Adaptive:** Given the right set of conditions, individuals organise themselves in a way that forms new, unexpected structures when looked at as a whole.
Internal: The energy that drives adaptation (innovation and change) comes from within — leadership, incentives, etc.	**Open:** The energy that drives adaptation (innovation and change) comes from outside the system.
Stable: Attempt to manage variables toward stability to ensure that organisation operates as planned.	**Bounded instability:** Need to operate with enough instability to allow change and enough stability to meet broad organisational objectives.
Linear: Cause and effect relationships allow control of target variables.	**Nonlinear:** Cause can have disproportionate effect or no effect at all due to positive and negative feedback loops.

Source: With thanks to Lesley Pan.

An example of the application of complexity theory to an innovation management problem is a study of an A&E improvement initiative in Scotland (Case study 7.1). This explored the concept of scale and the way this defines the boundaries of the A&E system, requiring both multiple levels of intervention and multiple levels of analysis (Dattée and Barlow, 2010). Another example is research on the role of 'simple rules' and organisational flexibility in a private clinic (Lemak and Goodrick, 2003). Running through all these studies is the idea that order naturally emerges in systems (Lewin, 1999), with the implication that such emergence can become the means for adaptation and change in the system.

Level, scale, boundaries and time

When considering a complex system, it can be useful to break it down into more manageable elements. Because of this, Dattée and Barlow (2010) argue that it is important to decide what *level* of analysis is appropriate — are we concerned about an innovative intervention that is focused largely at a *micro* level such as the individuals working in a hospital ward or patients, the *meso* level such as a hospital as an organisation or the local acute and primary care system within which it is located, or are we focusing at the *macro* level on the impact of a new policy across a local health system or even the entire national health system?

The *scale* of analysis, on the other hand, refers to how we calibrate the tools we use for observing and measuring the system. We can reduce the perceived complexity of a system by choosing an appropriate scale since this will identify the limits of the *boundaries* around the problem in question — in other words we have to make a choice about what to include and what to leave out. The level of analysis, the scale at which the observations are calibrated and the boundaries around what to include are therefore all interrelated.

Our chosen level of analysis also informs the *temporal* scale over which the dynamics of a system can be captured. The notion of time — as duration, rate of change, frequency, delays, timing or sequence — has a central place in the study of complex systems and in organisation science (Kaplan and Orlikowski, 2013). Scale influences the timescale over which the dynamics of the system can be perceived.

To take an analogy from physical geography, imagine a river basin. The speed at which we can observe things evolving depends on the scale of our analysis — very slowly at the level of the river basin as a whole, but fast if we take a square metre of ground where there are daily changes resulting from rainfall, temperature differentials or plant growth (see Figure 7.1).

Or compare the impact of a change or innovation being introduced into the micro processes taking place in a single hospital ward or a doctor's surgery, with those at the level of a hospital as an organisation. To observe the former, the micro processes, we may have to adopt a scale of observation which captures changes over a period of days. On the other hand, the impact of changes that take place at the level of the hospital as a complex organisational system, or the local health authority, with all its constituent parts and interactions between them, might require observation to be made over months or longer. Those at the level of the whole national health system may require annual observations. Events and processes take place at all these levels at different speeds and with different degrees of impact.

An important aspect of time in relation to managing complex organisational systems is the notion of *delays*. The consequences of a change may not be immediately noticeable. Cause and effect may be lagged because of inertia in a system, especially where the number of interdependencies between its components is high. An effect of this is that corrective actions made by managers or policy makers, which are often based on their perceptions of the *current* dynamics of the system, may be inappropriate (Dattée and Barlow, 2010). They may perceive a discrepancy between the target for the system and its observed current state and rate of change. But if the perception is based on a limited understanding of the system, including its inertia, they may respond with hasty or ill-considered corrections that fail to recognise the effect of previous corrections, to which the system is already responding (Sterman, 2000).[1] This is one reason why organisations or systems often go through a 'worse before better' period after a change

---

[1] MIT professor John Sterman's Management Flight Simulator allows us to play with managing a complex system with built-in time lags: http://web.mit.edu/jsterman/www/timedelay/index.html

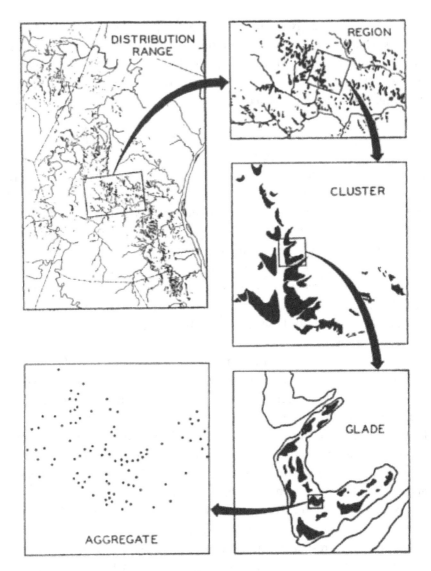

Figure 7.1.   Scale and levels in a complex system.

Source: Erickson R (1945) The Clematis fremontii Var. Riehlii Population in the Ozarks. *Annals of the Missouri Botanical Garden* 32: 413–460.

(Forrester, 1971). Deciding how long to wait before evaluating the impact of a previous correction needs to take into account the level and scale of analysis, because the time taken for the impact of changes to become observable varies, as the river basin example shows.

As well as the potential impact of time delays, policy makers or managers concerned with identifying how to intervene to deliver desirable changes need to understand where the leverage points in the system lie (see Innovation in Action 7.1). To control the dynamic behaviour of a complex system, we need to target the points in the system which have sufficient leverage to achieve the required system behaviour, rather than inadvertently triggering counterintuitive consequences. So when an innovative intervention is being designed, not only must policy and other decision-makers (as well as researchers) take into account the interdependencies in the healthcare system and time delays, they also need to understand the concept of scale, and its implications for the way we view whole system behaviour.

Together, the characteristics of complex systems — emergence, nonlinear change, interconnectivity between different components at different levels and so on — present challenges for those seeking to evaluate the economic impacts of interventions or the introduction of innovations. And not only

> ➔ *Chapter 5 discusses the complex nature of many healthcare innovations due to their mix of organisational and technology elements*

are they being deployed within complex health systems, interventions or innovations may themselves display the properties of complex systems. As we have seen, it can be hard to specify what the intervention (or innovation) is, what works and in what context, and how to replicate it beyond a trial. Box 7.2 describes the implications of this for designing evaluations.

Box 7.2   CONCEPTS: Implications of complexity for economic evaluation

Typically, economists compare the value of what goes in (the resources) with what comes out (the outcomes) of an intervention. If these can be specified with sufficient clarity to ensure that changes can be measured and valued, then it is not necessary to understand how the intervention works. But evaluating the economic efficiency of interventions which themselves display the properties

(Continued)

Box 7.2   (*Continued*)

of complex systems presents big challenges. These arise from the defining characteristics of complex systems, such as emergence and nonlinear change, properties that are a feature of the evolving system itself, rather than a summation of its individual components. Since everything is interconnected, changes in one part of the system impact elsewhere in the system and may be amplified. Moreover, the assumption that the value people assign to an intervention is unchanging may well be incorrect as the system undergoes evolution and change. Small differences in baseline conditions can lead to very large differences in the outcomes, so randomisation may not eliminate all causes of bias, even if it removes all observable differences between groups.

Outcomes of an intervention will therefore need to be measured at multiple levels and probably over longer time periods then those typical of most intervention studies. Without carefully designed studies, there is high risk of missing important outcomes and drawing premature conclusions about the impact of the intervention.

Shiell *et al.* (2008) argue that the methodological challenges are huge, and point to the need for extensive prospective data collection alongside cluster trials to capture signs of nonlinear change, unintended consequences, and multiplier effects. They also argue for greater use of modelling to assess the sensitivity of economic evaluations to the inclusion of these effects.

Source: Shiell *et al.* (2008).

Applying complexity theory to healthcare

In 2001, a series of articles in the British Medical Journal (BMJ) highlighted the importance of applying complexity theory to healthcare management. Since then, there have been many calls for more systems thinking in healthcare research and practice.

"*The science of complex adaptive systems brings new concepts that can provide fresh understandings of troubling issues in the organisation and management of delivery of health care.*"
(Plsek and Wilson, 2001)

The fact that healthcare is a complex system is aired so often that it has now more or less become received wisdom, but it is important to stop and think about why this might be the case and what it means in practice.

INNOVATION IN ACTION 7.1: The system fights back — introducing the Additional Duty Hours Allowance in Ghana

An example of the way interventions in a healthcare system are sometimes defeated by the system's response to the policy can be seen in Ghana's attempts to introduce the Additional Duty Hours Allowance (ADHA). In response to a strike by public sector doctors who were unhappy about a salary award to their counterparts in the military hospital, the government introduced an allowance over and above the standard 40 hours per week public sector salary level. This seemingly small decision became a trigger for events — cycles of reaction and counter-reaction — that would dominate, and periodically bring Ghana's health services to a near halt, over almost the next decade before uneasily settling down.

The introduction of the ADHA for doctors intensified the existing dissatisfaction of nurses about their pay. This triggered a strike which ended when nurses were included in the agreement. However, this decision in turn became the trigger for reduced satisfaction and strike action by other health sector workers. Eventually the agreement was extended to include virtually all permanent workers in Ghana's health sector. But this failed to end the instability in the system. Repeated delays in payment of the allowance and further strikes by doctors and nurses established yet another cycle of feedback. Collectively, this seems to have had the additional side effect of leading health workers and their unions to believe that industrial action was the only language government responded to. Under scrutiny for its failings in healthcare more generally, the government eventually began to review all health sector job portfolios and the ADHA payments were integrated into salaries. After another series of crippling strikes demanding a single pay scale and higher consolidated salaries, the system finally began to stabilise.

It may have been hard to anticipate all the positive and negative effects of policy decisions, the differing stakeholder interests and power, and the interactions between multiple actors. But in this example, the failure to appreciate these aspects of Ghana's health system resulted in a reductionist approach to interventions. 'Fixes' to a problem in turn initiated negative feedback loops that further complicated the situation. In this way, according to Agyepong *et al.* (2012) 'the solutions of yesterday became the problems of today'.

Source: Agyepong *et al.* (2012).

Box 7.3   BACKGROUND: A sceptical view on complexity theory

Not everyone is convinced by the value of applying complexity theory to healthcare, as this letter from Ian Reid to BMJ shows.

'Let them eat complexity: the emperor's new toolkit
Although Plsek and Greenhalgh's aim may have been to make some fairly abstract science more accessible, the result is misleading and potentially harmful. The series does not articulate honestly the background to the emerging study of complex adaptive systems by switching repeatedly between misapplied metaphor and empirically grounded science ... Greenhalgh's series continues the tradition of misusing scientific concepts by confusing technical terms (for example, nonlinear, attractor pattern) with "homey" everyday ideas (for example, hidden needs and motivations) ... This misuse of mathematical metaphor is hardly an original treatment and was regularly promulgated among business management organisations in the United States for at least a decade. Late and a bit stale, it is beginning to appear regularly in the BMJ ... The antirationalist outcome has more in common with 19th century romanticism than the sophisticated, postmodern thinking that proponents imagine they practise — serving political and careerist, rather than scientific, ends. There are useful applications of chaos theory (an established subset of the more speculative complexity theory) in the clinical sciences: the analysis of cardiac electrical rhythms; electroencephalography in epilepsy; sugar concentrations in diabetes patients; the behaviour of waiting lists; and so on. Unfortunately these ideas may be swamped by the intellectual snake oil of "complexity theory as metaphor", easily identified by the absence of mathematical modelling, which I fear we can expect to see spattered, expensively, across massed ranks of flip charts by healthcare administration faddists in the United Kingdom.'

Source: Reid (2002).

The applicability of complexity theory to healthcare is by no means universally accepted, as shown in one response to the BMJ special issue (see Box 7.3).

One problem is that 'complexity' has two meanings, although as Shiell *et al.* (2008) point out, this is rarely made explicit by health researchers or managers. In one, complexity is a property of the *intervention* (or innovation) itself; in the second it is a property of the *system* in which the intervention is implemented. The first view underpins the Medical Research Council's framework for evaluating of complex interventions (MRC, 2000; Craig *et al.*, 2006). This states that a complex intervention is 'built-up from a number of components, which may act both independently and inter-dependently', so it is hard to identify which component or combinations of components are influencing outcomes. Furthermore, some interventions can take on the characteristics of complex systems because they are adapted in use (see Chapter 5), hence displaying emergence, and a degree of human agency is required for their implementation (Pawson *et al.*, 2005).

The second view draws on the insights offered by complexity theory. Here, complexity is a property of the system, not the intervention (or innovation). An individual intervention may be simple or complex, but the setting into which it is introduced may be very complex. Researchers investigating the adoption or impact of healthcare innovations need to recognise the importance of

> ➜*In Chapter 5, we described how it is important to understand the interactions between components of intervention and the context in which it is being implemented*

context in influencing outcomes. The distinction between complexity in context and complexity in the intervention become especially important when we are evaluating the effectiveness of innovations in healthcare where the active elements of the intervention are subject to more variation because they comprise elements of organisational *and* technology change (see Box 7.2), rather than simple drugs or devices.

So what are the important concepts from complexity theory that are relevant to understanding innovation and change in healthcare systems? Developed healthcare systems certainly display many of the attributes of complex systems:

- They comprise interdependent constituent parts and structure spanning several scales. In other words, they are made up of many stakeholders, organisations, professional groups, supply chains, patients, government departments, and so on. These are arranged across different levels, from individuals in a doctor's surgery or hospital unit to regional and national health systems. Agents within these systems — whether as individuals, organisations or companies — can simultaneously be members of several parts of the overall systems. They co-evolve, as the evolution of one part of the system influences, and is influenced by, another part. Hence, the GP practice is part of a local primary care system which interacts with acute hospitals and is part of a broader regional or national health system and its institutions. Different activities and different groups or organisations across the system are subject to particular funding or regulatory models.

- Healthcare systems display adaptive and emergent behaviour, as interaction between agents takes place over time. Evolution in the face of policy change or the introduction of a new technology will trigger new interactions among the agents of the system, as the Ghana example shows (Innovation in Action 7.1).

- Nonlinear change and counterintuitive dynamics are clearly present in healthcare systems. Reducing admissions to hospital by frail elderly people may be designed to free beds and reduce costs, but in time costs may increase because more expensive cases for elective surgery are admitted. There are often inherent tensions between agents in healthcare systems, due to competing policy and operational targets. Another problem is that the actions of agents are driven by their own rules, which may not be shared, explicit or even logical when viewed by another agent. At a higher scale, the lifecycles between changes in crucial aspects of healthcare — its underlying science and technology, the prevailing models of care practice or services, its physical infrastructure, and policy context around healthcare — are mismatched, making coordination across the system hard. All these features mean that the observable outcomes of the interactions between elements and agents of the system will therefore be more than merely the sum of the individual parts.

Managing healthcare innovation in a world of complexity

Sometimes there is a high level of certainty and agreement about what is required to deliver high quality, effective healthcare — a surgical team undertaking a routine operation knows precisely what they need to do to achieve this. Under these circumstances, agents will relinquish some autonomy in order to accomplish a common and undisputed goal and the system will display less emergent behaviour. But beyond a certain level, we may need to embrace a wider range of stakeholders to achieve this. All this might lead us to think that the attributes of healthcare systems as complex systems — the nonlinear relationships, the emergent behaviour and so on — present those responsible for managing change and innovation in healthcare with a near impossible task. The behaviour of the system could be seen as fundamentally unpredictable, yet this is not the case. Much of healthcare fits into what has been termed 'the edge of chaos' (Langton, 1989), where there may be insufficient agreement and certainty to make the choices and decisions obvious, but not so much disagreement and uncertainty that the system tips into chaos.

Our learnt instinct, as Plsek and Greenhalgh (2001) put it, is based on reductionist thinking — we wish to troubleshoot and fix things by trying to move into the simple system zone in Figure 7.2, and achieve more certainty and agreement. But when we sit 'at the edge of chaos', perhaps a significant part of healthcare management, it is important not to be overly reductionist and deterministic by adopting the traditional management paradigm of 'reduce and resolve'. Rather, our management approach needs to incorporate a more dynamic, emergent and intuitive perspective. Complexity science directs us towards a model that involves experimentation with different approaches, allowing us to see what direction to take

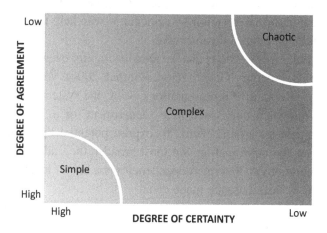

Figure 7.2. Complexity, simplicity and chaos in healthcare.

Source: Based on Stacey (1996). In Plsek and Greenhalgh (2001).

by gradually shifting our attention towards what seems to work best (Davis *et al.*, 2009; Sull and Eisenhardt, 2012). When seeking to achieve a difficult goal in healthcare, minimum specifications — a few flexible, simple rules — are seen as more effective than highly specified and consistently implemented plans (Plsek and Wilson, 2001). Yet it is the latter that dominates healthcare management thinking, resulting in a failure to take advantage of natural creativity and allow for the inevitable unpredictability of events. In a management environment where deliberate strategy and control processes dominate, it can be hard to accept the principle of 'equifinality', that by devolving authority and empowering local actors a given end-state in a system may be achieved from different starting conditions and in different ways (Gresov and Drazin, 1997).

How to ensure that change is seen as attractive, rather than trying to battle resistance is a key organisational task for management or policy makers at all levels (Plsek and Wilson, 2001). This means making self-interested agents, with different and often competing goals, aware of their interdependencies, and inducing cooperative behaviour and influencing adaptive actions across levels and boundaries (Levinthal and Warglien, 1999; Gavetti and Levinthal, 2000). An important task is to create a shared representation and understanding of what constitutes better performance, giving agents the freedom and ability to search for the most mutually attractive options (Levinthal and Warglien, 1999). Asking what changes and innovative practices have been successfully adopted or pioneered, and sharing meaningful information — evidence — can help those within the systems feel they must and can evolve.

One problem, however, is that we tend to simplify even our immediate organisational structure (Gavetti and Levinthal, 2000). We have our own perceptions — cognitive representations — of 'the system'. This may be based on functional units such as a 'department' or a 'hospital', with implicit boundaries around them. To expose potential opportunities for collaboration and coordination, we must broaden the scale of our cognitive representations so that interdependencies at a higher level (e.g. across departments or hospitals) are made clear.

Another problem is that actors in a system must manage twin tensions: a horizontal tension for coordination across boundaries — sometimes called 'landscape coupling' in complexity theory (Levinthal and Warglien,

1999) — and a vertical tension for self-organisation — balancing the simple top–down rules that guide local actions and the conditions for enabling bottom-up emergence. This tension between 'blueprint' planning approaches (i.e. deliberate strategy and control) and adaptive approaches informed — whether explicitly or not — by complexity theory has permeated many areas of management and policy. International development policy, for example, saw such a confrontation in the 1980s (see Box 7.4).

Box 7.4 CONCEPTS: Complexity and international development policy and practice

For policy makers, complexity poses challenges in designing interventions in socio-economic systems such as public health. These can be categorised as:

1. Problems where the capacity to act comes from well-defined, smoothly operating hierarchies, compared to those which cannot be controlled by one actor, and involve distributed capacities and a variety of dynamics at different levels.
2. Issues where there is relatively stable knowledge on cause and effect, or the means to address issues, compared to those where this is less well-understood or straightforward.
3. Issues where there is consensus on the questions policy must address, or the goals it must work towards, compared to those involving many plausible and equally legitimate interpretations and perspectives.

Different types of knowledge are required for decision-making about the design of policies and interventions. These are influenced by: *where* decision-making takes place (e.g. national versus. local level), *when* to derive knowledge about action and make decisions about how to act (e.g. before an intervention versus during it), and *how* decision-making can fruitfully take place and how knowledge should be integrated (e.g. instrumental and technocratic vs. dialogue-based).

Complex problems are characterised by limited knowledge of the different hierarchical levels and distributed capacities across the system, limited knowledge of cause and effect and high unpredictability, and/or limited consensus on the questions for policy to address or the overarching goals.

Source: Jones (2011).

Complexity and whole system change in healthcare

In recent years, interest in systems thinking and the application of complexity theory has grown in healthcare policy and practice. These ideas have been applied in different ways, ranging from the small scale — informing the way innovative healthcare products are developed — through the introduction of innovations into local health systems right up to large scale national transformation programmes.

Policy innovation — pilots, pilots and more pilots … and modelling

Where innovations and the environments in which they exist are complex, the extent to which we can plan and manage them grow less certain. Cause and effect are unclear, and outcome-based project management and scientific methods for evaluation and analysis do not work well. Viewing the world through a complex systems lens can help to provide us with tools to inform the development and implementation of innovations, from the early stages of the innovation pipeline to the adoption and diffusion processes.

We saw in Chapter 4 how some companies use a strategy of 'safe-fail' (or 'fast-fail' or 'pivoting') in their approach to new product development. This involves experimentation, adaptation and evolution, in which variations of initial product prototypes are sequentially tested, and the most effective ones are eventually whittled down to an optimum design. The trick is to ensure that failures are survivable — that mistakes do not amplify disastrously across the system as a whole, whether we are talking about an individual company or a local health system. The approach is all about allowing the weakest ideas to fail in ways that are tolerable, so that critical risks are contained and good outcomes are quickly arrived at without wasting resources. In complexity theory language, this can be seen as a process of emergence, allowing possibilities to become visible, discovering unexpected new sources of value,

> ➔ *Chapter 4 discusses the notions of 'fast-fail', 'safe-fail' and 'pivoting' in new product development. Chapter 5 discusses issues around piloting healthcare innovations*

identifying options for routes to market or implementation, and adapting the business or health system accordingly.

Chapter 4 also described how there is some debate about the value and applicability of 'fast-fail', which some regard as a fashionable, but not necessarily useful, approach since it may simply be an excuse for repeated failures that reveal how a company does not really know what it is doing. At its heart, this issue is really one which positions experimentation against planning, customer feedback against intuition, and

> ➜*See Chapter 4 for discussion on emerging approaches to new product such as open innovation, increased collaboration, more flexible stage-gate models, and technologies for rapid drug development*

iterative design against design 'up front' approaches. Complexity theory tells us that it is important to create safe spaces for failure, to move forward in small steps by experimentation within the boundaries of the system over which an organisation or policy makers have direct control. This allows direction to emerge as we begin to understand more about the innovation and its implications, and we gradually shift our attention towards what works best.

So how do these ideas play out within a healthcare context? When it comes to new product development, echoes of this approach can be seen in the new approaches used by pharmaceutical and medical device companies use to speed the process of developing new products. But for governments or health service organisations responsible for maintaining consistently high quality health services, trial and error experimentation — and fast or even safe fail — may in fact feel rather unsafe. 'Pivoting' when you have to keep services going is not likely to be possible. And when it comes to the introduction of health service innovations involving complex hybrids of technologies and organisational change, large-scale rapid experimentation is unlikely to be feasible. Apart from the cost of setting up a trial of small variations on an innovative intervention in the healthcare system, the complex environment places limits on *ex-ante* evaluation — there is limited knowledge of likely cause and effect, limited consensus on the existing evidence base, or there may be several objectives for a specific innovation, making it hard to predict what might happen and why.

Under these circumstances, different approaches are needed, but which still retain the useful lessons from a safe-fail, fast-fail model (Jones, 2011). First, better ways of experimenting are needed when a problem or innovation reaches a certain level of complexity. In these circumstances, the intervention itself becomes an opportunity for learning, as do 'natural experiments' where the same innovation is introduced into different health systems or local contexts. System thinking can help here, encouraging those responsible for implementing innovations to work collaboratively to create a shared vision of the problem, facilitating decentralised action and self-organisation by creating the space for interventions to be flexible, and building adaptive capacity (see Box 7.5).

Box 7.5   CONCEPTS: Injecting systems thinking into policy innovation

A report for the Overseas Development Institute (Jones, 2011) summarises when, where and how systems thinking can help to address complex policy problems. Also see Box 5.8, in Chapter 5.

Implementing agencies need to work collaboratively, facilitating decentralised action and self-organisation through:

- Decentralisation and autonomy, distributing power in decision-making and allowing increased autonomy for agents lower down the hierarchy.
- Engaging local institutions and anchoring interventions at different scales.
- Boundary management, facilitating processes that build trust and collaboration between key stakeholders.
- Building adaptive capacity to enable actors to capitalise on any autonomy for addressing problems and stimulate emergent responses.
- Removing barriers to self-organisation such as national legislation or issues of power and social capital.
- Supporting networked governance, focusing on holding units accountable for their mission or role.
- Leadership and facilitation, enabling working through attraction rather than coercion.

(Continued)

Box 7.5 (*Continued*)

- Incremental intervention, starting from existing networks and taking an evolutionary approach rather than trying to implement idealistic blueprints.

Implementing agencies need to deliver adaptive responses to problems, building space for interventions to be flexible to emerging lessons by:

- Appropriate planning, with light and flexible *ex ante* analysis, enhancing awareness of key risks, and tying accountability to clear principles for action rather than to unpredictable results or inflexible activity plans.
- Implementation as an evolutionary learning process, where experimentation through intervention becomes a central driver of learning.
- Creating short, cost-effective feedback loops, where there is transparency about who and what is being monitored.
- Iterative impact-oriented monitoring that promotes understanding of how change can be achieved, rather than simply recording progress.
- Stimulating autonomous learning, because actors are more likely to be responsive to evidence where it emerges in a context of trust and ownership.
- Accountability for learning, where policies place explicit value on learning and not just delivery and meeting performance goals. Promoting innovation in service delivery may require valuing redundancy and variety.

Implementation systems and processes must draw on an eclectic mix of sources of knowledge. Tools which allow for the negotiation between, and synthesis of, multiple perspectives are especially important:

- Decisions from deliberation, embedded in inclusive, face-to-face forums which focus on eliciting reasoned and legitimate inputs to action.
- Focusing on how change happens in implementation processes by ensuring that ideas and assumptions are made explicit so they can be purposefully tested; planning tools such as 'theory of change' and theory-based evaluation may assist.
- Realistic foresight and futures techniques to provide forward-looking analysis and create shared perspectives on implementation; scenario

(*Continued*)

Box 7.5   (*Continued*)

planning can be invaluable in enabling organisations to be both resilient and nimble.

- Peer-to-peer learning, rather than technocratic knowledge-transfer processes, to enable adaptation and learning.
- Broadening dialogues through contestation and argument, seeking out critical voices, rather than avoiding them and promoting reflexivity.
- Sense making to create a shared vision of the problem held by key stakeholders, perhaps involving the use of boundary objects such as shared models or standards.
- Facilitation and mediation to combine different sources of knowledge in a way that treads carefully and manages power across stakeholders.

Second, it is important for policy makers operating at a higher level in a system to capitalise on the effectiveness of actions at the lower levels — supporting small-scale interventions, but allowing for considerable variation in approach, evaluating their effectiveness, and providing mechanisms to select successful characteristics or interventions. Creating the right feedback loops for sharing the lessons arising from experiments is crucial. Making sure that monitoring is transparent and carried out at the local level helps to ensure that those responsible for implementation appreciate the role of local dynamics of interventions — putting monitoring in the hands of those who stand to benefit or lose from the intervention ensures that feedback loops are short and strong. We see an example of this in the use of rapid evaluation (PDSA cycles) in Case study 7.1.

Trying things out in pilot projects has, therefore, become an important approach when it comes to healthcare innovation. Pilot projects have been defined as:

'a programme or policy introduced on a limited basis — for example limited in time or geographical scope with the expressed purpose of producing evaluation evidence to inform a decision on whether or not to proceed to full implementation' (HM Treasury, 2011).

The underlying premise is one of deliberate intervention in a system in order to test a hypotheses on how to address a problem — in other words to try out an innovative approach on a small scale to understand if it works.

CASE STUDY 7.1 Top–down change with local experimentation — reforming unscheduled care services in Scotland

The policy to improve the quality of unscheduled (i.e. not elective) care in the UK's National Health Service (NHS) provides a good example of the challenges in designing and enacting change at a whole system level. It shows how performance targets, along with learning networks, can be useful in driving change and innovation; but an ability to exert leverage across the different parts of the health and social care systems is also needed for interventions to work.

Designing a programme informed by system thinking

In 2004, Scotland introduced a national target to assess and admit or discharge 98% of patients attending accident and emergency department (A&E) within four hours. This had been introduced in England two years previously, so Scotland was able to benefit from the lessons from this earlier programme. One lesson was the need to avoid 'gaming' the system, for example redefining hospital trolleys as 'beds' so that a patient could be deemed to have been 'discharged' from A&E, thus meeting the four-hour target. NHS Scotland realised the importance of addressing interactions between health and social care organisations across different system levels — that it was not enough to simply improve the performance of A&E processes within a hospital, but also to address the flows of patients into and out of the hospital.

The Unscheduled Care Collaborative Programme (UCCP) was set up to support the 14 local health boards across Scotland to put in place new initiatives to meet the target. A national programme team was established, along with local implementation teams in each of the health boards. It was expected that the four-hour target would induce innovation and behaviour change by 'concentrating the mind', allowing stakeholders to come up with new ideas or adapt ones that were working elsewhere.

Initiatives drew partly on lean thinking concepts to control the movement of patients into and out of A&E, by better management of patient flows such as minor injury and illness or medical admissions. In itself the introduction of

"There is strong evidence to suggest that change will not be delivered by issuing guidance and directives and that one size does not fit all. Solutions must meet local need and circumstance and

(Continued)

CASE STUDY 7.1   (*Continued*)

lean thinking was innovative within the context of many Scottish hospitals, although it had been deployed in the English four-hour programme. What was new was Scotland's focus on the *out-of-hospital* flow, relating to a hospital's relationship with parts of the care system outside its organisational boundaries. This meant attention needed to be paid especially to ambulance services, GPs and social services for elderly people. Better control of patient flows through improved coordination between in-hospital and out-of-hospital teams were expected to result in reduced A&E waits.

A powerful rhetoric on the need for whole system change permeated the UCCP, explicitly drawing on lessons from complexity theory. This tried to highlight to all relevant actors in local unscheduled care systems that they were interdependent, as the quotes show.

more importantly actively engage staff in the change process if significant and sustainable improvement is to be achieved."
(NHS Scotland, 2005).

"*The target is a recognized measure of whole-system design and capacity. This means all elements of the service in hospitals and in the community are involved in meeting the target — it is not just accident and emergency departments. Engagement across whole health and care systems is needed to make the necessary improvements — all parties are encouraged to think about the way the whole service delivery system works, rather than focusing only upon their own service.*"
(NHS Scotland, 2006)

Balancing top–down direction and local flexibility

There was much emphasis on the importance of empowering local actors to give them freedom of choice over actions, which could be adapted to local circumstances. This was coupled with national support and oversight. The national team recognised that there was no single change or 'magic bullet' that could deliver the required performance improvement alone. Proven high-impact improvement tools and techniques were recommended by the national team, which could be tried out by local teams for short periods using a 'plan-do-study-act' model (PDSA). By testing each action and tailoring it to suit local need and circumstances, teams gained ownership over the programme.

(*Continued*)

CASE STUDY 7.1 (*Continued*)

The PDSA model allowed teams to understand what worked and did not work. Thus a form of local experimentation to design and try out incremental changes, monitor their effects on performance, and then adopt or abandon them was put in place across the UCCP sites.

Reducing the 'cognitive distance' in the system

A major task for the UCCP was to reduce the cognitive distance between individuals and groups at different levels in the system, i.e. the gap between various representations of the system held by local actors. This required engagement across organisational boundaries. The greater the cognitive distance, for example between someone working in a social services department and one in the A&E department in a given hospital, the harder it was to begin to design activities to coordinate patient flows more effectively. Even within a hospital, it initially proved hard for some people in different departments to engage because their perception was that the problem lay elsewhere and they could not to see how any actions they undertook — such as changing the order in which clinicians conducted their ward round routines — could affect it.

Conveying credible evidence, in the form of data arising small-scale experiments and PDSA activities, was a very important aspect of this process of reducing cognitive distance and encouraging people to cooperate. Participants in the programme reported how some actions were not accepted until data measuring their impact were collected and analysed. Data were also important in convincing colleagues in other parts of the hospital of the magnitude of the problem and how improvements could make a difference to them.

One initiative involved empowering nurses to arrange diagnostic tests and initiate IV fluid replacement. This reduced the need for patients to experience excessive delays before a treatment plan was started. Prior to the introduction of new 'emergency nurse practitioners', decisions about every patient beyond the initial assessment and treatment were delegated to a doctor. One hospital reported how there was resistance to change from staff concerned about nurses encroaching on what was perceived as traditional medical territory. Bringing in the new model required careful engagement across the hospital, including senior managers to support the initiative and provide the budget for training, medical and radiography staff to agree changes to referral pathways, A&E nurses to agree to the new protocols, and senior nurses to help with protocol design.

(*Continued*)

CASE STUDY 7.1   *(Continued)*

Learning workshops were an integral part of the collaborative methodology. These provided opportunities for participants to share and spread new ideas and lessons. Informal learning networks emerged from these workshops, reinforcing the more formal process. The UCCP also developed a web-based tool to enable interactive problem solving and access to programme resources.

Outcomes

Over time, coordination between organisations within local health boards grew. This was guided partly by the national team recommending where to focus improvement efforts and how best to sequence interventions, and partly through the learning events organised by the national team. In these events, organisations and individuals from across the entire Scottish healthcare system could share knowledge of successful actions. The effort put into collaborative learning and the underlying whole systems perspective of the overall programme created a process of local emergence. This enabled A&E departments to coordinate with other parts of the hospital system; initial improvements in achieving the four-hour target were quite rapid. The quote from a doctor describes how she felt she was now equipped to see where changes in the system could lead to improved unscheduled care.

"The Unscheduled Care Collaborative has given me the opportunity as a clinician to help to address and solve some of the system problems which have frustrated me on a day to day basis when caring for emergency patients. It has equipped me with tools to identify where there is room for improvement in the system, and the confidence to take ownership of the solutions. I have had the opportunity to step outside my own clinical area, work with other clinicians and managers as part of a team, and gain a wider perspective of the needs of emergency patients as a group." (Staff grade doctor, emergency department, reported in NHS Scotland, 2007)

The collaborative approach was successful in moving those involved in delivering improvements to unscheduled care from a 'blame culture' to one of mutual understanding and greater awareness of the interdependencies between different hospital functions. There was whole system working *within* hospitals, leading to improved patient flows. However, the out-of-hospital patient flow was more of a problem. This was the result of two types of interdependencies

(Continued)

CASE STUDY 7.1   (*Continued*)

between the sub-systems — acute hospitals, primary care, social services and ambulance services — which became salient when stakeholders tried to engage with each other. These were information dependencies (e.g. A&E waiting for social care packages for elderly patients to be agreed) and competition over resources, exacerbated by conflicting targets distributed across the wider healthcare system.

Hospital teams experienced problems in fully engaging, incentivising and coordinating stakeholders from outside the hospital, or maintaining any initial momentum for their involvement. They had difficulty convincing out-of-hospital stakeholders of the significance of the various interdependencies and their impact on the A&E subsystem. Moreover, there was no incentive for stakeholders from outside the hospital to risk changes, because the formulation of the target in terms of A&E waiting time meant it was perceived solely as an acute care target.

Key lessons

The organisational structure, approach and experience of the UCCP provide several lessons on the use of complexity theory in a practical context. Taken at a whole system level, what we can see is the problem of coordinating actions at multiple scales:

- The local flexibility allowed by the overall programme design made it easier to test small changes. But even at the level of individual hospitals the existence of interdependencies in the system sometimes made it hard for local programme managers to isolate individual causation. This was exacerbated by time lags between the introduction of interventions and their effects — it was not always obvious what was responsible for cause and effect, especially at higher levels in the system.
- The project managers responsible for specific patient flows (e.g. within A&E, from A&E to medical admissions units or surgery) were able to stimulate actions within their own domain of authority, but they lacked authority over other parts of the system, especially the organisations involved in out-of-hospital patient flows. Whole system change could therefore be achieved within each hospital, but a whole system approach did not hold at a higher scale.

(*Continued*)

CASE STUDY 7.1   (*Continued*)

- The UCCP demonstrates importance of allowing experimentation in a safe context to stimulate innovation in healthcare. Staff working in A&E departments found that the four-hour target focused attention and gave them permission to try out small-scale local actions that they had already been thinking about and led to experimentation and innovative thinking. The programme therefore became the safe context in which new ideas could be tried out. Feedback and learning was shared with the national team and local teams, regional leaders and representatives from other parts of the healthcare system at national events.

The UCCP embraced some key principles of innovation development — we need to try new things, but expect some will fail, we need to ensure that failure is survivable, and we need to make sure we know when we have failed and learn from that failure.

Questions for discussion:

- What were the critical factors that contributed to the initial success of the UCCP programme?
- To what extent do you think the lessons about new product development (see Chapters 2 and 4) be applied to organisational innovations such as the UCCP?
- What does the UCCP story tells us about challenges of coordinating interventions in health systems across different system levels?

Source: Based on research carried out with Brice Dattée, including Dattée and Barlow (2010).

The use of pilot projects has grown in parallel to increased commitment to evidence-based policy making, to the extent that some have suggested that the approach ➜ *See Chapter 5 on the use of pilot projects in health policy* is now 'uncontroversial to the point of triviality' (Cartwright and Hardie, 2012). In the USA, the Coalition for Evidence-Based Policy was established in 2001 to advance evidence-based reforms in various social programmes. In the UK, faith in the ability of research to help policy makers became prominent under the Labour government in the 1990s, which stated that it wanted to end ideologically-led policy making. This commitment to evidence-based policy making was backed by support for research to evaluate specific policy initiatives and guidance for policy makers on how best to use evidence from research (e.g. Cabinet Office, 2003).

In the UK, a large number of pilots and demonstration projects of policy innovations have been initiated by the Department of Health. In theory, these should have informed policy learning, but they have been less influential than anticipated (Webb, 2005). A House of Commons Health Committee (2009) report concluded that evaluations of pilot projects suffer because insufficient thought is given to their design and implementation. A combination of weak study designs such as the absence of comparison groups, weak methods such as a lack of outcome indicators and baseline measurements, and evaluations that end before the innovation has time to 'bed down' all conspire to impair learning. This is sometimes compounded by changes to initiatives and their objectives during the evaluation period itself. Other problems are described in Box 7.6.

Box 7.6   CONCEPTS: Methodological problems of pilot projects

- Methods that imitate standard practices in medicine like randomised controlled trials may be inappropriate in the case of some complex or hard-to-define interventions (see Case study 7.2).
- Problems arise from site selection for pilots, where there may be a tension between picking enthusiastic sites — which might make implementation and evaluation easier — and piloting innovations in a wider and more realistic range of settings. It may be hard to find willing sites to act as 'controls' that are not receiving what may be perceived as a beneficial intervention.
- Finding the right scale at which to conduct and evaluate a pilot project can be hard. The intervention needs to be sufficiently ambitious to make a difference and provide real understanding of the impact at relevant levels in the system, but not so risky that any detrimental impact amplifies disastrously across the system as a whole. The duration of evaluations is also important. A problem with pilot projects and trials in healthcare is that politicians are often in a hurry and seek answers too early for the intervention to deliver meaningful results.

Source: House of Commons Health Committee (2009).

The policy environment may not help with learning from pilot projects. A study of pilot healthcare projects identified several factors detrimental to learning, including the extent to which commissioners and evaluators engage in effective dialogue, mismatched timing between evaluation and the policy process, and multiple — and sometimes methodologically conflicting objectives — within specific evaluations (Webb, 2005). Salisbury *et al.* (2009) examined the use of 21 evaluations specifically arising from the 2006 White Paper *Our Health, Our Care, Our Say*. The report concluded that findings would have been more useful if research had been commissioned at an earlier stage in the policy process, if more time had been available for evaluation, and if methods and study designs were more transparent. Rapid turnover of policy personnel and changing priorities also meant that some evaluations were less useful than expected.

Case study 7.2, on the experience of the Whole System Demonstrators programme, shows how there can be tensions between policy goals and a desire for evidence to support scale-up and inform policy. In this example, the rigidities of the evaluation approach clashed with the initial

---

CASE STUDY 7.2 Gathering the evidence for technology-driven whole system change — the Whole System Demonstrators programme

The 2006 Department of Health policy paper *Our Health, Our Care, Our Say* set out a broad objective to deliver new models of integrated care and move healthcare towards community-based patient-centred services. Remote care technology — telehealth and telecare — was seen both as a tool to help support people with longer term, complex health and social care needs, and also as a vehicle for stimulating whole system redesign, a 'glue' to bring together different parts of the care system (Department of Health, 2007; Goodwin, 2010).

Against this backdrop and in line with notions of evidence-based policy and practice, the Whole System Demonstrators (WSD) programme was set up to try out remote care at scale, investigate the evidence for its benefits, and make recommendations about its future deployment. The programme, which

(Continued)

CASE STUDY 7.2 (*Continued*)

ran from 2008 to 2011, is believed to be the largest evaluation of the implementation, impact and acceptability of telehealth and telecare technologies, involving over 6000 patients and 238 general practitioner practices in three localities in England (Bower *et al.*, 2011).

To take part in the programme, local health and social care authorities had to demonstrate 'a history of successful partnership working across health and social care, for example joint health and social care teams which provide comprehensive and integrated packages', and show 'evidence of a clear plan for a whole system approach' (Department of Health, 2007).

The experience of the WSD programme provides lessons on the tensions involved in introducing an innovation to promote whole system working in the messy world of health and social care, while at the same time trying to gather evidence to support scale-up and inform policy.

Early problems in defining 'whole system' working

Despite the objectives and the requirement on health and social care authorities to demonstrate a degree of prior collaboration in order to take part, whole system working was not in fact a large part of the culture in the selected sites. There was little evidence of any previous moves towards integration, with services largely operating within traditional cultural, structural and financial silos, and no strategic vision of integrated services in the three localities. The idea of a whole system approach lacked operational clarity, with no shared definition of what this meant in practice and ambiguity around how it might be achieved.

For many, whole system working was an integrated care model, placing emphasis on the holistic needs of patients and a 'seamless' service experience (i.e. the micro level in Curry and Ham's definition in Box 7.7), rather than a transformational change process focused on wider system benefits (the meso or macro levels). Overall, WSD programme managers and clinicians were more concerned with the local development of remote care services than a rather vague goal of increased integration, and there was a feeling of a lack of 'organisational readiness' for whole system working. From the first days of the programme, the vision of a technology-driven approach to whole system transformation emerged as flawed. The overall perception from policy makers was that change would largely happen organically as remote care was introduced,

(Continued)

CASE STUDY 7.2   *(Continued)*

but in the three localities it was clear that unless data sharing structures and strategic level leadership, were in place, achieving this task was unlikely. In the early stages of the WSD programme, there was a shift in strategic focus from a transformational programme to a research programme focused on delivering evidence of the clinical and cost effectiveness of remote care.

Tensions between evidence collection and iterative learning

As the WSD programme developed, it became clear that any moves towards an integrated model around new combined telecare and telehealth services were inhibited by the evaluation methodology and trial design itself. The selection criteria for participants in the randomised controlled trial (RCT) originally included a mixed group comprising those with both social and health needs, i.e. requiring both telecare and telehealth. However, early in the trial, it became clear there were problems recruiting participants into this mixed group due to the strict RCT recruitment conditions, and this trial arm was abandoned. This meant that the goal of demonstrating the advantages of telecare and telehealth together, as a driver for the redesign of care services and new levels of integration between health and social care, was no longer pursued. According to one senior manager, 'I would describe it actually *not* as being a whole system … because of the segregation between telehealth and telecare. I think we've called it "whole system" and it's not. I think it is two separate systems that have the *potential* of being the whole.'

"As an organisation, are they ready to change completely the way they work? And are there clinicians ready for that? … I think we have proved often that they aren't." Clinician, WSD programme.

"(WSD has) made me realise about the limitations of RCTs, that whilst they are the gold standard in evidence, to some extent they don't allow flexibility in terms of what you'd offer. Some of these sites have been working for two or three years, and I think … if left alone … they would be offering something different now than they were when they started, but we've restricted them from doing that." Manager, WSD programme.

"You have to unpick all the processes and procedures we put in place to deliver the RCT because they're not good business processes. They're too constrained so we've had to take everybody in that mind-set out of the programme environment." Senior manager, WSD programme.

(Continued)

CASE STUDY 7.2 (*Continued*)

The trial design also impeded organisational learning. To preserve the robustness of the RCT, remote care had to be delivered largely as originally planned, with no prospect for evolution. This trade off between iterative learning and ensuring the evidence was robust did not allow local experimentation and system responsiveness to the lessons learned during implementation. As the programme progressed, the requirements of the RCT meant that aspects of the remote care service model that were identified as sub-optimal during implementation could not be changed.

Once the trial was completed, many of the organisational processes that had been developed within the WSD programme to deliver remote care were replaced by new models, or health and social care authorities reverted back to old ones because it was perceived that the trial models were too rigid.

The WSD programme may not have led to the Department of Health objectives of whole system change, in terms of 'truly integrated services' and a 'radical and sustained shift in the way in which services are delivered', as stated in its proposed objectives. The introduction of remote care did, however, make some inroads in achieving increased collaborative working in the three localities. It was successful in helping to break down boundaries by increasing awareness of the interdependencies between and within the different actors in the system. Collaboration between care organisations was said to have improved and professional tribalism was suspended — at least temporarily — by the need to plan and implement the local remote care initiatives. Existing links between health and social care across the trial sites were strengthened and the programme helped to identify duplications in existing services.

Key lessons

- The WSD gives some insight into the extent to which technology innovation — remote care — can be used as a catalyst for large-scale transformational change around whole system working. On its own, this innovation was insufficient. It needed to be accompanied by senior management support from all the care organisations that were involved, as well as mechanisms for effectively sharing the financial costs and benefits, integrated data systems, and new joint working practices and hybrid roles.
- The programme shows how a reductionist approach to evidence gathering, in this case the use of an RCT model, does not allow us to take into account the unexpected or emergent order in the care system, or the possibility of developing an innovation through experimentation and trial and error.

(*Continued*)

CASE STUDY 7.2   (*Continued*)

Questions for discussion:

- To what extent would you judge the WSD programme to be a success or failure? Why?
- Would a more flexible approach to collecting evidence for the impact of remote care have prevented some of the WSD's implementation problems and its wider impact on the progress of this technology? Why?
- Did the lack of integration across different parts of the health and social care system mean that the technology was doomed to failure in any event?

Source: Based on research carried out with Jane Hendy and Theti Chrysanthaki, including Chrysanthaki *et al.* (2013) and Hendy *et al.* (2012).

programme goal of introducing an innovation to promote whole system working across health and social care.

Simulation and modelling

Pilot projects and trials can be hard to set up and may require substantial time and financial resources to implement. Nor do they necessarily provide sufficient insight into the potential impact of a healthcare innovation in a 'real-life' context, where resources may be more constrained and impacts may unfold at an unpredictable pace or

> "*You can always learn something from a model, even if you have no data ... (Modelling is) a smart way to squeeze the last drop of value from your data!.*"
> Sally Brailsford, professor of operational research at the University of Southampton (Brailsford, 2014).

unpredictable way. Where complex interventions are proposed — perhaps addressing multiple goals or involving many stakeholders — and where the precise design of the proposed intervention doesn't yet exist, simulation and modelling can be useful because they allow risk-free experimentation with different courses of action in a way that is far quicker and cheaper than trying them out for real (Barlow and Bayer, 2011) (Table 7.2). Models help to enable context, process, costs and outcomes of potential interventions to be linked at different levels in the care system. They can also provide a neutral framework for discussion. Engaging stakeholders from the relevant parts of the system directly in the development of the model and encouraging dialogue between them can force clarity by making their

Table 7.2.   *Choosing the right simulation technique.*

	Yes	No
Can behaviour be aggregated?	SD	DES & ABM
Are dynamic rules of behaviour within individual?	ABM	DES
Is variability/randomness important?	DES & ABM	SD
Do changes to the system happen over time?	SD & ABM	DES & ABM
Is the timeframe of interest long?	SD	DES & ABM
Is the number of entities large?	SD & ABM	DES
Is feedback important?	SD	DES & ABM
Is the scope more operational rather than strategic?	DES & ABM	SD
Is understanding more important than optimisation?	SD	DES

Source: Cravo-Oliveira (2014).

SD — system dynamics; DES — discrete event simulations; ABM — agent-based modelling.

assumptions more explicit. This can help to create support for any subsequent decisions that are taken on the basis of the modelling experiments.

Simulation models have been developed for healthcare planning since the mid 1960s, but have yet to be fully accepted and embedded within mainstream decision making by clinicians, health managers and policy makers. One important reason is that the approach provides a very different form of evidence from randomised controlled trials or other standard statistical methods, and therefore requires a culture shift for people immersed in those methods. Two of the most widely used modelling methodologies also have their own inherent shortcomings — discrete event simulation models can be time-consuming to develop and run, and are data-hungry, while system dynamic models do not capture individual variability, but are fast to run. Both require expertise and specialist software. Despite these features, simulation can still provide insight into a problem and 'what if' scenarios around it, even if it will never give the optimal answer to a problem.

Tackling health service challenges through 'whole system change'

At the other end of the spectrum from small-scale pilot projects and experiments are large flagship transformation projects designed to tackle major health service delivery challenges such as productivity, safety or quality. These sometimes draw on lessons about complex

➜ *See Chapter 5 for more on integrated care*

adaptive systems — not always explicit — and in recent years a policy rhetoric on the need for 'whole system change' has emerged, i.e. one which purports to account for the structure of key parts of the health system and its important interdependencies. In practice, this 'whole system' is usually defined in relation to a small part of the wider health system, such as the parts responsible for frail elderly people, the care pathway for people with stroke, or emergency care. The common thread is a quest for coordination and service integration around the patient. However, one of the problems with the notion of whole system working is identifying what it actually entails in practice (Box 7.7). There is no single or shared operational definition (Chrysanthaki *et al.*, 2013; Hudson, 2006) — terms such as 'partnership working', 'joint working', 'seamless services' and 'integrated care' all permeate policy and managerial discourse and are associated with whole system working. This ambiguity means the evidence base for the benefits of whole system working is also ambiguous. Nevertheless, the problem of silo thinking around aspects of health and social care such as budget allocations, performance targets and professional interests has ensured that a goal for policy makers and others seeking to improve services is to find ways of increasing collaboration between diverse healthcare groups and organisations in complex settings.

There is little research on how professional groups and their organisations make sense of the concept of whole system working, whether they are willing and ready to embrace this idea, and how this impacts on initiatives to implement innovations or engage in improvement programmes. Previous work indicates that the idea of making decisions in a 'joined up' manner may be viewed as threatening (Glendinning, 2003).

The Scottish example of unscheduled care reform (Case study 7.1) shows that whole system thinking, combined with performance targets and suitable support for sharing lessons, can be useful in driving change and innovation. However, it also shows that an ability to exert leverage across the different parts of the health and social care systems is needed for interventions to work — the Scottish approach was unable to adequately tackle the more complex out-of-hospital interactions between different stakeholders in the wider care system. The Apoteket-Medco example (Case study 7.3) from Sweden shows how whole system change at a national level can be made, providing the right conditions are in place. These apply across system levels, from individual patient and staff right up to the fit with national policy, and include a clear understanding of the key stakeholders and the potential costs and benefits for them.

Box 7.7 BACKGROUND: Integrated care programmes

The challenges posed by an ageing population and rising numbers of people with chronic, complex health needs are exacerbated by fragmentation, duplication and poor coordination across care services, hence the interest in integrating services where appropriate. 'Integrated care' is suffused with systems thinking. One classification splits integrated care into three types according to the scope and level of integration (Curry and Ham, 2010):

- '*Macro-level* models deliver integrated care to the whole populations served by an organisation (e.g. Kaiser Permanente and the Geisinger Health System in the USA).
- *Meso-level* integrated care is targeted at a particular care group or population with the same disease or health condition (e.g. integrated care for older people or chronic disease management programmes).
- *Micro-level* models focus on individual service users and their carers (e.g. care co-ordination and planning).

How we observe the impact of integrated care initiatives is therefore partly a function of the scale we choose because it influences our choice over where to draw the boundaries around the system and timescale over which the dynamics are captured. This choice will affect our observations of the success or otherwise of initiatives.

A major problem with the discussion about the benefits of integrated care is that the lack of consensus over the definition of 'integrated care' and variety of approaches make it hard to identify transferable best practice or causality (Singer *et al.*, 2011). There is little evidence that integrated care saves money (Øvretveit, 2011), but some approaches might lead to an overall reduction in

(Continued)

Box 7.7   (*Continued*)

secondary care costs. This lack of observable data may partly be a function of our choice of scale. Several Canadian provinces have implemented integrated care initiatives for the frail elderly population and primary care. These aim to improve population health, increase patient satisfaction and substitute institutional for community based services. While there has been some success in achieving these objectives, it is not clear whether this success is due to mechanisms to incentivise the stakeholders or to other factors.

In the UK, policy has increasingly advocated that the design of services should adopt an integrated care approach, underpinned by whole system thinking. A programme of fourteen integrated care 'pioneer' schemes is being implemented. Some of these involve very large system transformations. One of these is the North West London Whole System Integrated Care Programme (WSICP), covering 2 million people and bringing together the National Health Service, local authority social services and the voluntary sector, along with patients, carers and services users. The WSICP is explicitly informed by systems thinking:

'*Today, health and social care is delivered by different organisations that work separately. Organisational boundaries can prevent professionals from working together to provide the kind of high quality, joined up support that people expect and want. We want to change this so people and their goals are at the centre of a team of health and care professionals who work together smoothly. This will mean unlocking the social capital in our communities, viewing the energy, compassion, skills and learning of local people as valuable assets. We want to enable individuals, community groups, charities, local organisations and services to work effectively together. Integrated care means integrated care teams that are focused on individual people and their needs. Bringing together all the different parts of the health and social care system will provide better communication and sharing of relevant information to reduce duplication and confusion for individuals, carers and staff. This will mean one set of goals agreed by the individual, supported by one team, one approach.*'

The programme was launched by bringing together more than 150 representatives from across the local health and social care system, including service users and carers, to work together and define a framework. Through a process of co-design drawing on the collective knowledge and expertise of the

(*Continued*)

Box 7.7 (*Continued*)

partners, the WSICP developed local plans, which were aligned with the overall Department of Health integrated care programme goals and their own local strategic aims and direction. These are now being refined and rolled out.

Source: http://integration.healthiernorthwestlondon.nhs.uk/

CASE STUDY 7.3 Introducing 'drug utilisation reviews' (DURs) developed in the USA into Sweden's pharmacy sector — Apoteket and Medco

Pharmacy benefits managers (PBMs) originated in the USA during the 1970s as intermediaries between purchasers and payers to adjudicate prescription drug claims. Since then they have evolved into organisations that aggregate the buying power of people enrolled in health plans, negotiating price discounts from retail pharmacies and drug manufacturers. They also conduct DURs and create formularies for drug products. Today PBMs are sometimes separate services within a healthcare system such as Kaiser or the Veterans Administration, but usually they are a third party intermediary. This case focuses on the challenges faced by Sweden's healthcare services when attempting to develop a collaboration between Medco Health Solutions, a PBM from the USA, and Apoteket, Sweden's state owned pharmaceutical distribution monopoly.

Sweden's healthcare system — like all others in developed countries — has been undergoing intense pressure from an ageing population, the general rise in costs and a concern by governments to contain public expenditure. There was particular cost pressure in the rising consumption of drugs by patients. This was partly driven by an increasing range of therapeutic treatments becoming available, but also by prescribing patterns. By the mid-2000s, around 9% of Sweden's population was consuming 50% of the national drug budget, each person typically receiving over 10 separate prescriptions.

(*Continued*)

CASE STUDY 7.3   *(Continued)*

Shaking up Sweden's pharmacy market

The Apoteket–Medco story involves two parallel forces coming together in the mid-2000s. First, the government of the day was seeking to liberalise parts of the Swedish economy. Responding to consumer pressure for greater access to over-the-counter drugs, an improved range of services and lower cost drugs, a process of liberalisation began in Sweden's pharmacy market. One of the aims was to expose Apoteket to competition. When liberalisation began, Apoteket's core business consisted of sourcing drugs through wholesalers and distributing them in more than 900 retail pharmacies and hospital pharmacies. The company's mission was very much one of social obligation, combined with a concern to provide efficient pharmaceutical dispensing and distribution, at a modest profit. To facilitate other players entering the market, parts of Apoteket were sold off and by 2010 the number of newly established pharmacies had grown. Apoteket therefore needed to adapt to the transition from monopoly market to an open market.

At the same time, Apoteket was introduced to Medco through mutual contacts. Medco was the leading PBM in the USA, with 60 million members and managing approximately USD 36 billion in prescription drug expenditures each year. The company had 40 years' experience of prescription drug benefits management, extensive clinical resources and expertise, including 2,200 clinicians on its staff, a range of patents and intellectual property, and leading information systems technology in the PBM field. But it was also keen to tackle the limits to its organic growth within the US market. Under management and stock market pressure, it wanted to internationalise its operations. The Swedish opportunity was a chance to prove its ability to develop and manage new operations abroad.

The opportunity for innovation in Sweden's monopoly drug dispensing and fulfilment system and Apoteket's need to explore new avenues for business therefore aligned neatly with Medco's interest in bringing its processes for prescription management into fresh markets. Both companies were motivated to explore the possibility for a partnership and identify areas where Medco's innovative approach could be adopted in Sweden. But it was clear that simply transferring the Medco approach wholesale would not work — an understanding of Sweden's pharmacy ecosystem and the implications of any Medco intervention on its stakeholders and their work practices was essential. Successful innovation would require the societal and economic benefits to be

(Continued)

CASE STUDY 7.3 (*Continued*)

carefully defined — would an Apoteket-Medco joint venture make Sweden's health services better? And there would also need to be political and regulatory fit between Medco's solutions and Sweden's approach to healthcare.

Adapting the Medco model

Medco's model of PBM radically challenged traditional approaches to pharmacy dispensing processes. The company had moved this area of healthcare from a craft-based to an industrial process, changing work practices and the relationships between stakeholders. At the front end of the process, doctors' prescriptions were scanned within Medco's support centres and entered into a prescription database. Once an order had been instigated, a pharmacist would conduct a drug interaction review and either authorise the prescription or send it to a doctor for verification. The order would then be sent to an automated packaging plant, where the majority of orders were placed in the bag with no human interference, before despatch to the patient.

Medco had invested USD 600 million in the previous three years to support increased operating efficiencies and had introduced Six Sigma initiatives to achieve a 99.99994% accuracy rate in final prescription dispensing. Its DUR system allowed alerts to be triggered when potential problems in a prescription were identified, resulting in reduced medication errors and hospitalisations.

However, what was proven to be successful in one specific and very different healthcare system could not be transferred as a whole to Sweden. For example, differences in packaging regulations meant that Medco would not be able to introduce its automated packaging technology. Following a detailed analysis of its compatibility with Sweden's pharmacy processes and formulary, it was decided that Apoteket should license Medco's DUR system and establish it as part of prescription distribution and management in Sweden.

The DUR technology comprised an expert system, which reviewed prescriptions against a database containing the patient's prescription records. It employed several thousand clinical rules to evaluate the conformance of prescriptions to evidence-based medical practices. The technology gave both physicians and pharmacists a decision support system which identified drug cross interactions, potential errors in dosage levels and other adverse effects.

For Apoteket, licensing the Medco technology was a way of rapidly introducing a proven DUR approach and gaining knowledge and expertise in advanced drug management programmes. Introducing DUR was seen as a way

(*Continued*)

CASE STUDY 7.3 *(Continued)*

of creating a safety net for all stakeholders, lowering costs and improving the quality of prescribing decisions. For Medco, this was a potentially attractive licensing opportunity. Establishing a joint venture to introduce the DUR system potentially allowed the development time and risks to be reduced. There was therefore a strong rational case on both sides, but the healthcare ecosystem still had to be won over.

Implementing DUR — winning over the stakeholders

Although there were clear win–wins for both parties, the implementation of DUR was complex. Introducing the innovation required significant system change at many levels. It was necessary to introduce a new technology and adapt it for Sweden, at the same time changing work processes and the division of labour within the pharmacy sector. Engagement of different stakeholders at different levels in the system was needed — these ranged from individual pharmacists and doctors, through the country's 21 'Landsting' (the regional funders of healthcare), to the drug companies, national policy and regulatory bodies, and Apoteket itself. Implementation therefore meant creating a technical and economic case that was sufficiently compelling to a wide range of stakeholders.

Under the leadership of Michael Camitz, Apoteket developed both a technology and social implementation process. There were four core challenges and groups to convince.

- The first challenge was to prove the clinical and technical cases with the medical and pharmaceutical professionals, as well as drug manufacturers, who opposed the system on grounds of quality of information about drugs within the formulary. Creating a medical advisory council to assess the similarity between American and Swedish drug formularies helped to achieve buy-in from these groups. This concluded that there was sufficient similarity to allow adoption of Medco's US database, with minor modifications. Whilst not a simple process, over time a combination of technical trials and advocacy from leading clinicians won support from these key stakeholders, who eventually accepted the system as a useful way of supporting rather than challenging professional competences and decisions.
- The second challenge was the economic case. This was resolved by undertaking a trial using the American system to review 10,000 Swedish

(Continued)

CASE STUDY 7.3   (*Continued*)

high-user patients. The data showed sufficient evidence of suboptimal prescribing that a case could be made to show how patient safety would be significantly enhanced and that both direct and indirect savings of several billion Swedish kroner could be achieved. This created the business and investment case, which also suggested that the DUR system would rapidly cover its costs.

- The third challenge was political. This proved to be relatively simple. The patient safety and economic case won immediate support from the health minister, releasing central government funding for implementation costs. This meant that the Landsting were supportive. There was strong support from patient and elderly groups from the outset, who saw clear advantages in the DUR system.

- The final challenge was not about acceptance in principle but adoption in practice. This was achieved by modifying some of the features of Medco's US version of the system. The centralised checking of orders by specialists was not adopted; in Sweden this process was decentralised to pharmacists at the point of dispensing. This way the traditional working process and patient relationships of the local pharmacy were modified but not radically altered. Although this was possibly suboptimal in terms of time and cost savings, it was regarded as a suitable trade-off to ease acceptance, and was not seen to fundamentally weaken any aspects of the alert system.

Over a year or so, the Medco system was adopted not just by Apoteket but also became a systemic feature of the Swedish pharmacy market, such that all pharmacy companies were obliged to register and use the system as part of their license and regulatory conditions.

Since the introduction of the DUR system, Medco has been acquired by Express Scripts and Apoteket has been significantly restructured — two-thirds of its retail premises were sold off to new entrants and the running and maintenance of the DUR system was handed over to a separate government e-health agency. This now makes the system equally available to all pharmacy operators in Sweden. But although the core technology provider has been changed, and the two protagonist companies are no longer involved, system-wide innovation has been achieved and embedded as part of the infrastructure for Swedish healthcare.

(*Continued*)

CASE STUDY 7.3 *(Continued)*

Key lessons

The Apoteket–Medco case shows us how major innovation transfer across health systems is possible, driving change across the whole system, providing the right conditions are in place.

- Early **proof of concept** was critical in convincing stakeholders, including the minister for health, of the benefits of DUR. This required credible evidence not only of the economic case — in the form of savings for the Swedish health system and acceptable returns for the commercial participants — but a case in terms of clinical and quality of care benefits for patient case. A technical case, showing that Medco's DUR could be integrated into Sweden's pharmacy infrastructure, also needed to be made. Alongside this, it was important develop an understanding of the degree of fit between the innovation and the Swedish pharmacy system, and the elements that could be dropped or adapted to the local context without compromising the integrity of the innovation (see Chapter 5).

- Developing a clear **understanding of the core and other stakeholders**, and their ecosystem, was essential, along with an understanding of the potential costs and benefits for them. These were not necessarily immediately obvious or rational. The strength of opposition of the drug manufacturers, for example, was not foreseen. The industry was clearly concerned about the impact of DUR on its market, but expressed this in the form of criticism about the details of the DUR mechanism and quality of information about drugs. The key objection was that Swedish and US national formularies would be too different to enable leverage of Medco's clinical rules. This was overcome through research, which provided evidence that only 4% of drugs were sufficiently different to need updated rules.

- Putting in place the right **implementation and communications structure** was essential. The joint venture model emphasised openness in goals and aspirations, and allowed the level of patience required to create cultural understanding across the different companies. Early on, it was clear that winning the support of the core stakeholders would require an advisory board of sufficiently high seniority and a clinical reference committee nominated by Sweden's doctors association, responsible for helping to build the system rules. There was also a need for transparency on the mutual benefits and potential costs, along with the rationale for bringing in the DUR, which was communicated to all.

(Continued)

CASE STUDY 7.3   (*Continued*)

Exercise

- Map the stakeholders and their ecosystem — the organisations and institutions that you think would need to be involved in the introduction of DUR in your country's health system.

- Think about what changes, and who wins and loses. What might need to adapted to bring a DUR into the health system? What might be the unforeseen impacts of DUR across the different levels of the system?

Source: Case study prepared in collaboration with Adrian King. With thanks to Michael Camitz and Bengt Norin.

Systems thinking for global health

A failure to take into account the complexity of health systems is seen as a hindrance to efforts to achieve better and more equitable outcomes health systems in low- and middle-income countries (Adam and de Savigny, 2012). The general argument is that a systems approach reorients our perspective by allowing us to better understand the interconnected relationships among health system components. This in turn can help policy makers move away from linear and reductionist policy interventions that have bedeviled many global health initiatives.

"*We need new ways of thinking and of working in order to accommodate the complexity of the challenges in and urgent need for health system innovation and change.*" (Herbert and Best, 2011)

But such thinking is by no means embedded within mainstream approaches to global health innovation. One study found that few of a sample of over a hundred interventions designed to strengthen the health systems of low- and middle-income countries paid attention to their system-wide impacts (even though the interventions were often highly complex) and none incorporated concepts from theories about complex adaptive systems (Adam and de Savigny, 2012).

Nevertheless, in recent years, there have been calls for the use of such thinking in the design and evaluation of initiatives to strengthen health systems (Adam *et al.*, 2012; Adam and de Savigny, 2012; Paina and Peters, 2012). The World Health Organisation's Alliance for Health Policy and Systems Research devoted a flagship report to this topic (WHO, 2009), which along with other publications increased interest. The report noted that the timing for applying systems thinking was never better, given the efforts of many countries to scale-up successful pilot projects through major systems strengthening investments. It emphasised the untapped potential of systems thinking in the design and evaluation of interventions and argued that the approach delivers a range of benefits, including demonstration of the potential of solutions that work across sub-systems, the promotion of networks of diverse stakeholders and learning, and fostering more system-wide planning, evaluation and research.

So how have systems thinking and complexity theory been applied to global health challenges? The WHO report defines a health system as 'all organisations, people and actions whose primary intent is to promote, restore or maintain health'. It uses the WHO *Framework for Action* on health systems to identify six building blocks that together constitute a complete system:

1. service delivery,
2. health workforce,
3. information,
4. medical products, vaccines and technologies,
5. financing,
6. leadership and governance.

The report notes how

'The building blocks alone do not constitute a system, any more than a pile of bricks constitutes a functioning building. It is the multiple relationships and interactions among the blocks — how one affects and influences the others, and is in turn affected by them — that convert these blocks into a system.'

It also makes the point that a complex intervention is a system in itself, interacting with other building blocks of the system and triggering feedback that may sometimes be counterintuitive. Interventions range in complexity according to factors such as the number of stakeholders that need to be involved in adoption and implementation decisions, and the number of stakeholders which are affected by its introduction. The extent to which the intervention involves combinations of technological and organisational innovation will also influence its 'complexity' (see Chapter 5). Figure 7.3, based on the WHO report, maps various interventions according to the complexity of the intervention itself, its impact across the health system and the need for system thinking when designing or evaluating the intervention.

Designing interventions from a systems perspective requires us to think about how the different health system building blocks need to be combined and targeted. This will be shaped by our understanding of the problem and its dimensions. Because of the interactions between building blocks, interventions may have a wider impact outside their boundaries or at different levels in the system. An initiative such as pay-for-performance (see Chapter 5) is seen as a complex intervention with system-level effects on other building blocks of the health system.

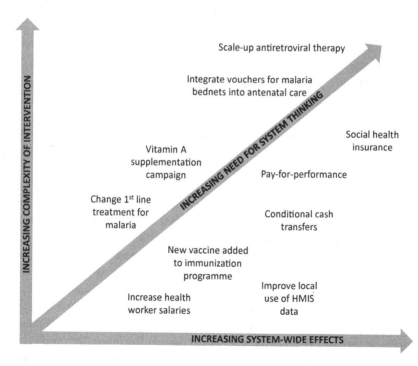

Figure 7.3.   Systems thinking in global health.
Source: WHO (2009).

INNOVATION IN ACTION 7.2:   Spreading the Tanzania Ministry of Health Essential Health Interventions Project

The Tanzania Ministry of Health Essential Health Interventions Project (TEHIP) was launched in 1996. It aimed to strengthen the health system by simultaneously applying a suite of interventions targeting each of its key building blocks (de Savigny *et al.*, 2008). These included:

- district decentralisation with increased ownership of the planning process and fiscal resources to target the governance building block;
- new approaches to financing to improve local resource allocation;
- improvements in information flows by introducing community-based surveillance systems;
- strengthening human resources through management training and better working conditions;
- increased authority to access and spend local financial resources on drugs and technologies;
- the adoption of service delivery innovations such as of 'integrated management of childhood illness' and insecticide treated bed nets to control malaria.

The programme could therefore be described as a highly complex innovation, across several dimensions (see Figure 5.1). While it is impossible to say which of these specific innovations were the most important, it was nevertheless clear that they all acted in an interdependent way:

'The financing intervention was essential — but funding alone would not have lead to such good performance outcomes… Without the governance change allowing decentralisation of responsibility with greater authority for spending, little would have changed. Without the new information sources that related spending priorities to health priorities, the subsequent resource re-allocations (which resulted in service delivery change) would not have occurred. Without the feedback on progress from their information system, there would have been little idea of what was working, and what not. Without further governance changes allowing ownership of planning and the flexibility to spend on human resource training, the new and more powerful interventions would not have been adopted so quickly.' (WHO, 2009)

(Continued)

INNOVATION IN ACTION 7.2 *(Continued)*

TEHIP showed how a coordinated and relatively low cost investment in interventions to strengthen healthcare on a system wide basis was able to lower the burden of disease (Masanja *et al.*, 2008). The programme essentially comprised a set of incremental, decentralised and sector-wide innovations, and a set of practical management, planning and priority-setting tools.

However, TEHIP has not become institutionalised and its benefits have proved hard to sustain. A combination of population growth and increasing health burdens from chronic and emerging diseases, shortages of health workers, and deficiencies in infrastructure and lack of medical supplies has overwhelmed the capacity of Tanzania's health system (Kwesigaboa *et al.*, 2012). Nor has the model in spread more widely in Africa. Although a delegation from Ghana came to observe TEHIP and introduce elements of the programme (de Savigny *et al.*, 2008), and despite the similarities in health system and other contexts between the two countries, experience of scaling up one of the interventions, insecticide treated bed nets, has proved somewhat different (de Savigny, 2012). Both countries tackled this issue by integrating consumer discount vouchers into the health system, a complex intervention requiring collaboration between the public, private and non-governmental sectors. In Tanzania, vouchers had become the main delivery system for insecticide treated bed nets by 2012. In Ghana, national implementation never progressed beyond initial discussions and piloting, and the approach was replaced by the alternative model of mass distribution. The different implementation pathways in the two countries result from the way the various health system building blocks and interactions played out. Factors that provided an enabling environment for the voucher scheme in Tanzania did not achieve this in Ghana — the voucher scheme was never seen as an appropriate national strategy, other delivery systems were not complementary and the private sector was underdeveloped. In Tanzania, the effort devoted to stakeholder engagement and consensus building was a key enabling factor, as was public sector support for the private sector. Together, these helped create a single coordinated strategy for service delivery which avoided the problems of competing delivery systems that occurred in Ghana.

Understanding the implications for adoption and sustainability, and the potential impact, therefore requires a collective systems thinking exercise among stakeholders and careful mapping of the potential system interactions, including any positive or negative feedback.

The WHO report also makes the point that while RCTs of large-scale interventions are often considered the best designs to evaluate efficacy, they need to be accompanied by other types of evaluation which better account for processes, context and wider effects. The example in Innovation in Action 7.2 describes how this thinking was applied in a Tanzania's health system and subsequently failed to spread to Ghana because of a failure to appreciate the effects of the different context.

Chapter summary

- Health systems display many of the attributes of complex systems, such as interconnected and interdependent elements, which can both influence and be influenced by any other element, and positive and negative feedback processes leading to counterintuitive behaviour.
- Complexity in healthcare can be a result of the property of the intervention (or the innovation) and also a property of the system in which the intervention is implemented.
- Interest in systems thinking and complexity in relation to healthcare has grown in recent years. Healthcare policy makers sometimes talk about the need for 'whole system change', implicitly drawing on ideas from complexity theory.
- Attempts to introduce change at a whole system level often fail to appreciate the interrelationships and their dynamics.
- It is important to consider the different levels of a system, for example from hospital ward to national health system. Interventions at one level can have ramifications at other levels or be constrained by features operating at another level. The scale at which we view a system is therefore important as it determines the timescale over which changes can be observed.

Questions for discussion

1. Healthcare is often described as a 'complex system'. Discuss why this is the case. What are the implications of this complexity for the introduction and spread of healthcare innovations?
2. Innovations in healthcare often have an impact outside the adopting organisation. What are the implications of this for the management of healthcare innovations?
3. Attempts to introduce 'whole system' change in healthcare require us to understand the interrelationships of the system and their dynamics. Discuss whether you agree with this statement, using examples.
4. To what extent do you agree that it is especially important to focus on stakeholder engagement when managing the introduction of healthcare innovation projects? Why might this be the case?
5. What aspects of a complex healthcare innovation might lead you to decide that careful planning and preparation was needed before its introduction?
6. What is it about a typical healthcare innovation that makes it hard to manage?

Selected further reading

Adam T, Hsu J, de Savigny D, Lavis J, Røttingen J-A, Bennett S (2012) Evaluating health systems strengthening interventions in low-income and middle-income countries: Are we asking the right questions? *Health Policy and Planning* 27: iv9–iv19.

Dattée B, Barlow J (2010) Complexity and whole-system change programmes. *Journal of Health Services Research & Policy* 15(S2): 12–18.

Plsek P, Greenhalgh T (2001) Complexity science: The challenge of complexity in health care. *British Medical Journal* 323: 625–628.

WHO (2009) *Systems Thinking For Health Systems Strengthening*. Geneva: World Health Organisation.

CHAPTER 08

CONCLUSIONS

Throughout this book, we have focused on the key themes which form the backdrop to innovation management within healthcare. These can be summarised as the following:

- *Technology and innovation are not the same — but they are connected.* We often see 'technology' in terms of physical artefacts to solve a particular problem or serve a particular need, but it is also about the knowledge that is embedded in those artefacts. That knowledge is the result of R&D and our experience of using those physical artefacts. 'Innovation' is both a process and also an outcome of this process, whether that outcome is a new physical artefact — a product — or some form of change. As a process, innovation embraces a series of steps from the creation of the initial idea to its adoption and diffusion. Within healthcare, it can often be unclear what the 'innovation' actually is because many innovations are not well-defined physical artefacts. They can bring together any combination of new products, processes, and services.

- *Whether an innovation is radical, incremental, disruptive, or some other type is something of a moot point.* It often depends on the context and perspective of those who are adopting it. Innovations may be new to an organisation that delivers healthcare, but widely used elsewhere, or they may be new to an entire health system, but practised in a neighbouring country. The task of managing the implementation of that innovation is no less difficult for that organisation or country than if they were the first adopter.

345

- *The environment into which innovations are adopted in healthcare is often quite unlike that of other industries or sectors of the economy.* Healthcare — even in countries with less developed health systems — is an immensely complex system. A wide range of organisations, institutions and regulations interact in ways that make the adoption of innovations unpredictable and challenging. This is as much the case for those involved in decisions to adopt them as it is for those creating and supplying them. The attributes of the innovation itself, the organisational, cultural and economic context for adoption, and the interpretation of the evidence for its prospective benefits and costs are all influential.

- *The economics of technological innovations in healthcare are unlike innovations in other industries.* This is something of a double-edged sword for health policy makers and managers. Often costs to the health system, or payers or governments, rise following the introduction of a new healthcare technology because it allows more care to be provided — more people can be treated and more problems can be diagnosed. The complexity of health systems also means that the effects — perhaps costs — of introducing an innovation can fall outside the immediate adopting organisation, perhaps in a way that was unintended or unpredicted.

- *Increasing attention is paid to the collection and use of evidence for the impact of innovations as a factor that drives decisions about the adoption of healthcare innovations.* However, it can still be hard to create a coherent case for investment of money, time and energy in adopting an innovation. This is partly due to the difficulty in gathering evidence, especially where a healthcare innovation combines organisational, service and technology change, and partly to the ways in which evidence is interpreted by different groups of care professionals.

- *There is a disconnection between the basic science and the creation of innovations that are taken-up into everyday use.* While the pace of scientific development remains intense, and ultimately the improvement in the performance of specific medical technologies or products can be dramatic, the average time taken for the science to be translated into new products is long. For companies developing technological innovations, the process of bringing them to market often requires considerable patience and deep pockets. This applies as much to global pharmaceutical and medical device companies as it does to small med tech start-ups.

- *Not all healthcare innovation involves the development of new high tech and high cost technologies.* We need to harness the potential of disruptive and frugal innovations to address the challenges of high cost healthcare systems in developed countries, as well as the lack of access to affordable healthcare in low- to middle-income countries. New technologies are certainly playing a part, but their implications for the infrastructure and organisations of healthcare are only just becoming clear. Making full use of the potential of disruptive and frugal innovations for shifting care from high-end, complex models towards simpler and more affordable solutions will severely challenge the incumbent institutions of healthcare in developed countries. For developing countries, they offer the prospect of leapfrogging old organisational models of healthcare and putting in place new ones.

The question we must ask ourselves is how these themes relate to the big global healthcare challenges described in Chapter 1. A key lesson is that managing innovation and technology in healthcare is not simply a matter of doing one or two things well. Innovation is not a simple magic bullet. Successfully embracing innovation in order to meet future healthcare challenges will require:

- *An innovation strategy that recognises path dependence.* The starting point — the current position of the different players within a healthcare system — closely influences the future paths that the system can take. The past accumulation of policies, institutions and physical and organisation infrastructure means that distinct sources and directions of change will be open to the organisations and governments involved in the provision of healthcare, while others may be closed to them. For all the talk of a need for disruptive innovation, fundamentally disrupting health systems often requires very considerable political and public willpower and engagement. Recognising the limitations as well as the possibilities is a crucial first step in creating any healthcare innovation strategy.
- Successful innovation requires the right mechanisms to enable change to happen. Mechanisms need to be put in place both to stimulate innovative

behaviour and ensure that a steady flow of new ideas, products and processes is available for adoption within the healthcare system. But while this is necessary, it is not a sufficient pillar for a truly innovative healthcare system. Support for the effective and sustainable *implementation* of innovation at both organisational and system levels, and sharing knowledge about what works and why, are also crucial for successful innovation management in healthcare.

The big challenges revisited

Chapter 1 described three healthcare innovation challenges for the 21st century:

- The need to balance resources, costs and changing patterns of demand. While this is clearly a universal feature of health systems, there are particular problems for the advanced health systems in achieving this.
- The need for the healthcare technology industries to evolve. Their products account for around a quarter of total global expenditure on healthcare but the changing type of demand for healthcare and the exigencies of health systems are making it harder for companies to find the right strategies for future growth.
- The need for lower-income countries to create and deliver universal high quality healthcare as far as possible. Ensuring that countries with emerging health systems do not merely seek to replicate the increasingly outmoded examples in developed countries is the trick here.

The background to these challenges is shared across much of the world. For the rest of this century and beyond, the long-term trends towards an ageing population and rising numbers of people with chronic diseases — diabetes, cancer, heart disease, stroke, chronic respiratory diseases and mental illness — will drive demand for healthcare services in both developed and emerging economies. Ageing populations and increasing life expectancies will place an increasing burden on many national healthcare systems. Europe is currently the region with the highest proportion of older individuals and this is projected to remain the case for at least the next half century. Projections by the UN suggest that by 2050, around 37% of Europeans will be aged 60 or over, compared to only 10% of Africa's population. Japan has long experienced the health and social care challenges associated with ageing; the country is a laboratory for the way technological innovation can be deployed to help. China is expected to see a combination of declining numbers of young people and an escalation in the number of elderly people. Across the world, there could be nearly two billion people aged 60 or above by 2050 (Deloitte, 2014b).

The spread of chronic diseases as a result of ageing and changing diet and lifestyles is the other great shared demographic trend leading to pressure on health systems. Chronic diseases are now by far the leading cause of mortality in the world, with some countries with emerging healthcare systems seeing a major growth in diabetes and cardiovascular illnesses. According to the International Diabetes Foundation, by 2010 China had overtaken India as the world leader in the absolute number of diabetes cases. And the numbers are huge — around 92 million diabetics in China and 80 million in India. There are an estimated 100 million hypertension sufferers in China, and three million new cases every year (Deloitte, 2014a). Not only does this pose a significant burden on national economies, the cost of treatment for chronic diseases is often out of reach for many of the world's poor.

While it plays out in different ways across the world, access to healthcare is another shared challenge. Worldwide, over a billion people lack access to a basic healthcare system (Deloitte, 2014b). Although economic growth across Asia and some other parts of the world has helped to improve access, coverage remains uneven between and within regions. This is partly a problem of resources allocated to healthcare. Even in middle income countries like Mexico less is spent on healthcare as a proportion of GDP — around 6.2% compared to the average 9.5% in OECD countries. But it is also a question of shortages of healthcare workers. Globally, the World Health Organisation estimates there is a shortage of 4.3 million doctors, nurses and other health workers. This is especially concentrated in developing countries (WHO, 2006). In 2010, of the 57 countries with critical shortages, where there are problems in delivering even the most basic immunisation and maternal health services, 36 are in sub-Saharan Africa. Other countries, including India and Pakistan, have critical shortages in their health workforce but are simultaneously amongst the countries with the highest number of doctors and nurses migrating to work elsewhere. Even the developed countries are experiencing workforce shortfalls in parts of their health systems such as rural and other underserved areas. The UK has severe shortages in the number of nurses and general practitioners. Across Europe, there will be a shortage of 230,000 doctors by 2020 (Lunghini, 2014).

The solutions

In the advanced health systems of developed countries, where costs are high, simply continuing to increase spending on healthcare is not an option. And in lower-income countries, in the short term, more money may not be an option either. Moreover, even if additional finance is available, ensuring it is deployed efficiently and fairly is not always the easy. But the ingredients of affordable high quality care systems are increasingly clear. The solutions are in fact not dissimilar across countries, but they need to recognise the cultural, social, economic and political circumstances of what are very different health systems and very different starting points. These have been described by Mark Britnell (2015) and are summarised in Box 8.1.

A focus on health promotion and illness prevention, based on a good understanding of populations and patients, can encourage and support people to achieve health and wellness; in time this can help to take demand out of the formal care system — the hospitals, primary care services and other institutional structures. Care services need to be redesigned (or designed in the first place) so that primary and secondary healthcare, and social care for elderly or vulnerable people, are integrated and incorporate care pathways built around the individual and their needs. Within this type of model, there should be a strong focus on strengthened primary care, but with tertiary healthcare centres acting as their own mini health systems.

Box 8.1 BACKGROUND: Essential ingredients for affordable high quality care systems

- Strong health promotion and illness prevention and good joined-up well-being policies and plans across the public and private sectors.
- Excellent population and patient segmentation and stratification techniques to encourage and support citizens and patients to live actively, all supported by the latest technology.
- Scaled-up primary care systems with access to speedy diagnostics and therapeutics provided in suitable facilities and supported through integrated community and pharmacy health teams.
- Simultaneously localised and centralised clinical services which put care in communities where possible and concentrate care when absolutely necessary, to improve patient outcomes and efficiency.
- Excellent care plans and pathways developed by clinicians and supported by improvement science, and which are accountable and transparent.
- Workforce motivation and development that looks at the sensible delegation and demarcation of skills from the patient's perspective and not just the producer's.
- Strong tertiary centres to act as health systems, linking secondary and primary care services and facilitated by leading-edge paramedic services that provide care on the spot.
- Integrated health and aged care provided seamlessly from the home and funded fairly through adequate financing from public and private sources, as necessary.
- Community-based mental health services which recognise the personal and economic importance of mental health.
- Above all else, a health system which treats patients as active partners in their care (and communities as carers), and allows individuals and carers control over their life and, ultimately, their death.

Source: Britnell (2015).

While there is considerable activity to put in place aspects of these essential ingredients in many health systems, progress in some areas — both countries and specific initiatives — is frustratingly slow. In particular, moves towards greater integration are impeded by the prevailing fragmented and silo-based systems, and the presence of hard-to-change legacy institutions and cultures. In countries which are still building their health systems, putting in place the essential ingredients will require a coordinated effort by payers and policy-makers, as well as providers. Payers — both insurers and governments — need to become active not only in shaping their care systems, but influencing the health behaviour of their populations. In the least well developed health systems, the best approach is generally felt to be to start from the ground up, to focus initially on breadth rather than depth (Britnell, 2015). This involves creating a critical mass of popular and political support for universal care by quickly providing a small number of benefits to all citizens to build support for community and primary care. This is easier said than done, given the challenges described in a KPMG report on developing affordable universal health coverage (KPMG, 2014):

'The individual building blocks of creating low-cost, high-quality health systems are well understood. Assembling them is difficult in environments that are shaped by immature insurance systems, unregistered private providers and widely held assumptions that high-tech and high prices automatically equal good quality. Successful low-cost systems require coordinated action across a wide range of areas. They also need markets that function effectively, with appropriate incentives for payers, providers and patients. Facilities need to be flexible, clinical quality must be routinely regulated and processes such as procurement should be standardised where possible. Above all, the focus on provision has to move beyond simply looking at "low cost per transaction" towards a system that seeks to create value along the whole care pathway and beyond this to managing population health.'

So what is the role of technology and innovation?

There is something of a disconnection between the pace of change in the science and technology of healthcare and the innovation needs that are implied by the challenges and solutions sketched out above. Moving the solutions from theory to policy to practice will require innovation, both in the form of new products and new organisational and business models. New technologies certainly play a part, but as we have noted elsewhere, there is an inverse relationship between much of the health technology that is created and the evolving health system needs. The bulk of technological innovation remains directed at health systems that can afford it. Islands of excellence exist in many developing countries, where there is healthcare that compares in quality with the best in developed countries using advanced technology. But only the few have access to this care. Every year large numbers of people in many countries risk falling below the poverty line because of the health costs they incur, or they receive dubious care from unregistered private providers.

Nevertheless, the development of appropriate and affordable health technologies, and ways of ensuring they are made available, is now firmly on the agenda in the form of frugal innovations and novel healthcare business models, as Chapter 6 describes. New uses for widely available technologies such as the mobile phone are also opening-up opportunities to create fundamentally new models of care, allowing elements of healthcare to be brought to hitherto hard-to-access populations or regions and breaking down the received wisdom about what primary and community-based care looks like.

In the high-income countries, the world of healthcare is also being reshaped through technological innovation. The picture is messy, with different trends occurring on several fronts. Some of these are the result of developments within the healthcare industries, while others are originating from outside healthcare such as mobile telecoms and gaming. The key technology innovation trends are:

- Developments in *biopharma*, resulting in drugs that are better targeted and personalised according to an individual's genetic profile.
- New *medical devices*, such as wearable and implantable systems allowing continuous monitoring or treatment.
- A revolution in *data capture and analysis*, providing a deeper understanding of population health trends, the impact of interventions, and personalised decision-making around medical care.

- Increasing interpenetration of *wireless and internet-enabled communications*, resulting in a proliferation of new health and lifestyle apps and devices for both the consumer and healthcare provider markets.

Increasingly, *technological convergence* — combinations of technology across manufacturing and service sectors — is creating new hybrid products and product-service combinations. An example we looked at in Chapter 6 is point-of-care testing, where new devices and services are developing rapidly. Developments in 'big data' are also generating opportunities for integrating physiological data with genetic data, advancing our understanding of the underlying basis of diseases and aiding the development of novel drugs. The trends towards technological convergence are already having an impact of the strategies and competitive position of companies supplying healthcare technologies, as we saw in Chapter 4.

Technological innovation is changing the models by which healthcare services are delivered. For example, innovations in medical and diagnostic equipment are increasing access to care close to or at home. Advances in surgery over the years have dramatically improved outcomes and reduced lengths of stay in hospital, while the introduction of new pharmaceuticals have reduced the requirement for in-patient care. All these innovations have an impact on healthcare practices and the way they are organised and delivered.

Despite the pace of change in the science and technology, a clear challenge for healthcare in developed health systems is to ensure that the best innovations are taken up more widely. Many 'innovations' have been around for two decades or more, such as computerised medical records, medication prescribing and PACS systems. They have all been deployed to varying degrees around the world, but are far from mainstream. There has also been widespread trialling of telehealth, the remote monitoring of vulnerable and elderly patients. But moving from trials to mainstream adoption has been slowed by organisational and business model considerations. We explored the reasons why it has proved hard to diffuse seemingly beneficial healthcare technologies in Chapters 5 and 7 especially.

What is on the horizon?

How will technological innovation change healthcare in the future and over what period? What will the healthcare services we consume look like in 20 years time? Prediction is hard and we never quite get it right. But there are ways of looking at the future potential effects of techno- logical innovation on healthcare. We can scan what is on the horizon and

"Prediction is very difficult, especially if it's about the future."
Niels Bohr

work through the implications, whether economic, political or social. Or we can pick specific technologies to look at their rate of perfor- mance improvement and think about when we might reach the limits or achieve breakthrough radical innovations that shift the performance S-curve described in Chapter 2.

Horizon scanning exercises are commonplace amongst policy mak- ers, industry and academics. Table 8.1, based on work carried out for the NHS Confederation (2008) report on disruptive technologies,

Table 8.1   Major trends in technological innovation in healthcare — 10–20 year horizon

Innovation area: biopharma	Implications
Genetics Better understanding of genetic implications of specific drugs leading to new generation of personalised medicine. Scale of impact and timing hard to predict.	• Cost, regulatory and supply chain challenges (smaller quantities of bespoke medicines for sub-groups of patients).
New drugs Fall in number of new molecular entities being registered, increasing importance of biotechnology-produced drugs and a shift towards 'personalisation.'	• Costs — higher costs per drug treatment and possibly very large numbers of patients involved. • Equity implications of drugs tailored to genetic profiles.
Regenerative medicine Growing new tissue outside the body and re-implanting it; stem cells used to generate re-growth *in situ.*	• Costs — relatively small numbers of patients compared to major chronic conditions? • New skills for the workforce, new laboratory disciplines?

(Continued)

Table 8.1 (Continued)

Innovation area: medical devices and equipment	Implications
Diagnostics Point-of-care testing ('lab on a chip'), cheaper imaging in the field.	• Significant reduction in overall costs of testing. • This may be offset by expansion of testing (increase costs for little health gain). • Change in location of testing (out-of-hospital) with implications for existing laboratory infrastructure and workforce/skills.
Surgery Minimally invasive/image-guided techniques, robotic surgery.	• Reduces time in hospital (hence lower infections rate) and risk of damage to surrounding tissues. • Increased access to specialists for patients in under-served regions.
Remote care (telecare/telemedicine) Monitoring people with diseases in the very early stages to allow earlier intervention when clinical or social signs deteriorate. Already in use but organisational challenges in mainstreaming.	• Shifts the location of care to the home/workplace, reduces time in hospital, nursing home etc. • Costs — relatively cheap to set-up and operate but may result in overall increased demand on health/social care systems.

Innovation: data, knowledge and processes	Implications
Understanding the risk of disease Genetic testing and data mining of electronic patient records and population health data.	• Helps population risk stratification and provision of tailored health advice. • Ethical concerns over insurance and data protection. • Big data and collaborative tools could be harnessed for medical research, product development and testing service model.
Managing knowledge Easier search and organisation of data, making information available to individuals across the world in easy to understand formats.	• Creates communities of interest allowing patients to exchange information, advice and support — potential to take some demand out of the system by enabling more self-care

(Continued)

Table 8.1   (Continued)

Improving decision-making and quality control Error-detection systems, safety thinking from other industries, process/supply chain management, decision support guidelines, risk-adjusted outcome measurement, rapid patient feedback.	• Merging of datasets for medical research and population health planning and intervention. • Improved patient safety/reduced risk, early feedback of impact of innovations. • Improvements to quality and efficiency.

Source: Based on NHS Confederation (2008).

discussed in Chapter 6, lists some of the important trends in healthcare innovation that are expected to unfold over the next 10–20 years, grouped by broad categories of technology. As well potentially improving the delivery of healthcare, all the innovations have important implications for access, equity, ethics, the healthcare workforce and work practices, and economics.

The last of these areas listed in Table 8.1 — data and knowledge — is where much of the action is at the moment. 'Big data' is a catch-all term for a variety of data-related innovations, but many see it as an opportunity to radically transform healthcare across several dimensions. These are shown in Figure 8.1. A series of converging trends is beginning to take effect, including a demand from governments, payers and providers for better data, the growing quantity of data becoming available from many sources and technical capabilities in data analytics (Groves *et al.* 2013). However, although the technology underpinning big data is evolving fast, this does not mean clinical and other health and wellbeing data — for example, data captured from fitness wearables — are becoming more 'liquid'. While moves to put in place interoperability standards and regulatory frameworks are underway, tensions remain over data ownership, access, ethics, and integration with current health and social care systems. These hinder the ability of individuals and organisations to readily share and access data.

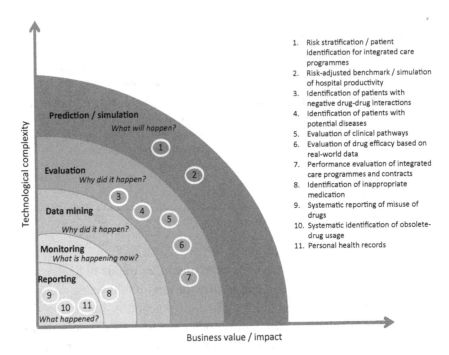

Figure 8.1.   Applications of big data in healthcare.
Source: Groves *et al.* (2013).

It is not just about medical devices and drugs

As we have seen, health technologies — devices, drugs, medical and surgical procedures, and the associated knowledge — are largely produced in high-income countries for high-income markets. There is a need to speed up the development and adoption of affordable health technologies, and embed them within moves to strengthen health systems and introduce universal coverage. But as well as the technological, financial and organisational innovations that must be put in place to achieve this, much can be done to improve the health of populations through innovative thinking in the *technologies for health* — in contrast to *health technologies* (Howitt *et al.*, 2012).

Technologies for health represent a much broader category than health technologies and are not usually the main concern of a health system. One example would be improvements in food production in low-income countries, which reduce hunger and malnutrition. Road traffic accidents are a leading and growing cause of death and disability, with ensuing effects on household incomes, earning capacity, and economic productivity. Technologies that improve road safety — perhaps as simple as motorcycle helmets — can do much to contribute to overall public health, along with investment in better road infrastructure.

The built infrastructure also needs innovative thinking in order to improve the housing conditions and access to water and sanitation for a large number of households. The challenges are huge — research by the McKinsey Global Institute (Woetzel *et al.*, 2014) estimates that globally some 330 million households are unable to find decent housing that they can afford without severe financial stress. By 2025, the number could reach 440 million or 1.6 billion people. Innovation in financing and construction, including use of frugal innovation concepts, to meet these basic needs will also be hugely beneficial for public health.

Better built infrastructure directed specifically at healthcare is also much needed. Creation of new facilities and replacement of outdated ones is underway. The challenge is to avoid models that involve creating large hospitals that are both expensive to run and need to attract patients to remain competitive. This requires a strong primary care infrastructure to be established. In India, many people living in areas where there is an underinvestment in primary care infrastructure, notably smaller towns and rural areas, either lack access to healthcare or have to travel to larger cities at a point when their medical condition is at a more advanced stage. This contributes to high out-of-pocket expenditures. Adding hospital beds — over 1.8 million — to achieve a target of two beds per 1000 people by 2025 is a target in India. In other parts of the world, the need for hospital infrastructure is even more acute — in 2011, there were 0.3 hospital beds per 1,000 population in Guinea (Deloitte, 2014b). While this signals that truly innovative thinking is needed to create appropriate and affordable hospitals, it is essential not to neglect development of primary care infrastructure as well.

Managing healthcare innovation — closing thoughts

Creating a healthcare system that is sustainable and affordable requires those responsible for leading, designing and managing innovation to play a central part. Understanding the complexity of health systems, and embracing this complexity and the interactions between the constituent parts, is essential if leaders are to manage the processes of change and innovation.

Occasionally, healthcare experiences major innovation driven by the emergence of new technology — a new vaccine against a significant health problem, for example. But most innovation does not attract headlines. Most innovation involves relatively minor changes to existing services or processes, which on their own only incrementally change the organisations and practices of healthcare. However, healthcare depends on successful innovation of all forms to develop better ways to meet needs, solve problems and use its resources more effectively. Innovation is not an optional luxury, but it is often seen as an added burden. Most healthcare organisations and systems find innovation difficult and tend to see it as disruptive. One way to deal with this is to focus not on innovation as such. Instead, governments and healthcare organisations need to agree on the desired outcome or the problem to be resolved, and then make sure the right organisational cultures, rewards and methods are in place to generate the solutions. Developing a dissident culture and encouraging — but also managing — a constant questioning of the status quo is an essential part of this process.

It is also important to beware 'best practice'. One size seldom fits all. Innovation in healthcare takes place in very variable contexts and creating sustainable models and systems must recognise this variety. The building blocks for good healthcare may be known, and some can be standardised, but the way they are put together to deliver healthcare has to be tailored to individual and local needs. And to sustain an innovative health system and create robustness against future unforeseen and unforeseeable circumstances, understanding the diversity of approaches around the world and sharing knowledge about them is essential.

REFERENCES

Abernathy W, Utterback J (1975) A dynamic model of product and process innovation. *Omega* 3(6): 639–656.

Abma I, Jayanti A, Bayer S, Mitra S, Barlow J (2014) Perceptions and experiences of financial incentives: a qualitative study of dialysis care in England. *BMJ Open* 4: e004249.

Adam T, de Savigny D (2012) Systems thinking for strengthening health systems in LMICs: Need for a paradigm shift. *Health Policy and Planning* 27: iv1–iv3.

Adam T, Hsu J, de Savigny D, Lavis J, Røttingen J-A, Bennett S (2012) Evaluating health systems strengthening interventions in low-income and middle-income countries: Are we asking the right questions? *Health Policy and Planning* 27: iv9–iv19.

Adamski J, Godman B, Ofierska-Sujkowska G, *et al.* (2010) Risk sharing arrangements for pharmaceuticals. Potential considerations and recommendations for European payers. *BMC Health Services Research* 10(1): 153.

Addicott R, McGivern G, Ferlie E (2007) The distortion of a managerial technique? The case of clinical networks in UK health care. *British Journal of Management*, 18(1): 93–105.

Agyepong I, Kodua A, Adjei S, Adam T (2012) When 'solutions of yesterday become problems of today': Crisis-ridden decision making in a complex adaptive system (CAS) — the Additional Duty Hours Allowance in Ghana. *Health Policy and Planning* 27: iv20–iv31.

Amadi H, Mokuolu O, Adimora G, *et al.* (2007) Digitally recycled incubators: Better economic alternatives to modern systems in low-income countries. *Annals of Tropical Paediatrics* 27: 207–214.

Amadi H, Azubuike J, Etawo U, *et al.* (2010) The impact of recycled neonatal incubators in Nigeria: A 6-year follow-up study. *International Journal of Pediatrics*: 269293.

Anand G (2009) The Henry Ford of heart surgery. *Wall Street Journal*. http://online.wsj.com/article/SB125875892887958111.html (Accessed on 19 August 2016).

Anderson P (1999) Complexity theory and organisation science. *Organisation Science* 10(3): 216–232.

Anderson S, Evers N, Griot C (2013) Local and international networks in small firm internationalization: Cases from the Rhône–Alpes medical technology regional cluster. *Entrepreneurship & Regional Development* 25(9–10): 867–888.

Appleby J (2015) How much has generic prescribing and dispensing saved the NHS? http://www.kingsfund.org.uk/blog/2015/07/how-much-has-generic-prescribing-and-dispensing-saved-nhs (Accessed on 19 August 2016).

Arnkil R, Järvensivu A, Koski P, Piirainen T (2010) Exploring the quadruple helix. Report on quadruple helix research for the CLIQ project. Työraportteja 85/2010 Working Papers Work Research Centre, University of Tampere.

Asghar R (2014) Why Silicon Valley' fail-fast mantra is just hype. http://www.forbes.com/sites/robasghar/2014/07/14/why-silicon-valleys-fail-fast-mantra-is-just-hype/ (Accessed on 19 August 2016).

Asthana P (1995) Jumping the technology s-curve. *IEEE Spectrum* 32(6): 49–54.

Atun R, McKee M, Drobniewski F, Coker R (2005a) Analysis of how the health systems context shapes responses to the control of human immunodeficiency virus: Case-studies from the Russian Federation. *Bulletin of the World Health Organisation* 83: 730–738.

Atun R, Samyshkin Y, Drobniewski F, Skuratova N, *et al.* (2005b) Barriers to sustainable tuberculosis control in the Russian Federation health system. *Bulletin of the World Health Organisation* 83: 217–223.

Atun R, Baeza J, Drobniewski F, Levicheva V, Coker R (2005c) Implementing WHO DOTS strategy in the Russian Federation: Stakeholder attitudes. *Health Policy* 74: 122–132.

Atun R, Menabde N, Saluvere K, Jesse M, Habicht J (2006) Introducing a complex health innovation — primary health care reforms in Estonia (multimethods evaluation). *Health Policy* 79: 79–91.

Atun R, Kyratsis I, Jelic G, Rados-Malicbegovic D, Gurol-Urganci I (2007) Diffusion of complex health innovations — implementation of primary health care reforms in Bosnia and Herzegovina. *Health Policy and Planning* 22: 28–39.

Atun R, de Jongh T, Secci F, Ohiri K, Adeyi O (2010) Integration of targeted health interventions into health systems: A conceptual framework for analysis. *Health Policy and Planning* 25: 104–111.

Avorn J (2015) The $2.6 billion pill. Methodologic and policy considerations. *New England Journal of Medicine* 372(20): 1877–1879.

Baker J (1999) *Creating Knowledge Creating Wealth: Realising the Economic Potential of Public Sector Research Establishments. A Report by John Baker to the Minister for Science and the Financial Secretary to the Treasury.* HM Treasury.

Balas E, Boren S (2000) Managing clinical knowledge for health care improvement. In van Bemmel J, McCray A (eds.), *Yearbook of Medical Informatics.* Stuttgart: Schattauer Verlagsgesellschaft mbH.

Barder O (2010) Development, complexity and evolution. https://www.owen.org/blog/4018 (Accessed on 19 August 2016).

Barley S (1986) Technology as an occasion for structuring. Evidence from observations of CT scanners and the social order of radiology departments. *Administrative Science Quarterly* 31(1): 78–108.

Barley S, Tolbert P (1997) Institutionalization and structuration: Studying the links between action and institution. *Organisation Studies* 18(1): 93–119.

Barlow J (2015) Changing the innovation landscape in the UK's National Health Service to meet its future challenges. *Innovation and Entrepreneurship in Health* 2: 59–67.

Barlow J, Venables T (2004) Will technological innovation create the true lifetime home? *Housing Studies* 19(5): 795–810.

Barlow J, Bayer S, Curry R (2006) Implementing complex innovations in fluid multi-stakeholder environments: Experiences of 'telecare'. *Technovation* 26: 396–406.

Barlow J, Singh D, Bayer S, Curry R (2007) A systematic review of the benefits of home telecare for frail elderly people and those with long-term conditions. *Journal of Telemedicine & Telecare* 13: 172–179.

Barlow J, Burn J (2008) *All Change Please. Putting the Best New Healthcare Ideas into Practice.* Policy Exchange. http://www.policyexchange.org.uk/publications/category/item/all-change-please (Accessed on 19 August 2016).

Barlow J, Köberle-Gaiser M (2009) Delivering innovation in hospital construction. Contracts and collaboration in the UK's Private Finance Initiative hospitals program. *California Management Review* 51: 126–143.

Barlow J, Bayer S (2011) Raising the profile of simulation and modeling in health services planning and implementation. *Journal of Health Services Research & Policy* 16(3): 129–130.

Barlow J, Curry R, Chrysanthaki T, Hendy J, Taher N (2012) *Remote Care plc. Developing the capacity of the remote care industry to supply Britain's future needs.* Report for WSD evaluation. www.haciric.org. Accessed on 19 August 2016.

Barlow J, Roehrich J, Wright S (2013) Europe sees mixed results from public–private partnerships for building and managing health care facilities and services. *Health Affairs* 32: 146–154.

Barnsley J, Lemieux-Charles L, McKinney M (1998) Integrating learning into integrated delivery systems. *Health Care Management Review* 23: 18–28.

Barratt C (2014) The 7 deadly sins of NHS innovation. https://www.linkedin.com/pulse/20140530085226-81796176-the-7-deadly-sins-of-nhs-innovation (Accessed on 19 August 2016).

Baru J, Bloom D, Muraszko K, Koop C (2001) John Holter's shunt. *Journal of the American College of Surgeons* 192(1): 79–85.

Barry A (2001) *Political Machines. Governing a Technological Society.* London: Athlone Press.

Basu R, Banerjee P, Sweeny E (2013) Frugal innovation. Core competencies to address global sustainability. *Journal of Management for Global Sustainability* 2: 63–82.

Bate P, Robert G (2003) Where next for policy evaluation? Insights from researching National Health Service modernisation. *Policy & Politics* 31(2): 249–262.

Baumol W (2012) *The Cost Disease. Why Computers get Cheaper and Health Care doesn't.* Yale University Press.

Bayer S, Barlow J, Curry R (2007) Assessing the impact of a care innovation: Telecare. *System Dynamics Review* 23: 61–80.

Beinhocker E (2006) *The Origin of Wealth. Evolution, Complexity and the Radical Remaking of Economics.* Cambridge: Harvard Business Press.

Bellal J, Morton J, Hernandez-Boussard T, Rubinfeld I, Faraj C, Velanovich V (2009) Relationship between hospital volume, system clinical resources, and mortality in pancreatic resection. *Journal of the American College of Surgeons* 208(4): 520–527.

Bennett D (2014) Clayton Christensen responds to New Yorker takedown of 'disruptive innovation'. *Business Week.* http://www.bloomberg.com/news/articles/2014-06-20/clayton-christensen-responds-to-new-yorker-takedown-of-disruptive-innovation#p1 (Accessed on 19 August 2016).

BERR (2008) *Medical Technology Metrics. Introduction and Commentary.* London: Department for Business Enterprise and Regulatory Reform.

Berwick D (2002) A user's manual for the IOM's 'quality chasm' report. *Health Affairs* 21: 80–90.

Berwick D, Hackbarth A (2012) Eliminating waste in US health care. *JAMA* 307(14): 1513–1516.

Bessant J, Francis D, Thesmer J (2004) *Managing Innovation Within Coloplast. Case study.* Cranfield School of Management.

Bessant J, Francis D (2005) Transferring soft technologies: Exploring adaptive theory. *International Journal of Technology Management & Sustainable Development* 4(2): 93–112.

Bessant J, Tidd J (2007) *Innovation and Entrepreneurship.* John Wiley & Sons.

Bienkowska-Gibbs T (2013) Integrated care programmes in Canada. *Eurohealth* 19(2): 13–14.

Bijker W, Hughes T, Pinch T (1987) *The Social Construction of Technological Systems. New Directions in the Sociology and History of Technology.* Cambridge: MIT Press.

Bijker W (1995) *Of Bicycles, Bakelites and Bulbs. Toward a Theory of Sociotechnical Change.* Cambridge: MIT Press.

BIS (2012a) Industrial strategy. UK sector analysis. *BIS Economics Paper* 18. September. http://www.bis.gov.uk/assets/biscore/economics-and-statistics/docs/i/12-1140-industrial-strategy-uk-sector-analysis (Accessed on 19 August 2016).

BIS (2012b) SME access to external finance. *BIS Economics Paper* 16. January. http://www.bis.gov.uk/assets/BISCore/enterprise/docs/S/12-539-sme-accessexternal-finance.pdf (Accessed on 19 August 2016).

BIS (2013) *Strength and Opportunity 2013 The Landscape of the Medical Technology, Medical Biotechnology, Industrial Biotechnology and Pharmaceutical Sectors in the UK.* London: Department of Business, Innovation & Skills.

Black N (2001) Evidence based policy: Proceed with care. *British Medical Journal* 323: 275–279.

Blackler F (1995) Knowledge, knowledge work and organisations. An overview and interpretation. *Organisation Studies* 16(6): 1021–1046.

Blank S (2013) Why the lean start-up changes everything. *Harvard Business Review* (May).

Bloom G, Ainsworth P (2010) Beyond scaling up. Pathways to universal access to health services. *STEPS Working Paper* 40. University of Sussex, STEPS Centre.

Blume S (1992) *Insight and Industry. On the Dynamics of Technological Change in Medicine.* Cambridge: MIT Press.

Bojke C, Castelli A, Laudicella M, Street A, Ward P (2010) Regional variation in the productivity of the English National Health Service. Report for the Department of Health. *CHE Research Paper* 57, University of York.

Bossuyt P (2006) New diagnostics can enter the clinical pathways in one of three ways, triage test, replacement test or add on test. *British Medical Journal* 332: 1089.

Bower J (2003) Innovation in healthcare delivery. In Tidd J, Hull F (eds.) *Service Innovation. Organisational Responses to Technological Opportunities and Market Imperatives*. London: Imperial College Press.

Bower P, Cartwright M, Hirani S, Barlow J, Hendy J, Knapp M, Henderson C, Rogers A, Sanders C, Bardsley M, Steventon A, Fitzpatrick R, Doll H, Newman S (2011) A comprehensive evaluation of the impact of telemonitoring in patients with long-term conditions and social care needs: Protocol for the Whole Systems Demonstrator cluster randomized trial. *BMC Health Services Research* 11: 184.

Brailsford S (2014) More bang for your buck: Using modelling & simulation to add value to healthcare evaluation studies. *Policy Innovation Research Unit (PIRU) conference, 'Evaluation — making it timely, useful, independent and rigorous*, London School of Hygiene and Tropical Medicine, 4 July 2014.

Britnell M (2015) *In Search of the Perfect Health System*. London: Palgrave.

Brown J, Duguid P (1991) Organisational learning and communities-of-practice: Towards a unified view of working, learning and innovation. *Organisation Science* 2(1): 40–57.

Brown T (2008) Design thinking. *Harvard Business Review* 86: 84–92.

Buntz B (2010) The race for open innovation. *European Medical Device Technology*. http://www.emdt.co.uk/article/race-for-open-innovation (Accessed on 19 August 2016).

Burfitt A, Macneill S, Gibney J (2007) The dilemmas of operationalizing cluster policy. The medical technology cluster in the West Midlands. *European Planning Studies* 15(9): 1273–1290.

Burns L, Nicholson S, Wolkowski J (2012) Pharmaceutical strategy and the evolving role of merger and acquisition. In Burns L. (ed.), *The business of healthcare innovation*. 2nd Edition. Cambridge: Cambridge University Press.

Busse R (2014) *Health systems in transition: Germany*. Health Systems Review, European Observatory on Health Systems and Policies.

Carlson J, Gries K, Sullivan S, Garrison L (2011) PHP146 current status and trends in performance-based schemes between health care payers and manufacturers. *ValueHealth* 14: A359–360.

Carlsson B, Jacobsson S, Holmen M, Rickne A (2002) Innovation systems: Analytical and methodological issues. *Research Policy* 31(2): 233–245.

Champagne F, Denis J-L, Pineault R, Contandriopoulos A-P (1991) Structural and political models of analysis of the introduction of an innovation in organizations: the case of the change in the method of payment of physicians in long-term care hospitals. *Health Services Management Research* 4: 94–111.

Charitou C, Markides C (2003) Responses to disruptive strategic Innovation. *MIT Sloan Management Review* 44(2): 55–63.

Chatterji A, Fabrizio K, Mitchell W, Schulman K (2008) Physician–industry cooperation in the medical device industry. *Health Affairs* 27(6): 1532–1543.

Chernew M (2010) Health care spending growth: Can we avoid fiscal Armageddon? *Inquiry* 47: 285–295.

Chesbrough H (2003) *Open Innovation. The New Imperative for Creating and Profiting from Technology.* Harvard Business School Press.

Chesbrough H (2006) *Open Business Models: How to Thrive in the New Innovation Landscape.* Harvard Business School Press.

Christensen C (1997) *The Innovator's Dilemma. When New Technologies cause Great Firms to Fail.* Cambridge: Harvard Business School Press.

Christensen C, Bohmer R, Kenagy J (2000) Will disruptive innovations cure healthcare? *Harvard Business Review* 78(5): 102–112.

Christensen C, Raynor M (2003) *The Innovator's Solution: Creating and Sustaining Successful Growth.* Cambridge: Harvard Business School Press.

Christensen C, Anthony S, Roth E (2004) *Seeing What's Next. Using the Theories of Innovation to Predict Industry Change.* Cambridge: Harvard Business School Press.

Christensen C, Horn M, Caldera L, Soares L (2011) *Disrupting College. How Disruptive Innovation can Deliver Quality and Affordability to Postsecondary Education.* Center for American Progress/Innosight Institute.

Chrysanthaki T, Hendy J, Barlow J (2013) Stimulating whole system redesign. Lessons from an organisational analysis of the Whole System Demonstrator programme. *Journal of Health Services Research & Policy* 18(1 Suppl.): 47–55.

CIHR (2015) Guide to knowledge translation planning at CIHR: Integrated and end-of-grant approaches. http://www.cihrirsc.gc.ca/e/45321.html#a1 (Accessed on 19 August 2016).

Cilliers P (1998) *Complexity and Postmodernism. Understanding Complex Systems.* London: Routledge.

Clark A (2015) With no low-hanging fruit, pharma turns to new crop of medicines. *The Times* 13 January 2015, 40.

Clark K (1985) The interaction of design hierarchies and market concepts in technological evolution. *Research Policy* 14(5): 235–251.

Cochrane A (1972) *Effectiveness and efficiency. Random Reflections on Health Services.* Nuffield Trust. http://www.nuffieldtrust.org.uk/publications/effectiveness-and-efficiency-random-reflections-health-services (Accessed on 19 August 2016).

Cohen W, Levinthal D (1990) Absorptive capacity. A new perspective on learning and innovation. *Administrative Science Quarterly* 35(1): 128–153.

Coker R, Atun R, McKee M (2004) Health-care system frailties and public health control of communicable disease on the European Union's new eastern border. *The Lancet* 363: 1389–1392.

Coker R, Dimitrova B, Drobniewski F, *et al.* (2003) Tuberculosis control in Samara Oblast, Russia: Institutional and regulatory environment. *International Journal of Tuberculosis and Lung Disease* 7: 920–932.

Cook D, Brown D, Alexander R, March R, Morgan P, Satterthwaite G, Pangalos M (2015) Lessons learned from the fate of AstraZeneca's drug pipeline. A five-dimensional framework. *Nature Reviews Drug Discovery* 13: 419–431.

Cooksey D (2006) *A Review of UK Health Research Funding.* London: HM Treasury.

Coombs R, Harvey M, Tether B (2003) Analysing distributed processes of provision and innovation. *Industrial and Corporate Change* 12(6): 1125–1155.

Cooper R (2001) *Winning at New Product Development. Accelerating the Process from Ideas to Launch.* Basic Books.

Cooper R (2013) Where are all the breakthrough new products? Using portfolio management to boost innovation. *Research-Technology Management* 56(5): 25–32.

Cooper R, Edgett S, Kleinschmidt E (2000) New problems, new solutions. Making portfolio management more effective. *Research-Technology Management* 43(2): 18–33.

Corr P, Williams D (2009) The pathway from idea to regulatory approval: Examples for drug development. In Lo B, Field M (eds.), *Conflict of Interest in Medical Research, Education, and Practice.* Institute of Medicine (US), Committee on Conflict of Interest in Medical Research, Education and Practice. Washington, DC: National Academies Press.

Cosh A, Hughes A, Bullock A, Milner I (2008) *Financing UK Small and Medium-sized Enterprises. The 2007 Survey.* Centre for Business Research, University of Cambridge.

Craig P, Dieppe P, Macintyre S, Michie S, Nazareth I, Petticrew M (2006) *Developing and Evaluating Complex Interventions: New Guidance.* London: Medical Research Council.

Crasemann W, Lehto P, Starzer O, van der Zwan A (2012) *ERAC Peer Review of the Danish Research and Innovation System Outcomes Report 2012.* European Commission.

Cravo Oliveira T (2014) *Accounting for behaviours and context in evaluations of complex health interventions.* PhD thesis, Imperial College, London.

Cravo Oliveira T, Barlow J, Bayer S (2015) The association between general practitioner participation in joint teleconsultations and rates of referral: A discrete choice experiment. *BMC Family Practice* 16:50.

Crilly T, Jashapara A, Trenholm S, Peckham A, Currie G, Ferlie E (2013) *Knowledge Mobilisation in Healthcare Organisations. Synthesising the Evidence and Theory using Perspectives of Organisational Form, Resource Based View of the Firm and Critical Theory.* NIHR Health Services and Delivery Research programme.

Crisp N (2010) *Turning the World Upside Down: The Search for Global Health in the Twenty First Century.* London: CRC Press.

Crowley D (2014) The role of social impact bonds in pediatric health care. *Pediatrics* 134(2): e331–e333.

Currie G, Grubnic S, Hodges R (2011) Leadership In public services networks: Antecedents, process and outcome. *Public Administration* 89(2): 242–264.

Currie G, Lockett A, El Enany N (2013) From what we know to what we do. Lessons learnt from the translational CLAHRC initiative in England. *Journal of Health Services Research and Policy* 13(S3): 27–39.

Curry N, Ham C (2010) *Clinical and Service Integration. The Route to Improved Outcomes.* London: The King's Fund.

Cusano D (2014) Soapbox: How healthcare disruption can be sidetracked, Telehealth & Telecare Aware, 10 April 2014. http://telecareaware.com/soapbox-how-healthcare-disruption-can-be-sidetracked/

Cutler D, McClellan M (2001) Is technological change in medicine worth it? *Health Affairs* 20(5): 11–29.

Damanpour F, Schneider M (2006) Phases of the adoption of innovation in organisations: Effects of environment, organisation and top managers. *British Journal of Management* 17(3): 215–236.

Danneels E (2004) Disruptive technology reconsidered. A critique and research agenda. *Journal of Product Innovation Management* 21(4): 246–258.

Danzon P, Nicholson S, Pereira N (2005) Productivity in pharmaceutical-biotechnology R&D. The role of experience and alliances. *Journal of Health Economics* 24(2): 317–339.

Dattée B, Barlow J (2010) Complexity and whole-system change programmes. *Journal of Health Services Research & Policy* 15(S2): 12–18.

David P (1985) Clio and the economics of QWERTY. *American Economic Review* 75(2): 332–337.

Davis D, Evans M, Jadad A, Perrier L, Rath D, Ryan D, *et al.* (2003) The case for knowledge translation: Shortening the journey from evidence to effect. *British Medical Journal* 327(7405): 33–35.

Davis J, Eisenhardt K, Bingham C (2009) Optimal structure, market dynamism, and the strategy of simple rules. *Administrative Science Quarterly* 54(3): 413–452.

Deloitte (2013) *Impact of Austerity on European Pharmaceutical Policy and Pricing. Staying Competitive in a Challenging Environment.* Centre for Health Solutions, Deloitte LLP.

Deloitte (2014a) *Global Life Sciences Outlook. Resilience and Reinvention in a Changing Marketplace.* Deloitte LLP.

Deloitte (2014b) *2014 Global Health care Outlook. Shared Challenges, Shared Opportunities.* Deloitte LLP.

Denis J, Hébert Y, Langley A, Lozeau D, Trottier L (2002) Explaining diffusion patterns for complex health care innovations. *Health Care Management Review* 27: 60–73.

Department of Health (2002) *The NHS as an Innovative Organisation. A Framework and Guidance on the Management of Intellectual Property in the NHS.* London: Department of Health.

Department of Health (2007) *White Paper Pilots: Whole System Long Term Conditions (Telecare) Demonstrator Programme.* London: The Stationery Office.

Department of Health (2008) *High Quality Care for All. NHS Next Stage Review Final Report.* London: Department of Health.

Department of Health (2011) *Innovation, Health and Wealth. Accelerating Adoption and Diffusion in the NHS.* London: Department of Health.

De Sanctis G, Poole M (1994) Capturing the complexity in advanced technology use. Adaptive structuration theory. *Organisation Science* 5(2): 121–147.

De Savigny D, Kasale K, Mbuya C, Reid G (2008) *Fixing Health Systems.* Ottawa: International Development Research Center.

De Savigny D (2012) Introducing vouchers for malaria prevention in Ghana and Tanzania: Context and adoption of innovation in health systems. *Health Policy and Planning* 27: iv32–iv43.

Dhankhar A, Evers M, Møller M (2012) *Escaping the Sword of Damocles. Towards a New Future for Pharmaceutical R&D*. McKinsey.

Di Masi J, Hansen R, Grabowski H (2003) The price of innovation: New estimates of drug development costs. *Journal of Health Economics* 22(2): 151–185.

Di Masi J, Grabowski H (2007) The cost of biopharmaceutical R&D: Is biotech different? *Managerial and Decision Economics* 28(45): 469–479.

Di Masi J, Feldman L, Seckler A, Wilson A (2010) Trends in risks associated with new drug development: Success rates for investigational drugs. *Clinical Pharmacology Therapeutics* 87(3): 272–277.

Di Masi J, Grabowski H, Hansen R (2015) The cost of drug development. *New England Journal of Medicine* 372: 1972.

Doering D, Parayre R (2000) Identification and assessment of emerging technologies. In Day G, Schoemaker P, Gunther R (eds.), *Wharton on Managing Emerging Technologies*. Hoboken, NJ: Wiley.

D'Oliveira Vieira R, Hueb W, *et al.* (2012) Cost-effectiveness analysis for surgical, angioplasty, or medical therapeutics for coronary artery disease. 5-year follow-up of Medicine, Angioplasty, or Surgery Study (MASS) II Trial. *Circulation*, 126: S145–S150.

Dodgson M, Gann D, Salter A (2008) *The Management of Technological Innovation*. Oxford: Oxford University Press.

Dopson S, FitzGerald L, Ferlie E, Gabbay J, Locock L (2002) No magic targets! Changing clinical practice to become more evidence based. *Health Care Management Review* 27(3): 35–47.

Drucker P (1985) The discipline of innovation. *Harvard Business Review* 63: 67–72.

DTI (2004) *Succeeding Through Innovation, Creating Competitive Advantage Through Innovation. A Guide for Small and Medium Sized Businesses*. London: Department of Trade and Industry.

DTT (2014) *Global Life Sciences Sector Outlook*. Deloitte Touche Tohmatsu Ltd.

Ecker G, Williams-Jones B (2012) Open innovation in drug discovery. *Molecular Informatics* 31(8): 519–520.

Eddy D (1993) Three battles to watch in the 1990s. *JAMA* 270(4): 520–526.

Edgerton D (1999) From innovation to use. Ten eclectic theses on the historiography of technology. *History & Technology* 16(2): 111–136.

Edmonson A, Bohmer R, Pisano G (2001) Disrupted routines, Team learning and new technology implementation in hospitals. *Administrative Science Quarterly* 46(4): 685–716.

Edquist C (2001) Innovation policy — a systemic approach. In Archibugi D, Lundvall B (eds.), *The Globalizing Learning Economy*. Oxford: Oxford University Press.

Eggers W, Baker L, Vaughn A (2013) *Public Sector, Disrupted. How Disruptive Innovation can help Government Achieve More for Less*. Deloitte University Press.

Eichler H, Baird L, *et al.* (2014) From adaptive licensing to adaptive pathways. Delivering a flexible life-span approach to bring new drugs to patients. *Clinical Pharmacology & Therapeutics* 97(3): 234–246.

EIU (2013) *World Healthcare Outlook*. Economist Intelligence Unit.

Ellerman D (2004) Parallel experimentation. A basic scheme for dynamic efficiency. University of California at Riverside, Department of Economics.

Ettelt S, Mays N, Allen P (2015) Policy experiments. Investigating effectiveness or confirming direction? *Evaluation* 21(3): 292–307.

Etzkowitz H, Leydesdorff L (2000) The dynamics of innovation. From national systems and 'mode 2' to a triple helix of university–industry–government relations. *Research Policy* 29(2): 109–123.

Eucomed (2012) *Medical technology in Europe. Key facts and figures*. http://archive.eucomed.org/medical-technology/facts-figures

European Commission (2009) *Interim evaluation of the entrepreneurship and innovation programme*. Final Report. DG Enterprise and Industry.

Fairfax-Clay R (2013) Health impact bonds: Will investors pay for intervention? *Environmental Health Perspectives* 121(2): a45.

Ferlie E, Gabbay J, Fitzgerald L, Locock L, Dopson S (2001) Evidence based medicine and organisational change: An overview of some recent qualitative research. In Ashburner L (ed.), *Organisational Behaviour and Organisational Studies in Health Care Reflections on the Future*. Basingstoke: Palgrave.

Ferlie E, Fitzgerald L, Wood M, Hawkins C (2005) The nonspread of innovation: The mediating role of professionals. *Academy of Management Journal* 48(1): 117–134.

Ferlie E, Fitzgerald L, McGivern G, Dopson S, Exworthy M. (2010). *Networks in Health Care: A Comparative Study of their Management, Impact and Performance*. Report for the National Institute for health research service delivery and organisation programme.

Ferlie E, Fitzgerald L, McGivern G, Dopson S, Bennett C (2011) Public policy networks and 'wicked problems': A nascent solution? *Public Administration* 89(2): 307–424.

Fernandes A, Melo Mendes P (2003) Technology as culture and embodied knowledge. *European Journal of Engineering Education* 28(2): 151–160.

Fitzgerald L, Ferlie E, Wood M, Hawkins C (2002) Interlocking interactions, the diffusion of innovations in health care. *Human Relations* 55: 1429–1449.

Fleuren M, Wiefferink K, Paulussen T (2004) Determinants of innovation within health care organisations: Literature review and Delphi study. *International Journal of Quality Health Care* 16(2): 107–123.

Fonseca J (2002) *Complexity and Innovation in Organisations*. London and New York: Routledge.

Foreman L (2014) What's the best way to tap the crowd to commercialize your invention? http://www.entrepreneur.com/article/238885 (Accessed on 19 August 2016).

Forrester J (1971) Counterintuitive behavior of social systems. *Theory and Decision* 2(2): 109–140.

Foss N, Pedersen T, Pyndt J, Schultz M (2012) *Innovating Organisation and Management. New Sources of Competitive Advantage*. Cambridge: Cambridge University Press.

Foster R (1986) *Innovation: The attacker's Advantage*. Macmillan.

Foy R, MacLennan G, Grimshaw J, Penney G, Campbell M, Grol R (2002) Attributes of clinical recommendations that influence change in practice following audit and feedback. *Journal of Clinical Epidemiology* 55: 717–722.

Free M (2004) Achieving appropriate design and widespread use of health care technologies in the developing world. Overcoming obstacles that impede the adaptation and diffusion of priority technologies for primary health care. *International Journal of Gynecology & Obstetrics* 85(S1): S3–13.

Freel M, De Jong J (2009) Market novelty, competence-seeking and innovation networking. *Technovation* 29(12): 873–884.

Frey J (2010) Little things mean a lot. *British Journal of General Practice* 60(572): 225.

Friese C, Lake E, Aiken L, Silber J, Sochalski J (2008) Hospital nurse practice environments and outcomes for surgical oncology patients. *Health Services Research* 43(4): 1145–1163.

Fuchs V (1986) *The Health Economy*. Harvard University Press.

Fulmer T (2012) Paper point of care. *SciBX* 5(39); doi: 10.1038/scibx.2012.1021.

Garber S, Gates S, Keeler E, Vaiana M, Mulcahy A, Lau C, Kellermann A (2014) Redirecting innovation in US health care: Options to decrease spending and increase value. Santa Monica: Rand Corporation. http://www.rand.org/pubs/research_reports/RR380.html (Accessed on 19 August 2016).

Gardiner P, Rothwell R (1985) Tough customers: Good designs. *Design Studies* 6(1): 7–17.

Gardner C, Acharya T, Yach D (2007) Technological and social innovation: A unifying new paradigm for global health. *Health Affairs* 26(4): 1052–1061.

Garrison L, Towse A, Briggs A, de Pouvourville G, *et al.* (2013) Performance-based risk-sharing arrangements. Good practices for design, implementation, and evaluation: Report of the ISPOR good practices for performance-based risk-sharing arrangements task force. *Value in Health* 16(5): 703–719.

Gartner (2015) Gartner says worldwide IT spending across vertical industries to decline 3.5 percent in 2015. http://www.gartner.com/newsroom/id/3135718 (Accessed on 19 August 2016).

Garud R, Rappa M (1994) A sociocognitive model of technology evolution. The case of cochlear implants. *Organisation Science* 5(3): 344–362.

Gassmann, O, Enkel, E, Chesbrough, H (2010) The future of open innovation. *R&D Management* 40(3): 213–221.

Gatrell A (2005) Complexity theory and geographies of health: A critical assessment. *Social Science & Medicine* 60(12): 2661–2671.

Gavetti G, Levinthal D (2000) Looking forward and looking backward: Cognitive and experiential search. *Administrative Science Quarterly* 45(1): 113–137.

GE/BLIHR (2009) Promoting Ethical Ultrasound Use in India. A BLIHR Emerging Economy Case Study from GE.

Gelijns A, Rosenberg N (1994) The dynamics of technological change in medicine. *Health Affairs* 13(3): 28–46.

Geroski P (2000) Models of technology diffusion. *Research Policy* 29(4–5): 603–625.

Gestrelius S, Oerum M (2006) Cluster formation as a tool for development in Medicon Valley. *IEEE Engineering In Medicine and Biology Magazine* 1: 102–105.

Glanville J, Duffy S, Mahon J, Cardow T, Brazier H, Album V (2010) *Impact of hospital treatment volumes on patient outcomes.* York Health Economics Consortium, Cooperation and Competition Panel Working Paper Series 1. University of York.

Glasgow R, Emmons K (2007) How can we increase translation of research into practice? Types of evidence needed. *Annual Review of Public Health* 28(1): 413–433.

Glendinning C (2003) Breaking down barriers; integrating health and care services for older people in England. *Health Policy* 65: 139–151.

Godin B (2006) The linear model of innovation. The historical construction of an analytical framework. *Science Technology & Human Values* 31(6): 639–667.

Gold A (2014) Global healthcare IT market projected to hit USD 66 billion by 2020. http://www.fiercehealthit.com/story/global-healthcare-it-market-projected-hit-66-billion-2020/2014–04-01 (Accessed on 19 August 2016).

Goodwin N (2010) The state of telehealth and telecare in the UK: Prospects for integrated care. *Journal of Integrated Care* 18: 3–9.

Govindarajan V (2010) Tea with Vijay Govindarajan. *The Economist*. http://www. youtube.com/watch?v=FYIwa3Y1KAo&NR=1 (Accessed on 19 August 2016).

Govindarajan V, McReary L (2010) How U.S. businesses can really win in India. *Bloomberg Businessweek*, 23 November.

Govindarajan V, Trimble C (2012) *Reverse Innovation. Create Far From Home, Win Everywhere.* Boston: Harvard Business Review Press.

Grabowski H, Long G, Mortimer R (2014) Recent trends in brand-name and generic drug competition. *Informa Healthcare* 17(3): 207–214.

Greenhalgh T, Robert G, Macfarlane F, Bate P, Kyriakidou O (2004a) Diffusion of innovations in service organisations. Systematic review and recommendations. *Milbank Quarterly* 82: 581–629.

Greenhalgh T, Robert G, Bate P, Kyriakidou O, Macfarlane F, Peacock R (2004b) *How to spread good ideas. A systematic review of the literature on diffusion, dissemination and sustainability of innovations in health service delivery and organisation.* National Co-ordinating Centre for NHS Service Delivery and Organisation R&D (NCCSDO).

Gresov C, Drazin R (1997) Equifinality: Functional equivalence in organisation design. *Academy of Management Review* 22(2): 403–428.

Grimshaw J, Thomas R, MacLennan G, Fraser C, Ramsay C, Vale L, Donaldson C (2004) Effectiveness and efficiency of guideline dissemination and implementation strategies. *Health Technology Assessment* 8(6): 1–72.

Groves P, Kayyali B, Knott D, Van Kuiken S (2013) *The 'Big Data' Revolution in Healthcare. Accelerating Value and Innovation.* Center for US Health System Reform, McKinsey & Company.

Hadjimanolis A (2003) The barriers approach to innovation. In Shavinina L (ed.), *The International Handbook on Innovation*, Abingdon, UK: Elsevier Science.

Haines A, Kuruvilla S, Borchert M (2004) Bridging the implementation gap between knowledge and action for health. *Bulletin of the World Health Organisation* 82: 724–732.

Hansen M (1999) The search-transfer problem: The role of weak ties in sharing knowledge across organisation subunits. *Administrative Science Quarterly* 44(1): 82–111.

Harford T (2011) *Adapt. Why Success always Starts with Failure.* London: Abacus.

Harrison S (2002) New labour, modernisation and the medical labour process. *Journal of Social Policy* 31(3): 465–485.

Hart S (2005) Capitalism at the crossroads: the unlimited business opportunities in solving the world's most difficult problems. Upper Saddle River, NJ, Wharton School.

Health Affairs (2012) Policy briefs: Pay-for-performance. New payment systems reward doctors and hospitals for improving the quality of care, but studies to date show mixed results. 11 October 2012. 10.1377/hpb2012.19.

Henderson R, Clark K (1990) Architectural innovation. The reconfiguration of existing product technologies and the failure of established firms. *Administrative Science Quarterly* 35: 9–30.

Hendy J, Barlow J (2012) The role of the organisational champion in achieving health system change. *Social Science and Medicine* 74(5): 348–355.

Hendy J, Chrysanthaki T, Barlow J, *et al.* (2012) An organisational analysis of the implementation of telecare and telehealth: The whole systems demonstrator. *BMC Health Services Research* 12: 403.

Herbert C, Best A (2011) It's a matter of values: Partnership for innovative change. *Healthcare Papers* 2: 31–37.

Herper M (2012) The truly staggering cost of inventing new drugs. (Forbes 10 February 2012) http://www.forbes.com/sites/matthewherper/2012/02/10/the-truly-staggeringcost-of-inventing-new-drugs/2/ (Accessed on 19 August 2016).

Higgins M, Rodriguez D (2006) The outsourcing of R&D through acquisitions in the pharmaceutical industry. *Journal of Financial Economics* 80(2): 351–383.

Hinsch M, Stockstrom C, Lüthje C (2014) User innovation in techniques: A case study analysis in the field of medical devices. *Creativity and Innovation Management* 23(4): 484–494.

Hirai Y, Kinoshita H, Kusama M, Yasuda K, Sugiyama Y, Ono S (2010) Delays in new drug applications in Japan and industrial R&D strategies. *Clinical Pharmacology & Therapeutics* 87(2): 212–218.

Hirschler B (2015) New analysis underscores improving pharma R&D productivity. http://www.reuters.com/article/us-pharmaceuticals-r-d-idUSKCN0Q909620150804. Accessed on 19 August 2016.

HITF (2004) *Better Health Through Partnership: A Programme for Action.* Health Industries Task Force.

HMRC (2012) *CIRD80150. R&D tax relief: Overview.* London: HM Revenue & Customs.

HM Treasury (2011) *The Magenta Book. Guidance for evaluation.* London: HM Treasury.

Hollmer M (2012) GE wants to share ideas to accelerate development of ultrasound tech, 24 September 2012. http://www.fiercebiotech.com/medical-devices/ge-wants-to-share-ideas-to-accelerate-development-ultrasound-tech (Accessed on 19 August 2016).

House of Commons Health Committee (2009) *Health Inequalities. Third Report of Session 2008–09. Volume 1.* HC-286-1. London: The Stationery Office.

Howitt P, Darzi A, Yang G-Z, Ashrafian H, Atun R, Barlow J, *et al.* (2012) Technologies for global health. *The Lancet Commissions.* http://dx.doi.org/10.1016/S0140-6736(12)61127-1 (Accessed on 19 August 2016).

HSR-Europe (2011) *Health Services Research into European Policy and Practice. Final Report of the HSREPP Project.* Utrecht: NIVEL.

Hudson R (2006) *Whole Systems Working: A Guide and Discussion Paper.* London: Integrated Care Network.

Hurt D (2014) *Unleashing the Potential of Reverse Innovation for the NHS.* http://www.polygeia.com/unleashing-the-potential-of-reverse-innovation-for-the-nhs (Accessed on 19 August 2016).

Hutton J, McGrath C, Frybourg J, Tremblay M, Bramley-Harker E, Henshall C (2006) Framework for describing and classifying decision-making systems using technology assessment to determine the reimbursement of health technologies (fourth hurdle systems). *International Journal of Technology Assessment Health Care* 22(1): 10–18.

Hutton J, Trueman P, Henshall C (2007) Coverage with evidence development: An examination of conceptual and policy issues. *International Journal of Technology Assessment in Health Care* 23(4): 425–432.

Ibrahim M, Bhandari A, Sandhu J, Balakrishnan P (2007) Making sight affordable (part 1). Aurolab pioneers production of low-cost technology for cataract surgery. *Innovations: Technology, Governance, Globalization* 2(4): 53–57.

IHI (2010) Institute for Healthcare Improvement conference to advance the science and practice on scale-up and spread of effective health programs 25–26 June 2010. Washington DC.

Immelt J, Govindarajan V, Trimble C (2009) How GE is disrupting itself. *Harvard Business Review* (October).

Imison C (2011) *Reconfiguring Hospital Services.* The King's Fund.

IMS (2012) *IMS Market Prognosis International 2012–2016.* IMS Health.

Izsak K (2014) *Cross-sectoral Trends and Geographic Patterns in the Medical Devices Industry.* European Commission: European Cluster Observatory.

Jackson T (2012) Let's be less productive. *New York Times Sunday Review,* 26 May. http://www.nytimes.com/2012/05/27/opinion/sunday/lets-be-less-productive.html (Accessed on 19 August 2016).

Jennings K, Miller K, Materna S (1997) *Changing Health Care. Creating Tomorrow's Winning Health Enterprise Today.* Santa Monica Knowledge Exchange.

Jones H (2011) *Taking responsibility for complexity. How implementation can achieve results in the face of complex problems.* Overseas Development Institute, Working Paper 330.

Judd D (2013) Open innovation in drug discovery research comes of age. *Drug Discovery Today* 18: 315–317.

Kanani R (2011) Jaipur Foot. One of the most technologically-advanced social enterprises in the world. *Forbes,* 8 August 2011. http://www.forbes.com/sites/rahimkanani/2011/08/08/jaipur-foot-one-of-the-most-technologically-advanced-social-enterprises-in-the-world/ (Accessed on 19 August 2016).

Kaplan H, Provost L, Froehle C, Margolis P (2011) The model for understanding success in quality (MUSIQ): building a theory of context in healthcare quality improvement. *BMJ Quality and Safety* 21: 13–20.

Kaplan R, Porter M (2011) How to solve the cost crisis in health care. *Harvard Business Review* (September).

Kaplan S, Orlikowski W (2013) Temporal work in strategy making. *Organisation Science* 24(4): 965–995.

Karnani A (2007) The mirage of marketing to the bottom of the pyramid: How the private sector can help alleviate poverty. *California Management Review* 49(4): 90–111.

Karsh B-T (2004) Beyond usability: Designing effective technology implementation systems to promote patient safety. *Quality and Safety in Health Care* 13(5): 388–394.

Kibasi T, Teitelbaum J, Henke N (2012) *The Financial Sustainability of Health Systems. A Case for Change.* World Economic Forum and McKinsey & Company.

Kim M, Harris T, Vusovic S (2008) Efficiency analysis of the US biotechnology industry: Clustering enhances productivity. *AgBioForum* 12(3&4): 422–436.

Kirkup J (2006) *The Evolution of Surgical Instruments: An Illustrated History from Ancient Times to the Twentieth Century.* San Francisco: Jeremy Norman Co.

Klenner P, Hüsig S, Downling M (2013) Ex-ante evaluation of disruptive susceptibility in established value networks. When are markets ready for disruptive innvoations? *Research Policy* 42: 914–927.

Kleyn D, Kitney R (2007) Partnership and innovation in the life sciences. *International Journal of Innovation Management* 11(2): 323–347.

Kogut B, Zander U (1992) Knowledge of the firm, combinative capabilities and the replication of technology. *Organisation Science* 3(3): 383–397.

Kruger K, Kruger M (2012) The medical device sector. In Burns L. (ed.), *The Business of Healthcare Innovation*. 2nd Edition. Cambridge: Cambridge University Press.

Kwesigaboa G, Mwangua M, Kakokoa D, Warrinerb I, Mkonyc C, Killewoa J, Macfarlaned S, Kaayac E, Freemane P (2012) Tanzania's health system and workforce crisis. *Journal of Public Health Policy* 33: S35–S44.

Lagarde M, Wright M, Nossiter J, Mays N (2014) *Challenges of Payment-for-performance in Health care and Other public Services Design, Implementation and evaluation*. London School of Hygiene and Tropical Medicine, London: PIRU.

Langton C (1989) *Artificial life (Volume 6)*. Proceedings of the Santa Fe Institute studies in the sciences of complexity. Reading: Addison-Wesley.

Lanham H, Leykuma L, Taylord B, McCannon C, Lindbergg C, Lesterh R (2012) How complexity science can inform scale-up and spread in health care: Understanding the role of self-organisation in variation across local contexts. *Social Science & Medicine* 93: 194–202.

Lansisalmi H, Kivimaki M, Aalto P, Ruoranen R (2006) Innovation in healthcare: A systematic review of recent research. *Nursing Science Quarterly* 19(1): 66–72.

Lanza G (2009) Building today's platform company. *Nature Biotechnology* 27(8). doi:10.1038/bioe.2009.6.

Lave J, Wenger E (1991) *Situated Learning. Legitimate Peripheral Participation*. Cambridge Cambridge University Press.

Lavis J, Robertson D, Woodside J, McLeod C, Abelson J (2003) How can research organisations more effectively transfer research knowledge to decision makers? *Milbank Quarterly* 81(2): 221–248.

Leadbeatter C (2014) *The Frugal Innovator. Creating Change on a Shoestring Budget*. London: Palgrave-MacMillan.

Legurreta A, Silber J, Costantino G, Kobylinski R, Zatz S (1993) Increased cholecystectomy rate after the introduction of laparoscopic cholecystectomy. *Journal of the American Medical Association* 270: 1429–1432.

Lehto M (2009) Whole system limited companies in a national health system. European Observatory meeting, 26 November 2009, Berlin.

Lemak C, Goodrick E (2003) Strategy as simple rules: Understanding success in a rural clinic. *Health Care Management Review* 28(2): 179–188.

Leonard-Barton D (1988) Implementation as mutual adaptation of technology and organisation. *Research Policy* 17(5): 251–267.

Lepore J (2014) The disruption machine. *The New Yorker*. http://www.newyorker.com/magazine/2014/06/23/the-disruption-machine?currentPage=all (Accessed on 19 August 2016).

Lettl C (2005) The emergence of radically new health care technologies: Inventive users as innovation networkers. *Technology & Healthcare* 13(3): 169–183.

Lettl C, Herstatt C, Gemünden H (2006) Users' contributions to radical innovation: Evidence from four cases in the field of medical equipment technology. *R&D Management* 36(3): 251–272.

Levinthal D, Warglien M (1999) Landscape design: Designing for local action in complex worlds. *Organisation Science* 10(3): 342–357.

Lewin A (1999) Application of complexity theory to organisation science. *Organisation Science* 10(3): 215.

Lewis G, Georghiou T, Steventon A, Vaithianathan R, Chitnis X, Billings J, Blunt I, Wright L, Roberts A, Bardsley M (2013) *Impact of 'Virtual Wards' on hospital use: A research study using propensity matched controls and a cost analysis.* Final report, NIHR Service Delivery and Organisation programme.

Lewis L, Seibold D (1993) Innovation modification during adoption. *Academy of Management Review* 18(2): 322–354.

Lichtenthaler U (2010) Technology exploitation in the context of open innovation. Finding the right 'job' for your technology. *Technovation* 30(7–8): 429–435.

LIF/Vasco Advisers (2013) *Innovation in European healthcare — what Can Sweden Learn? An Analysis of the Systems for Innovation in Five European Countries.* LIF/Vasco Advisers. http://www.vascoadvisers.com

Lindqvist G, Sölvell O (2011) *Organising clusters for innovation: Lessons from city regions in Europe.* CLUSNET final report.

Llano R (2013) The 'Gesundes Kinzigtal' integrated care initiative in Germany. *Eurohealth* 19(2): 7–8.

Locock L, Dopson S, Chambers D, Gabbay J (2001) Understanding the role of opinion leaders in improving clinical effectiveness. *Social Science & Medicine* 53(6): 745–757.

Lomas J (2007) The in-between world of knowledge brokering. *British Medical Journal* 334: 129–132.

Love T, Burton C (2005) General practice as a complex system: A novel analysis of consultation data. *Family Practice* 22(3): 347–352.

Lunghini R (2014) Europe's ageing population will face doctor shortage. http://www.west-info.eu/europes-ageing-population-will-face-doctor-shortage/ (Accessed on 19 August 2016).

Lüthje C (2003) Customers as co-inventors. An empirical analysis of the antecedents of customer-driven innovations in the field of medical equipment. Proceedings of the 32nd EMAC Conference.

Lüthje C, Herstatt C (2004) The lead user method: an outline of empirical findings and issues for future research. *R&D Management* 34(5): 553–568.

MacFarlane A, Harrison R, Murray E, Berlin A, Wallace P (2006) A qualitative study of the educational potential of joint teleconsultations at the primary–secondary care interface. *Journal of Telemedicine & Telecare* 12(S1): 22–24.

Mackenzie M, O'Donnell C, Halliday E, Sridharan S, Platt S (2010) Evaluating complex interventions: one size does not fit all. *British Medical Journal* 340 (7743): 401–403.

Maguerez G, Erbault M, Terra M, Maisonneuve H, Mafillon Y (2001) Evaluation of 60 continuous quality improvement projects in French hospitals. *International Journal of Quality in Health Care* 13(2): 89–97.

Maguire S, McKelvey B, Mirabeau, Ötzas N (2006) Complexity science and organisation studies. In Clegg S, Hardy C, Lawrence T, Nord W (eds.), *The SAGE Handbook of Organisation Studies*. London: Sage.

Mair F, May C, Murray E, Finch T (2009) *Understanding the Implementation and Integration of e-Health Services*. National Institute for Health Research Service Delivery and Organisation programme.

Malerba F (2004) *Sectoral Systems of Innovation: Concepts, Issues and Analyses of Six Major Sectors in Europe*. Cambridge: Cambridge University Press.

Malloch K (2011) Creating the organisational context for innovation. In Porter-O'Grady T, Malloch K (eds.), *Innovation Leadership. Creating the Landscape of Health care*. Sudbury, MA, USA: Jones and Bartlett.

Markides C (2006) Disruptive innovation: In need of better theory. *Journal of Production Innovation Management* 23: 19–25.

Markides C (2012) How disruptive will innovations from emerging markets be? *Sloan Management Review* 54(1): 23–25.

Martellia N, van den Brink H (2014) Special funding schemes for innovative medical devices in French hospitals. The pros and cons of two different approaches. *Health Policy* 117: 1–5.

Masanja H, De Savigny D, Smithson P *et al.* (2008) Child survival gains in Tanzania: Analysis of data from demographic and health surveys. *Lancet* 371(9620): 1276–1283.

May C, Finch T, Mair F, Ballini L, Dowrick C, Eccles M, *et al.* (2007) Understanding the implementation of complex interventions in health care: The normalization process model. *BMC Health Services Research* 7(1): 148.

May C, Finch T (2009) Implementing, embedding and integrating practices. An outline of normalization process theory. *Sociology* 43(3): 535–554.

May C, Murray E, Finch T, Mair F, *et al.* (2010) Normalization process theory on-line users' manual and toolkit. http://www.normalizationprocess.org (Accessed on 19 August 2016).

Maynard A (2007) Translating evidence into practice: Why is it so difficult? *Public Money and Management* 27(4): 251–256.

McKelvey B (1999) Avoiding complexity catastrophe in coevolutionary pockets: Strategies for rugged landscapes. *Organisation Science* 10(3): 294–321.

McKinsey (2011) Innovation in Healthcare delivery: The power of technology. The Future of Healthcare in Europe Conference, London, May 2011.

Menchik D, Meltzer D (2010) The cultivation of esteem and retrieval of scientific knowledge in physician networks. *Journal of Health and Social Behavior* 51(2): 137–152.

Mestre-Ferrandiz J, Sussex J, Towse A (2012) *The R&D Cost of a New Medicine.* London: Office of Health Economics.

Metcalfe J, James A, Mina A (2005) Emergent innovation systems and the delivery of clinical services: The case of intra-ocular lens. *Research Policy* 34(9): 1283–1304.

Metcalfe J, Pickstone J (2006) Replacing hips and lenses. Surgery, industry and innovaton in post-war Britain. In Webster A (ed.), *New Technologies in Health Care. Challenge, Change, and Innovation.* London: Palgrave Macmillan.

Meyer A, Goes J (1988) Organisational assimilation of innovations. A multi-level contextual analysis. *Academy of Management Review* 31: 897–923.

MIT Technology Review (2013) A new approach to medtech R&D. http://www. technologyreview.com/about/views-from-the-marketplace/ (Accessed on 19 August 2016).

Mitcham C (1994) *Thinking through technology. The path between engineering and philosophy.* Chicago: University of Chicago Press.

Moldoveanu M, Bauer R (2004) On the relationship between organisational complexity and organisational structuration. *Organisation Science* 15(1): 98–118.

Monheim T (2011) Maximizing profit capture for medical device manufacturers: Gain control over pricing strategies, value stories, and profit visibility. http://www.mdtmag.com/article/2011/07/maximizing-profit-capture-medical-device-manufacturers-gain-control-over-pricing-strategies-value (Accessed on 19 August 2016).

Morison E (1966) *Men, Machines and Modern Times.* Cambridge, MA, USA: MIT Press.

Moore G (1991) *Crossing the Chasm.* HarperBusiness.

Morrisey M (2008) *Health care.* The Concise Encyclopedia of Economics. http://econlib.org/library/Enc/HealthCare.html

MRC (2000) *MRC Framework for the Development and Evaluation of RCTs for Complex Interventions to Improve Health.* London: Medical Research Council.

Munos B (2009) Lessons from 60 years of pharmaceutical innovation. *Nature Reviews Drug Discovery* 8(12): 959–968.

Muir Gray J (2011) *How to Get Better Value Healthcare.* Oxford: Offox Press.

Naran S (2011) *An analysis of the transferability of frugal innovations to the healthcare industry, from less developed countries to high income countries.* MSc dissertation, Centre for Environmental Policy, Imperial College London.

Nadvi K, Halder G (2005) Local clusters in global value chains: Exploring dynamic linkages between Germany and Pakistan. *Entrepreneurship & Regional Development* 17: 339–363.

National Joint Registry (2013) *10th Annual Report. National Joint Registry for England, Wales and Northern Ireland.* http://www.njrcentre.org.uk/njrcentre/Implantprocurement/tabid/380/Default.aspx. Accessed on 19 August 2016.

Nelson R, Peterhansi A, Sampat B (2004) Why and how innovations get adopted: A tale of four models. *Industrial and Corporate Change* 13(5): 679–699.

NESTA (2009) Reshaping the UK economy. The role of public investment in financing growth. June 2009. http://www.nesta.org.uk/assets/documents/reshaping_the_uk_economy (Accessed on 19 August 2016).

Neumann P, Drummond M, Jonsson B, Luce B, Schwartz J, Siebert U, *et al.* (2010) Are key principles for improved health technology assessment supported and used by health technology assessment organisations? *International Journal of Technology Assessment in Health Care* 26(1): 71–78.

Newhouse J (1992) Medical care costs: How much welfare loss? *Journal of Economic Perspectives* 6(3): 3–21.

Newhouse J (1993) An iconoclastic view of cost containment. *Health Affairs* 12 (Suppl. 1): 152–171.

NHS Confederation (2008) *Disruptive innovation. What does it mean for the NHS?* Futures Debate, Paper 5, NHS Confederation.

NHS Confederation (2011) *The Search for Low-cost Integrated Healthcare. The Alzira Model — from the Region of Valencia.* NHS Confederation.

NHS Confederation (2012) Integrating research into practice: The CLAHRC experience. *Health Services Network Briefing,* Issue 245 (June).

NHS Scotland (2005) *An Introduction to the Unscheduled Care Collaborative Programme.* Scottish Executive.

NHS Scotland (2006) *Building the foundations for delivery. The first year progress report of the Unscheduled Care Collaborative Programme.* Scottish Executive.

NHS Scotland (2007) Unscheduled Care Collaborative Programme. *Local changes for improvement: The journey, ideas and accomplishments.* Scottish Executive.

Niccolini D, Powell N, Conville P, Martinez-Solano L (2008) Managing knowledge in the healthcare sector: A review. *International Journal of Management Reviews* 10(3): 245–263.

NICE (2011) Centre for Health Technology Evaluation. Diagnostics assessment programme. Consultation on DA Programme manual. National Institute for Health and Clinical Excellence.

Nicholl J, West J, Goodacre S, Turner J (2007) The relationship between distance to hospital and patient mortality in emergencies. *Emergency Medicine Journal*, 24, 665–668.

Nichols D (2007) Why innovation funnels don't work and why rockets do. *Market Leader* (Autumn): 26–31.

Normand C (1998). Ten popular health economic fallacies. *Journal of Public Health*, 20, 129–132.

Northern Ireland Health and Social Care Board (2011) *Transforming Your Care. A Review of Health and Social Care in Northern Ireland.*

Northrup J, Tarasova M, Kalowski L (2012) The pharmaceutical sector: Rebooted and reinvigorated. In Burns L. (ed.), *The Business of Healthcare Innovation.* 2nd Edition. Cambridge: Cambridge University Press.

OECD (2001) *Measuring Expenditure on Health–related R&D.* Paris: Organisation for Economic Co-Operation and Development.

OECD/EUROSTAT (2005) *Oslo Manual: Guidelines for Collecting and Interpreting Innovation Data.* 3rd edition. Paris: OECD Publishing.

Orlikowski W (1992) The duality of technology: Rethinking the concept of technology in organisations. *Organisation Science* 3(3): 398–427.

Orlikowski W (2000) Using technology and constituting structures: A practice lens for studying technology in organisations. *Organisation Science* 11(4): 404–428.

Øvretveit J (2011) *Does clinical coordination improve quality and save money? Volume 2: A detailed review of the evidence.* The Health Foundation.

Paina L, Peters D (2012) Understanding pathways for scaling up health services through the lens of complex adaptive systems. *Health Policy and Planning* 27: 365–373.

Paley J (2010) The appropriation of complexity theory in health care. *Journal of Health Services Research & Policy* 15(1): 59–61.

Pammolli F, Magazzini L., Riccaboni M (2011) The productivity crisis in pharmaceutical R&D. *Nature Reviews Drug Discovery* 10(6): 428–438.

Pannenborg O (2010) *Medical technology & device financing & health systems, strengthening in the twenty first century. A summary: Options for thought.* http://www.who.int/medical_devices/01_health_systems_strengthening_financing_charles_ok_pannenborg.pdf (Accessed on 19 August 2016).

Papadopoulos M, Hadjitheodossiou M, Chrysostomou C, Hardwidge C, Bell B (2001) Is the National Health Service at the edge of chaos? *Journal of the Royal Society of Medicine* 94(12): 613–616.

Parmar A (2015a) Can Medtronic still be called a device maker? *Medical Device Business*, 3 April 2015. http://www.mddionline.com/blog/devicetalk/can-medtronic-still-called-device-maker-04-03-15 (Accessed on 19 August 2016).

Parmar A (2015b) Medtronic launches pilot program to improve OR efficiency. *Medical Device Business*, 2 June 2015. http://www.mddionline.com/blog/devicetalk/medtronic-launches-pilot-program-improve-or-efficiency-06-02-15 (Accessed on 19 August 2016).

Paul S, Mytelka D, Dunwiddie C, Persinger C, Munos B, Lindborg S, Schacht A (2010) How to improve R&D productivity: the pharmaceutical industry's grand challenge. *Nature Reviews Drug Discovery* 9(3): 203–214.

Pawson R, Greenhalgh T, Harvey G, Walshe K (2005) Realist review. A new method of systematic review designed for complex policy interventions. *Journal of Health Services Research & Policy* 10: 21–34.

Pawson R, Tilley N (1997) *Realistic Evaluation.* London: Sage.

Persson U (2012) Value based pricing in Sweden: Lessons for design? Office of Health Economics briefing 12. http://www.ohe.org/publications/article/value-based-pricing-insweden-122.cfm (Accessed on 19 August 2016).

Persson U, Willis M, Ödegaard K (2010) A case study of ex ante, value-based price and reimbursement decision-making: TLV and rimonabant in Sweden. *European Journal of Health Economics* 11(2): 195–203.

Petrick I, Juntiwasarakij S (2011) Special issue: Innovation in emerging markets. The rise of the rest: Hotbeds of innovation in emerging markets. *Research-Technology Management* 54(4): 24–29.

Pettigrew A, Ferlie E, McKee L (1992) *Shaping strategic change: making change in large organizations. The case of the National Health Service.* London: Sage.

Pfeffer G (2012) The biotechnology sector: therapeutics. In Burns L (ed.), *The Business of Healthcare Innovation*. 2nd Edition. Cambridge: Cambridge University Press.

Picard J, Ward S, Zumpe R, Meek T, Barlow J, Harrop-Griffiths W (2009) Guidelines and the adoption of 'lipid rescue' therapy for local anaesthetic toxicity. *Anaesthesia* 64(2): 122–125.

Pierce J, Delbecq A (1977) Organisation structure, individual attitudes and innovation. *Academy of Management Review* 2(1): 27–37.

Pigott R, Barker R, Kaan T, Roberts M (2014) *Shaping the Future of Open Innovation. A Practical Guide for Life sciences Organisations*. Wellcome Trust.

Plsek P, Greenhalgh T (2001) Complexity science: the challenge of complexity in health care. *British Medical Journal* 323: 625–628.

Plsek P, Wilson T (2001) Complexity science: complexity, leadership, and management in health care organisations. *British Medical Journal* 23: 746–749.

Porter-O'Grady T, Malloch K (eds.) (2011) *Innovation Leadership. Creating the Landscape of Health care*. Sudbury, MA, USA: Jones and Bartlett.

Powell A, Goldsmith J (2012) The healthcare information technology sector. In Burns L (ed.), *The Business of Healthcare Innovation*. 2nd Edition. Cambridge: Cambridge University Press.

Prahalad C (2006) The innovation sandbox. *Strategy + Business* 44 (autumn). http://www.strategy-business.com/article/06306?gko=caeb6 (Accessed on 19 August 2016).

Prahalad C (2010a) Column: Best practices get you only so far. *Harvard Business Review* April. https://hbr.org/2010/04/column-best-practices-get-you-only-so-far

Prahalad C (2010b) *The fortune at the bottom of the pyramid: Eradicating Poverty through profits*. Pearson Education.

Prime Faraday Partnership (2003) *Medical devices. The UK industry and its technology development*. Prime Faraday Technology Watch.

Provines C (2010) Overcoming organisational barriers to implementing value-based pricing in the medical devices and diagnostics industry. *Journal of Medical Marketing* 10(1): 37–44.

Pullen A, de Weerd-Nederhof P, Groen A, Fisscher O (2012) Open innovation in practice: Goal complementarity and closed NPD networks to explain differences in innovation performance for SMEs in the medical devices sector. *Journal of Product Innovation Management* 29(6): 917–934.

PwC (2010) *Build and Beyond. The Revolution of Healthcare PPPs*. PwC Health Research Institute.

PwC (2011a) *Pharma 2020: Supplying the future. Which path will you take?* https://www.pwc.com/gx/en/pharma-life-sciences/pdf/pharma-2020-supplying-the-future.pdf (Accessed on 19 August 2016).

PwC (2011b) *Pharma 2020: Virtual R&D. Which path will you take?* https://www.pwc.com/gx/en/pharma-life-sciences/pdf/pharma2020_virtualrd_final2.pdf (Accessed on 19 August 2016).

PwC (2011c) *Medical Technology Innovation Scorecard: The race for global leadership.*

PwC (2013) *Medtech companies prepare for an innovation makeover.* http://www.pwc.com/us/en/health-industries/medical-technology-innovation/downloads.html (Accessed on 19 August 2016).

Radjou N, Prabhu J, Ahuja S (2010) Jugaad: A new growth formula for corporate America. *Harvard Business Review.* http://blogs.hbr.org/cs/2010/01/jugaad_a_new_growth_formula_fo.html (Accessed on 19 August 2016).

Rae-Dupree J (2008) Eureka! It really takes years of hard work. *New York Times,* 3 February. http://www.nytimes.com/2008/02/03/business/03unbox.html (Accessed on 19 August 2016).

Rangan V, Ravilla T (2007) Making sight affordable (Innovations case narrative: The Aravind Eye Care System). *Innovations: Technology, Governance, Globalization* 2(4): 35–49.

Ravilla T (2009) *How low-cost eye care can be world-class.* TED India. http://www.ted.com/talks/lang/eng/thulasiraj_ravilla_how_low_cost_eye_care_can_be_world_class.html (Accessed on 19 August 2016).

Ravindran R, Venkatesh R, Chang D, Sengupta S, Gyatsho J, Talwar B (2009) Incidence of post-cataract endophthalmitis at Aravind Eye Hospital: Outcomes of more than 42,000 consecutive cases using standardized sterilization and prophylaxis protocols. *Journal of Cataract and Refractive Surgery* 35(4): 629–636.

Raynal J (2015) Open innovation: Roche s'associe au biohackerspace La Paillasse. 8 July 2015. http://www.industrie-techno.com/open-innovation-roche-s-associe-au-biohackerspace-la-paillasse.39105 (Accessed on 19 August 2016).

Raynor M (2014) *Of Waves and Ripples. Disruption Theory's Newest Critic tries to Make a Splash.* Deloitte University Press.

Reid I (2002) Let them eat complexity: The emperor's new toolkit. *British Medical Journal* 324: 171.

Richman B, Udayakumar K, Mitchell W, Schulman K (2008) Lessons from India in organisational innovation: A tale of two heart hospitals. *Health Affairs* 27(5): 1260–1270.

Robert G, Greenhalgh T, MacFarlane F, Peacock R (2009) *Organisational factors influencing technology adoption and assimilation in the NHS: A systematic literature review.* Report for the National Institute of Health Research, SDO Project (08/1819/223).

Roberts K, Grabowksi M (1996) Organisations, technology and structuring. In Clegg S *et al.* (eds.) *Handbook of Organisation studies.* London: Sage.

Rogers E (2003) *Diffusion of Innovations.* New York: Free Press.

Rogers H, Silvestor K, Copeland J (2004) NHS Modernisation Agency's way to improve health care. *British Medical Journal* 328: 463.

Rogowski W, Hartz S, John J (2008) Clearing up the hazy road from bench to bedside: A framework for integrating the fourth hurdle into translational medicine. *BMC Health Services Research* 8: 194–205.

Roland D (2014) AstraZeneca reinforces pipeline with 'open innovation'. *The Telegraph.* http://www.telegraph.co.uk/finance/newsbysector/pharmaceuticalsandchemicals/10775160/AstraZeneca-reinforces-pipeline-with-open-innovation.html (Accessed on 19 August 2016).

Romley J, Goldman D, Sood N (2015) US hospitals experienced substantial productivity growth during 2002–11. *Health Affairs* 34(3): 511–518.

Rowe A, Hogarth A (2005) Use of complex adaptive systems metaphor to achieve professional and organisational change. *Journal of Advanced Nursing* 51(4): 396–405.

Rupp S (2015) CVS and the rise of the MinuteClinic. *NueMD*, 11 September 2015. http://www.nuemd.com/news/2015/09/11/cvs-rise-minute-clinic (Accessed on 19 August 2016).

Rushmer R, Kelly D, Lough M, Wilkinson J, Davies H (2004) Introducing the learning practice. 1. The characteristics of learning organisations in primary care. *Journal of Evaluation in Clinical Practice* 10 (3):375–386.

Rye C, Kimberly J (2007) The adoption of innovations by provider organisations in healthcare. *Medical Care Research Review* 64: 235–278.

Sahni N, Chigurupati A, Kocher B, Cutler D (2015) How the U.S. can reduce waste in health care spending by $1 trillion. *Harvard Business Review* 13 October. https://hbr.org/2015/10/how-the-u-s-can-reduce-waste-in-health-care-spending-by-1-trillion

Sammut S (2012) Biotechnology business and revenue models. In Burns L. (ed.), *The Business of Healthcare Innovation.* 2nd Edition. Cambridge: Cambridge University Press.

Sanderson I (2002) Evaluation, policy learning and evidence-based policy making. *Public Administration* 80(1): 1–22.

Savory C (2006) Does the UTTO model of technology transfer fit public sector healthcare services? *International Journal of Innovation and Technology Management* 3(2): 171–187.

Savory C (2009a) *User-led innovation in the UK National Health Service.* PhD thesis, The Open University.

Savory C (2009b) Building knowledge translation capability into public-sector innovation processes. *Technology Analysis & Strategic Management* 21(2): 149–171.

Savory C, Fortune J (2013) *NHS adoption of NHS-developed technologies. Final report.* NIHR Service Delivery and Organisation programme.

Schell M, Barcia A, Spitzer A, Harris H (2008) Pancreaticoduodenectomy: Volume is not associated with outcome within an academic health care system. *HPB Surgery* 2008: 825940.

Scannell J, Blanckley A, Boldon H, Warrington B (2012) Diagnosing the decline in pharmaceutical R&D efficiency. *Nature Reviews Drug Discovery* 11(3): 191–200.

Schon D (1967) *Technology and Change. The New Heraclitus.* Delacorte Press.

Schuhmacher A, Germann P, Trill H, Gassmann O (2013) Models for open innovation in the pharmaceutical industry. *Drug Discovery Today* 18: 1133–1137.

Seddon M, Marshall M, Campbell S, Roland M (2001) Systematic review of studies of quality of clinical care in general practice in the UK, Australia and New Zealand. *Quality in Health Care,* 10: 152–158.

Sehgal V, Dehoff K, Panneer G (2010) The importance of frugal engineering. *Strategy and Business* 12: 1–5.

Shetty D (2011) Disruptive innovation: new delivery models. In *A Lot more for a Lot Less. Disruptive Innovation in Healthcare,* Reform conference, 8 June 2011.

Shiell A, Hawe P, Gold L (2008) Complex interventions or complex systems? Implications for health economic evaluation. *British Medical Journal* 336: 1281–1283.

Shortell S, Bennett C, Byck G (1998) Assessing the impact of continuous quality improvement on clinical practice: What it will take to accelerate progress? *Milbank Quarterly* 76: 593–624.

Singer S, Burgers J, Friedberg M, Rosenthal M, Leape L, Schneider W (2011) Defining and measuring integrated patient care: Promoting the next frontier in health care delivery. *Medical Care Research Review* 68: 112–27.

Smith M (2007) Disruptive innovation. Can health care learn from other industries? A conversation with Clayton M. Christensen. *Health Affairs* 26(3): w288–w295.

Smith D (2010) *Exploring Innovation*. McGraw Hill Education.

Smith S, Newhouse J, Freeland M (2009) Income, insurance, and technology: Why does health spending outpace economic growth? *Health Affairs* 28(5):1276–1284.

Snowden D (2010) Safe-fail probes. http://cognitive-edge.com/blog/safe-fail-probes/

Snowdon A, Bassi H, Scarffe A, Smith A (2015) Reverse innovation: An opportunity for strengthening health systems. *Globalization and Health* 11: 2.

Sole D, Edmondson A (2002) Situated knowledge and learning in dispersed teams. *British Journal of Management* 13(s2): S17–S34.

Salisbury C, Stewart K, Purdy S *et al.* (2009) Lessons from evaluation of the NHS white paper Our Health, Our Care, Our Say. *British Journal of General Practice* 61(592): e766–e771.

Spurgeon P, Cooke M, Fulop N, Walters R, *et al.* (2010) *Evaluating Models of Service Delivery. Reconfiguration Principle.* National Institute for Health Research Service Delivery and Organisation programme. London: HMSO.

Spyridonidis D, Hendy J, Barlow J (2015) Leadership for knowledge translation: The case of CLAHRCs. *Qualitative Health Research* 25(11): 1492–1505.

Stacey R (1996) *Strategic Management and Organisational Dynamics*. Financial Times/Prentice Hall.

Sterman J (2000) *Business Dynamics: System Thinking and Modeling for a Complex World*. New York: Irwin McGraw-Hill.

Steventon A, Bardsley M, Billings J, Dixon J, Doll H *et al.* (2012) Effect of telehealth on use of secondary care and mortality: Findings from the Whole System Demonstrator cluster randomised trial. *British Medical Journal* 344: e3874.

Storey J, Fortune J, Johnson M, Savory C (2011) The adoption and rejection patterns of practitioner-developed technologies: A review, a model and a research agenda. *International Journal of Innovation Management* 15(5): 1043–1067.

Street A (2013) What has been happening to NHS productivity? http://www.nuffieldtrust.org.uk/blog/what-has-been-happening-nhs-productivity (Accessed on 19 August 2016).

Suchman L (1987) *Plans and situated actions. The Problem of Human–machine communication*. Cambridge: Cambridge University Press.

Sull D, Eisenhardt K (2012) Simple rules for a complex world. *Harvard Business Review* 90(9): 68–74.

Sussex J, Towse A, Devlin N (2013) Operationalizing value-based pricing of medicines: A taxonomy of approaches. *PharmacoEconomics* 31: 1–10.

Swamidass P, Nair A (2004) What top management thinks about the benefits of hard and soft manufacturing technologies. *IEEE Transactions on Engineering Management* 51(4): 462–471.

Teich A (2003) *Technology and the Future.* Thomson Wadsworth, Belmont, CA, USA.

Tether B (2005) Do services innovate (differently)? Insights from the European Innobarometer survey. *Industry and Innovation* 12(2): 153–184.

The Economist (2009) Health care in India. Lessons from a frugal innovator. http://www.economist.com/node/13496367?story_id=13496367 (Accessed on 19 August 2016).

The Economist (2011) Frugal healing. http://www.economist.com/node/17963427 (Accessed on 19 August 2016).

Thorpe K, Florence C, Joski P (2004) Which medical conditions account for the rise in health care spending? *Health Affairs* Web Exclusive doi: 10.1377/hlthaff.w4.437.

Tidd J, Bessant J (2014) *Strategic Innovation Management.* John Wiley & Sons.

Towse A, Garrison L, Puig-Peiró R(2012) The use of pay-for-performance for drugs: Can it improve incentives for innovation? Office of Health Economics Occasional Paper 12/01

Transparency Market Research (2012) Knee implants market — global industry size, share, trends, analysis and forecasts 2012–2018. http://www.transparencymarketresearch.com/knee-implants-market.html (Accessed on 19 August 2016).

Trupin E, Weiss N, Kerns S (2014) Social impact bonds: Behavioral health opportunities. *JAMA Pediatrics* 168(11): 985–986.

Trist E (1981) The evolution of sociotechnical systems as a conceptual framework and as an action research program. In Van de Ven A, Joyce W (eds.), *Perspectives on Organisation Design and Behaviour.* Wiley.

Tsoukas H, Chia R (2002) On organisational becoming: rethinking organisational change. *Organisation Science* 13(5): 567–582.

Turner A, Fraser V, Muir Gray J, Toth B (2002) A first class knowledge service: Developing the ational electronic library for health. *Health Information and Libraries Journal* 19: 135–145.

Tushman M, Anderson P (1986) Technological discontinuities and organisational environments. *Adminstrative Science Quarterly* 31: 439–465.

USAID (2010) USAID conference on *Research and evaluation methods for scaling up evidence-based interventions.* 12 June 2010. US Agency for International Development.

Uzun Jacobson E, Bayer S, Barlow J, Dennis M, MacLeodd M-J (2015) The scope for improvement in hyper-acute stroke care in Scotland. *Operations Research for Health Care* 6: 50–60.

Van de Ven A (1999) *The Innovation Journey*. Oxford: Oxford University Press.

Villon de Benveniste G (2104) Why are pivoting and failing fast a failed innovation strategy? http://theinnovationandstrategyblog.com/2014/02/failing-fast-and-pivoting-are-not-an-innovation-strategy-says-tony-ulwick-ceo-of-strategyn-an-innovation-consultancy-based-in-san-francisco-22/

Vitry A, Roughead E (2014) Managed entry agreements for pharmaceuticals in Australia. *Health Policy* 117(3): 345–352.

Von Hippel E (2005) *Democratizing Innovation*. Cambridge: MIT Press.

Walshe K, Rundall T (2001) Evidence-based management: From theory to practice in health care. *Milbank Quarterly* 79(3): 429–457.

Webb D (2005) *Evaluation in a policy environment: Approaches to the evaluation of complex health policy pilots in the UK from 1994 to 2004*. PhD thesis, University of Southampton.

Webster A (2007) *Health, Technology and Society. A Sociological Critique*. Basingstoke: Palgrave Macmillan.

Weick K (1995) *Sensemaking in Organisations*. London: Sage.

Weick K (2001) *Making Sense of the Organisation*. Oxford: Blackwell.

Weiner B (2009) A theory of organisational readiness for change. *Implementation Science* 4:67.

Wenger E (1998) *Communities of Practice: Learning, Meaning, and Identity*. Cambridge: Cambridge University Press.

Wenger E (2000) Communities of practice and social learning systems. *Organisation* 7(2): 225–246.

Wessner C, William A (2012) Clusters and regional initiatives. In Wessner C, Wolff A (eds.), *Rising to the Challenge: U.S. Innovation Policy for the Global Economy*. Washington DC: National Academies Press.

West E, Barron D, Dowsett J, Newton J (1999) Hierarchies and cliques in the social networks of health care professionals: implications for the design of dissemination strategies. *Social Science & Medicine* 48: 633–646.

WHO (2006) *The World Health Report 2006: Working Together for Health*. World Health Organisation.

WHO (2009) *Systems Thinking for Health Systems Strengthening*. World Health Organisation.

WHO (2011) *Compendium of New and Emerging Health Technologies*. World Health Organisation.

WHO (2012) *Global Health Expenditure Atlas*. World Health Organisation.

WHO (2014) *A Universal Truth: No Health Without a Workforce*. Geneva: World Health Organisation/Global Health Workforce Alliance.

Williams C (2007) Transfer in context: replication and adaptation in knowledge transfer relationships. *Strategic Management Journal* 28: 867–889.

Williams I, Dickinson H (2010) Can knowledge management enhance technology adoption in healthcare? A review of the literature. *Evidence & Policy* 6(3): 309–331.

Woetzel J, Ram S, Mischke J, Garemo N, Sankhe S (2014) *A Blueprint for Addressing the Global Affordable Housing Challenge*. McKinsey Global Institute.

Wonder M, Backhouse M, Sullivan S (2012) Australian managed entry scheme. A new manageable process for the reimbursement of new medicines? *Value in Health* 15(3): 586–590.

Wooldridge A (2011) Adrian Wooldridge of The Economist on frugal innovation. http://www.youtube.com/watch?v=Wysf_gFC7W4 (Accessed on 19 August 2016).

Workman P (2014) *Five ways that NICE could help bring innovative cancer medicines into the NHS*. The Institute of Cancer Innovation. http://www.icr.ac.uk/blogs/the-drug-discoverer/page-details/five-ways-that-nice-could-help-bring-innovative-cancer-medicines-into-the-nhs (Accessed on 19 August 2016).

Worthington F (2004) Management, change and culture in the NHS: Rhetoric and reality. *Clinician in Management* 12 (2): 55–67.

Zachariah R, Reid S, Chaillet P, Massaquoi M, Schouten E, Harries A (2011) Viewpoint. Why do we need a point-of-care CD4 test for low-income countries? *Tropical Medicine & International Health* 16: 37–41.

Zahra S, George G (2002) Absorptive capacity. A review, reconceptualization and extension. *Academy of Management Review* 27(2): 185–203.

Zeschky M, Widenmayer B, Gassmann O (2011) Frugal innovation in emerging markets: The case of Mettler Toledo. *Research-Technology Management* 54(4): 38–45.

Zhou Y (2013) Designing for complexity: Using divisions and hierarchy to manage complex tasks. *Organisation Science* 24(2): 339–355.

Zhu K, Kraemer K, Xu S (2006) The process of innovation assimilation by firms in different countries. A technology diffusion perspective on Ebusiness. *Management Science* 52(10): 1557–1576.

INDEX

Printed in the United States
By Bookmasters